AT LAST! A BOOK THAT TELLS YOU
WHAT CHOICES ARE AVAILABLE,
WHERE YOU CAN TURN, AND HOW TO COPE—
EMOTIONALLY AND PHYSICALLY—
WITH TRYING TO HAVE A BABY.

If you have to give yourself fertility injections, this book shows you how to do it and when to do it. If you need to sign a contract with an ovum donor, this book has one to use. Written by two nationally recognized authorities on the subject, a married couple who have themselves struggled to conceive a child, this book uses a total approach to overcoming infertility—touching on psychological concerns, legal concerns, and medical concerns. Compassionate and empowering, it pulls together the latest research to lead you every step of the way through this swiftly changing field.

"A book like this is long overdue. . . . It presents a great deal of information in a sensitive, accessible, and thorough manner. It is essential for couples experiencing the emotional, physical, and financial trauma of infertility and miscarriage. This book will be comforting and give direction and hope for the future."
   —Dr. Jonathan Scher,
      Assistant Clinical Professor of Obstetrics and Gynecology,
      Mt. Sinai School of Medicine and author of *Preventing Miscarriage*

"This is a most compassionate and useful resource for infertile couples. It is filled with sound advice and helpful information."
   —Arnold A. Lazarus, Ph.D.,
      Distinguished Professor, Graduate School of Applied Medicine
      and Professional Psychology, Rutgers University

D0108083

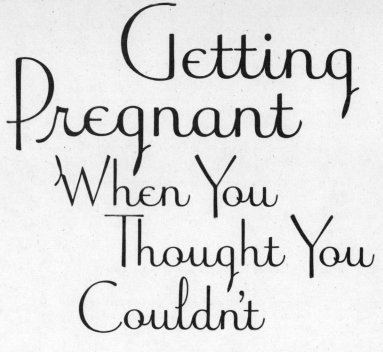

Getting Pregnant When You Thought You Couldn't

The Interactive Guide That Helps You Up the Odds

HELANE S. ROSENBERG, PH.D., AND
YAKOV M. EPSTEIN, PH.D.

FOREWORD BY BENJAMIN SANDLER, M.D.

WARNER BOOKS

A Time Warner Company

Copyright © 1993 by Helane S. Rosenberg and Yakov M. Epstein
All rights reserved.

Warner Books, Inc., 1271 Avenue of the Americas, New York, NY 10020

W A Time Warner Company

Printed in the United States of America
First Printing: June 1993
10 9 8 7 6 5 4 3 2

Library of Congress Cataloging-in-Publication Data

Rosenberg, Helane S.
    Getting pregnant when you thought you couldn't / Helane S.
Rosenberg and Yakov M. Epstein ; foreword by Benjamin Sandler.
        p.   cm.
    Includes bibliographical references and index.
    ISBN 0-446-39388-6
    1. Infertility, Female—Popular works.   2. Infertility, Female
—Psychological aspects.   3. Human reproductive technology—Popular
works.   I. Epstein, Yakov.   II. Title.
RG201.R67   1993
618.1'78—dc20   92-30888
                                                                          CIP

Book design by Giorgetta Bell McRee

Cover design by Cathy Saksa

To our families:
past, present, and future

ACKNOWLEDGMENTS

FEW PEOPLE have the opportunity to make a difference in other peoples' lives. In writing *Getting Pregnant,* we feel we have already been able to help others and, in the process, have been helped ourselves. And happily, as we worked on both "Getting Pregnant" projects—our baby (ies) and our book—our two ventures became intertwined. The people who helped us in either or both also entered our personal circle of friends and cheered us on. We gratefully acknowledge the contributions of the following people:

Jamie Raab, our enthusiastic, energetic editor at Warner Books, who believed in us and in the merits of our project. We thank her for cracking the whip at just the right time and providing the vision that is responsible for the merits of this book. Richard Cohen, Editorial Assistant at Warner Books, for listening to us and paying attention to every detail of the project.

Barbara Lowenstein, our agent, for putting up with our naivete ("only professors could write something like this," she said about our long-winded first draft proposal) and for guiding us skillfully in the right direction.

Robin Levinson who made an invaluable contribution to the substance and style of this book. We congratulate her on her pregnancy, which occurred while she was working on, and embracing, the principles of the book.

The wonderful physicians involved in both our pregnancy projects: Michael Darder, M.D. and Susan Treiser, M.D., Ph.D. of IVF New Jersey, who helped educate us about infertility, lent us their library (which we promise we'll return someday), allowed us to watch laboratory and surgical procedures, read and carefully critiqued the entire manuscript, got us pregnant, and became our good friends.

Benjamin Sandler, M.D. of Mount Sinai Medical Center, for his thoughtful comments on the manuscript. Daniel Navot, M.D., also of Mount Sinai, who believed in our project and made his patients available for our interviews. And Jonathan Scher, M.D., our long-time gynecologist, who, as well as cheering us on in both endeavors, shared his expertise about the medical aspects of miscarriage and ensured the accuracy of the medical information on this topic.

Other medical related personnel also provided needed information and first-hand experience that gave us the confidence to write about so many miraculous procedures. Cindy Elling and Greg Brennan, Embryologists at IVF New Jersey; Albert Anouna, President of Biogenetics Corporation; Marianne Williams, R.N. of Mount Sinai Medical Center; Marilyn Harris, Billing Coordinator of Mount Sinai, and Nancy Parker, Office Manager of IVF New Jersey.

We are also indebted to the clinical psychologists and researchers who offered feedback about our psychological material, both original and adapted: Cyril Franks, Ph.D., Professor Emeritus of Rutgers University; Violet Franks, Ph.D., Chief of Psychology at the Carrier Clinic; Donald Meichenbaum, Ph.D., Professor of Psychology at Waterloo University; and Annette Stanton, Ph.D., Professor of Psychology at the University of Kansas.

Members of the clergy helped us to be sensitive to a variety of religious issues. We thank Rabbi Yakov Hilsenrath of the Highland Park Conservative Temple who provided information on Jewish Halachic positions on third party procedures. Father Ron Stanley of the Rutgers University Catholic Center who shared his knowledge about the Catholic Church's perspective on assisted reproductive technology.

We needed a great deal of support in the early stages of our project.

We thank Esther Hautzig who was the first person to encourage us to pursue this project. Roth Wilkofsky and Cindy Cooper, who read our proposal for this book and helped us make the transition from academia to the real world of writing. Harriet Schweitzer, matchmaker extraordinaire, who helped us team up with the doctors at IVF New Jersey and with one another. And Donna Mancuso who is always our friend.

Our many clients and interviewees taught us about the emotional aspects of infertility. Our clients at the Infertility Counseling Center, members of our RESOLVE Inc. support groups, members of our IVF New Jersey support groups, and people we interviewed, all of whom provided us with stories that were compelling and life-affirming.

Our friends at Rutgers and at Congregation Ansche Chesed who supported us throughout this endeavor.

Members of our household, Jenny Epstein, our favorite teenager, and Fred, our favorite dog, whose many nights without home cooked meals are testimony to their good will and patience.

Finally, we offer our gratitude to God, our silent partner, who guided us throughout this project and brought our other project to wonderful fruition.

Helane S. Rosenberg and Yakov M. Epstein
Highland Park, NJ
September 1992

CONTENTS

FOREWORD

EVERY DAY in my work as a physician specializing in infertility, I see couples who are having trouble coping with their infertility treatment. They struggle to balance the demands of their careers with the rigorous treatment-monitoring schedule, to master the information necessary to understand what they're going through, to keep their marriage together, and, most importantly, to live as normal a life as possible while going through repeated attempts at getting pregnant. I'm often so busy managing their medical treatment that I don't have as much time as I would like to minister to their emotional needs. I am delighted to say that now there is a resource—Drs. Rosenberg and Epstein's splendid book *Getting Pregnant When You Thought You Couldn't*—that I can recommend every one of my patients read and use during both diagnosis and treatment.

For couples in any stage in their battle against infertility, this book has it all: well-researched medical information in easy-to-understand language; a compassionate outlook that reassures readers they are not alone in their struggle; and exercises that show the reader how to cope with virtually any type of infertility-related stress, ranging from an invitation to a baby shower to a miscarriage after years of treatment.

In my practice, I can point to the many successes modern medicine has enabled me to achieve, but unfortunately I also must personally confront the many cycles that don't result in pregnancy. I believe, however, that many of my patients would ultimately conceive with repeated attempts, but am hard-pressed to know what to do to help couples hang in there until they get the baby of their dreams. *Getting Pregnant When You Thought You Couldn't* provides the support and information these couples need to be vital participants in their medical treatment.

I am particularly impressed with the authors' emphasis on teamwork. They advise patients to work as a team with their physicians and they show how husbands and wives can unite to combat infertility. In some cases, patients can read this book and actually raise the level of their own treatment by becoming active partners with their physicians. I don't believe—and this book does not advocate—that patients should try to wrest from their physician complete control over their diagnosis and medical management. I have found, however, that the more my patients know about how their reproductive systems work, about why they may not be getting pregnant, and how medical intervention might solve their problem, the better equipped they are to ask me questions and understand my explanations.

Another strength of the book is the section on third party pregnancy and gamete donation, which reflects the authors' expertise in this area. As more and more women over the age of forty turn to ovum donation, they will need informed, up-to-date information that will enable them to make the appropriate decision about whether to use anonymous or known donors; and whether to tell or not to tell friends and relatives, or, at a later date, whether and how to tell their child. *Getting Pregnant* offers help in making these important decisions, suggests ways that couples can strengthen their relationship, and even provides tips about how they can tell their children when the time is appropriate.

Drs. Rosenberg and Epstein also reach out to patients with secondary infertility, a segment of the infertile population who, because they do have one child, fail to elicit the sympathy that society accords to couples with no children. For this population, the authors provide emotional validation and useful activities to help them cope.

What makes this book so empowering is its unique interactive approach. The authors have skillfully combined their professional knowledge, their research skills and personal experiences, and their compassion to create a book that couples can use as a sort of surrogate counselor to provide emotional support and trustworthy guidance.

Infertility specialists, too, can benefit by reading this book. I, for one, feel it has helped me become more sensitive to my patients' emotional needs and has given me unusual insight into the concerns and frequently unexpressed fears of the patients I treat.

In writing *Getting Pregnant When You Thought You Couldn't,* Drs. Epstein and Rosenberg fill an enormous void. Of the handful of infertility books in the lay literature, theirs is the only one that truly emphasizes and integrates both the emotional and medical aspects of this widespread problem. I view this book as the first in a new generation of books on infertility: one that acknowledges the patient as a feeling and thinking participant in medical treatment, not just someone on whom to measure blood level and conduct ultrasound scans, or someone who merely grieves and mourns. Fully researched, beautifully written, well organized, and brimming with compassion, *Getting Pregnant When You Thought You Couldn't* sets the standard for infertility books just as the field of infertility medicine enters a new phase of advancement and success.

Benjamin Sandler, M.D.
Assistant Professor of Obstetrics and Gynecology
Department of OB/GYN and Reproductive Science
Mount Sinai Medical Center, New York

INTRODUCTION

"*Everything in my life has always worked out," says Anne. "I went to the right college. I'm a partner in the best law firm in the city. I have the perfect husband. Maybe I met him a little later than I should have, but I did meet him. I work out every day. We have the perfect house and, until this, the perfect life. Why is this happening to me? I can't get pregnant. For two years we've been going from doctor to doctor. The most important thing to me now is to have a baby. And I can't do it. I just can't believe this is happening.*"

For the first time in her life, Anne has been unable to achieve what she wants. In the mini-baby-boom of the 1990s, Anne sees pregnant women everywhere, constant reminders of their good fortune and what Anne perceives as her failure. Their big bellies infuriate her; she finds it difficult to hide her feelings. Her carefully planned life, it seems, has turned out to be nothing more than a house of cards.

"*I already have a child," says Bea. "Susan is five. My husband, Sal, loves her a lot. I want another one. Sal said, 'Fine.' But then we started trying, and I didn't get pregnant fast, like before. Sal was disappointed, but I was really upset. We've been trying for three years. I'm so sad. Last year, I said we should go see a specialist. Sal said, 'Fine.' They did some tests and said I should take Pergonal shots to stimulate ovulation. That's when Sal drew the line. He said, 'I'm not giving shots. We've got one kid. That's enough for me.' So I go to the clinic by myself. My neighbor gives me the shots. I feel like I'm in this alone. Sal won't even talk about it anymore.''*

Bea is one of the many women experiencing *secondary* infertility, the inability to get pregnant after having one successful birth. Sal is typical of the husbands who are not supportive of their infertile wives. Bea loves being a mother and desperately wants another child. Sal can't deal with Bea's depression and her total involvement in the "pregnancy project." Infertility is difficult enough. Going through it alone is almost impossible. Life would be better, Bea sighs, if only they could unite in the face of this crisis.

"I always thought I'd have a large family just like my mother," says Grace. *"There are seven of us—five girls and two boys. We're very close. We get together all the time. But in recent years, it's been increasingly difficult for me. My kid brother and I are the only ones with no children. Last year, I suffered my third miscarriage. That time the doctors gave me progesterone. But it still didn't work. My brothers and sisters are warm and loving, but I'm starting to feel jealous of them. Sometimes I feel angry at them. And that makes me feel guilty. The terrible thing is I'm not sure who I'm angry at. I cry all the time.''*

Not all infertile women have trouble getting pregnant. Some, like twenty-eight-year-old Grace, get pregnant easily enough but seem unable to carry the pregnancy to term. For Grace, each miscarriage is another death to mourn; her developing babies seem so real to her. Once gregarious and outgoing, Grace feels guilty and confused by her sudden lack of interest in family events, and she is tormented by her negative feelings toward the people she loves. Grace needs to allow herself to grieve for her miscarriages; then she needs to tell her family what she is experiencing and ask for their support. But Grace is stuck. She fails to reach out and feels more and more ashamed and isolated as time goes on.

Anne, Bea, and Grace tell very different stories, but they share the same dream, giving birth to a new life—a dream being replaced by the nightmare of infertility. Every aspect of their lives is colored by their inability to conceive and deliver a baby.

Infertility is a crisis that affects one out of six—an estimated 2.6 million—couples in the United States.[1] As more and more people delay child-rearing until their mid-thirties or early forties, more and more find themselves engaged in a desperate struggle to cope with the physical and emotional traumas caused by infertility. Most couples assume they are fertile. However, if after six to twelve months of unprotected intercourse they have not conceived, they are classified as infertile and urged to seek medical tests and treatment. Unfortunately, most are given nowhere to turn for emotional support, which can be vital to the couple's ability to conquer infertility.

We know because we've experienced infertility ourselves. Our story is most like Anne's. We got married later in life and thought we would conceive and have a baby within the first year. It didn't work out that way. We went from our gynecologist to specialists to a famous clinic. Our label was "unexplained infertility"—the worst, from our perspective, because we were not sure what, if anything, would ever work. Each treatment buoyed our hopes. Each failure plummeted us to the depths of depression.

Because we are psychotherapists, we found that we could best help ourselves by helping others. Over the last few years, we have limited our private practice almost solely to people with fertility problems. And we have become support group leaders for RESOLVE Inc., a nationwide infertility support group, and counseling associates for IVF New Jersey, a medical practice specializing in infertility treatment.

Clients first come to our Infertility Counseling Center overwhelmed by negative feelings and confusing thoughts. They can't figure out what to do next. We start by telling them about infertility—why it's stressful and how it strains people's lives. We help them acquire the medical information they need to continue their quest to have a baby. We also counsel clients to become more aware of how they feel and think about their infertility. And most importantly, since so many infertile clients put their lives on hold, we help them regain a semblance of normalcy so they don't throw out the bathwater—their friends, family, self-esteem, and marriage—while trying to have a baby.

We do this by teaching our clients the skills necessary to lead satisfying lives and build strong marriages despite their infertility. We help them reframe their thinking. We teach them to relax. We help them practice talking with family, friends, and colleagues about what they are experiencing. We show them how to make a Getting Pregnant Plan. And we coach them to become more assertive with their doctors. Our goal is to equip our clients to help themselves through their infertility. Through this book, we'd like to do the same for you.[2]

Our own personal battle with infertility continued for over three years. And finally, after countless failures, in the summer of 1992, we became pregnant—with twins—through an ovum donor GIFT (Gamete IntraFallopian Transfer) procedure. Not coincidentally, in the year prior to the procedure we completed *Getting Pregnant When You Thought You Couldn't*. As we refined the Getting Pregnant Activities, we incorporated them, with gusto, into our lives. We believe that staying optimistic, gathering support, reducing stress, as well as securing the best medical care and being partners in our treatment, upped our odds. So, on this positive note, we hope we can be role models for you as you fight your own battles.

We count our blessings every day. We know how fortunate we are—that we had wonderful medical care, that we had insurance that covered much of our medical treatment, and that the treatment finally worked. But most of all, we are grateful that we found the strength and inspiration to keep trying until we succeeded. Our dream is that this book can give you the skills, the strength, and the inspiration to keep on trying until, like us, you get pregnant when you thought you couldn't.

CHAPTER ONE

NINE POINTERS TO GETTING PREGNANT WHEN YOU THOUGHT YOU COULDN'T

THIS BOOK presents our unique approach to helping our clients cope with their infertility. The people we work with come to us despondent, brokenhearted, and often on the verge of marital breakup. While helping them deal with their grief, we also teach them an active approach to treatment. We coach them in ways to develop and maintain an optimistic outlook while engaging in these treatments. We don't promise them that they'll get pregnant. But we do help them find a way to lead a satisfying life while fighting infertility.

Our method is based upon Nine Pointers to Getting Pregnant When You Thought You Couldn't and upon activities and exercises that put those Pointers into action. The Pointers stem from experience with scores of infertile couples we have counseled as well as our own experiences. Since these Pointers are an outgrowth of a healthy approach to any kind of problem-solving, you instinctively may have incorporated some of them into your daily life already.

We begin with The Getting Pregnant Quiz, a thirty-six-item questionnaire that can help you find out how *you* deal with your infertility. Your answers to the quiz will help you map out your Psychological Getting Pregnant Profile. Using this information you can pinpoint any attitudes and behaviors that stand in your way.

Please take a few minutes now to complete the quiz. Then score your answers. Finally, chart your results on the graph. Before you begin, we recommend that you photocopy the quiz so you can retake it after you have completed the book and begun to incorporate the Pointers into your life. By the time you finish this book, you will have two books: the one you bought and the one you create as you photocopy pages and make your own personal notebook.

Put a bookmark on the page that contains your profile and refer to this page as you read about each of the Nine Pointers. As you make your way through the infertility maze, keep in mind that your job is to help yourself through your infertility. By incorporating these Nine Pointers into your daily life, you can feel as though you have some control in a situation that is often considered uncontrollable. You can help yourself stay strong, active, and optimistic as you seek and undergo treatment. You can empower yourself. The following Nine Pointers can help you get pregnant when you thought you couldn't.

THE NINE POINTERS

1. Educate Yourself About Infertility

Familiarize yourself with the nature and use of diagnostic tests, procedures, and medications typical in infertility treatment. You need to understand what's happening to you. Most adults think they already know how to make babies. For infertile couples, making babies demands knowledge far beyond what the average person knows. There is much to learn but not so much as to be daunting. Learn about basal body thermometers, ovulation kits, laparoscopies, and infertility drugs. These topics are detailed in later chapters.

Make all the important infertility terms part of your vocabulary. Let the glossary at the end of this book be your guide. The glossary includes explanations of the alphabet soup of high-tech infertility treatment: GIFT, IVF, ZIFT, TET, PCT, HSG, IUI, among many. It also covers

THE GETTING PREGNANT QUIZ

The Getting Pregnant Quiz allows you to examine how you deal with your infertility. *There are no right or wrong answers.* Each question has four choices. Pick the one that best represents how you act or what you believe. Read the questions carefully. Then check the box that represents your choice.

1. My partner accompanies me to my doctor or clinic appointments.

0 ☐ Never   1 ☐ Rarely   2 ☐ Often   3 ☐ Always

2. I do just what the doctor says—no questions asked.

0 ☐ Always   1 ☐ Often   2 ☐ Rarely   3 ☐ Never

3. When I receive an invitation to an upsetting social event, I go even though it upsets me.

0 ☐ Always   1 ☐ Often   2 ☐ Rarely   3 ☐ Never

4. I have difficulty finding the receipts for my medical treatment.

0 ☐ Always   1 ☐ Often   2 ☐ Rarely   3 ☐ Never

5. I record the date of each medical test I have and the results of that test.

0 ☐ Never   1 ☐ Rarely   2 ☐ Often   3 ☐ Always

6. I have no idea how much longer I will continue to do the treatment I am now doing.

0 ☐ Strongly Agree   1 ☐ Agree   2 ☐ Disagree   3 ☐ Strongly Disagree

7. My partner and I help each other cope with stressful situations.

0 ☐ Never   1 ☐ Rarely   2 ☐ Often   3 ☐ Always

8. I consider myself a failure because I have not been able to get pregnant.

0 ☐ Strongly Agree   1 ☐ Agree   2 ☐ Disagree   3 ☐ Strongly Disagree

9. I would believe that I am at fault if I were not willing to do more advanced treatments.

0 ☐ Always   1 ☐ Often   2 ☐ Rarely   3 ☐ Never

10. I have a clear plan about what I will do to try to get pregnant during the next six months.

0 ☐ Strongly Disagree   1 ☐ Disagree 2 ☐ Agree   3 ☐ Strongly Agree

11. I let my doctor know that I understand what he or she says to me.

0 ☐ Never   1 ☐ Rarely   2 ☐ Often   3 ☐ Always

12. If my doctor suggests several choices of medical treatment, I pick the one he or she recommends rather than the one I feel most comfortable with.

0 ☐ Always   1 ☐ Often   2 ☐ Rarely   3 ☐ Never

13. I have a good understanding of the medical terms and concepts of infertility.

0 ☐ Strongly Disagree   1 ☐ Disagree 2 ☐ Agree   3 ☐ Strongly Agree

14. When I hear about a new book on infertility, I arrange to read it as soon as possible.

0 ☐ Never   1 ☐ Rarely   2 ☐ Often   3 ☐ Always

15. I permit myself to grieve when I have a failed treatment procedure.

0 ☐ Never   1 ☐ Rarely   2 ☐ Often   3 ☐ Always

16. My outlook for getting pregnant is optimistic but also realistic.

0 ☐ Strongly Disagree   1 ☐ Disagree 2 ☐ Agree   3 ☐ Strongly Agree

17. My partner encourages and supports me during difficult and upsetting times.

0 ☐ Never   1 ☐ Rarely   2 ☐ Often   3 ☐ Always

18. When I hear about a conference or lecture about infertility, I try to attend it.

0 ☐ Never   1 ☐ Rarely   2 ☐ Often   3 ☐ Always

19. I tell my close friends that I am having infertility treatment.

0 ☐ Never   1 ☐ Rarely   2 ☐ Often   3 ☐ Always

20. If a friend or relative asks an embarrassing question, I am ready with an answer.

0 ☐ Never   1 ☐ Rarely   2 ☐ Often   3 ☐ Always

21. I try to find out from other people how they've gotten insurance coverage for their treatment procedures.

0 ☐ Never   1 ☐ Rarely   2 ☐ Often   3 ☐ Always

22. I have a good support system to help me handle the emotional and logistical problems caused by infertility.

0 ☐ Strongly Disagree   1 ☐ Disagree 2 ☐ Agree   3 ☐ Strongly Agree

23. During this year, I have calculated, as precisely as possible, how much money I will spend for infertility treatment.

0 ☐ Strongly Disagree   1 ☐ Disagree 2 ☐ Agree   3 ☐ Strongly Agree

24. I try to psych myself up when I am going to have a particularly difficult infertility test or treatment.

0 ☐ Never   1 ☐ Rarely   2 ☐ Often   3 ☐ Always

25. I permit myself to get angry when acquaintances tell me they got pregnant by accident.

0 ☐ Never   1 ☐ Rarely   2 ☐ Often   3 ☐ Always

26. I believe that my infertility is a punishment for all the past bad things I have done.

0 ☐ Strongly Agree   1 ☐ Agree   2 ☐ Disagree   3 ☐ Strongly Disagree

27. Despite all our problems, infertility has strengthened my relationship with my partner.

0 ☐ Strongly Disagree   1 ☐ Disagree 2 ☐ Agree   3 ☐ Strongly Agree

28. I have a system for keeping track of the information about the money I've spent and the amounts I've been reimbursed for my infertility treatments.

0 ☐ Strongly Disagree   1 ☐ Disagree 2 ☐ Agree   3 ☐ Strongly Agree

29. I've experienced new and strong emotions as a result of my infertility.

0 ☐ Strongly Disagree   1 ☐ Disagree 2 ☐ Agree   3 ☐ Strongly Agree

30. Even though I am not yet pregnant, I still have hope that I will succeed.

0 ☐ Never   1 ☐ Rarely   2 ☐ Often   3 ☐ Always

31. If my doctor uses a medical term that I don't understand, I ask him or her to please explain it to me.

0 ☐ Never   1 ☐ Rarely   2 ☐ Often   3 ☐ Always

32. As long as I am physically and financially able to pursue treatment, I will keep trying.

0 ☐ Strongly Disagree   1 ☐ Disagree 2 ☐ Agree   3 ☐ Strongly Agree

33. I have a system for keeping track of the medical information I've accumulated about my diagnosis and treatment.

0 ☐ Strongly Disagree   1 ☐ Disagree 2 ☐ Agree   3 ☐ Strongly Agree

34. My treatment during the next six months has been planned to create the best odds of success balanced against the least expensive treatment cost that I can afford.

0 ☐ Strongly Disagree   1 ☐ Disagree 2 ☐ Agree   3 ☐ Strongly Agree

35. Infertility has caused me to experience feelings that have sometimes surprised me.

0 ☐ Strongly Disagree   1 ☐ Disagree 2 ☐ Agree   3 ☐ Strongly Agree

36. My repeated failures to get pregnant make me want to give up.

0 ☐ Always   1 ☐ Often   2 ☐ Rarely   3 ☐ Never

Scoring Key

This test provides you with a score for each of the Nine Getting Pregnant Pointers. There are four questions for each Pointer. For example, you can find out your score for the first pointer, Work as a Team, by adding up your points for questions 1, 7, 17, and 27. Likewise, you get your score for the second pointer, Educate Yourself About Infertility, by adding up your points for questions 13, 14, 18, and 21. Use the table below to fill in the number of points you scored for each of the questions. Then add up your total score for each Pointer.

Pointer	Question No.	Points	Question No.	Points	Question No.	Points	Question No.	Points	Total:
Work as a Team	1		7		17		27		
Educate Yourself About Infertility	13		14		18		21		
Get Organized	4		5		28		33		
Make a Plan	6		10		23		34		
Manage Your Social Life	3		19		20		22		
Change Your Thinking	8		9		24		26		
Don't Give Up	16		30		32		36		
Be a Partner in Your Treatment	2		11		12		31		
Get in Touch With Your Feelings	15		25		29		35		

PREGNANCY POINTERS PROFILE

Look up your score for each Pointer. Then blacken in the box for that score in the appropriate column.

Score	Work as a Team	Educate Yourself About Infertility	Get Organized	Make a Plan	Manage Your Social Life	Change Your Thinking	Don't Give Up	Be a Partner in Your Treatment	Get in Touch with Your Feelings
12									
11									
10									
9									
8									
8									
7									
6									
5									
4									
3									
2									
1									
0									

procedures that sound more akin to construction or animal husbandry than to the lexicon of human medical care: cryopreservation, egg retrieval, embryo transfer. Other terms, such as luteal phase defect, endometrial biopsy, sperm morphology, varicocelectomy, and anticardiolipin antibodies sound ominous but are less frightening when you know their meaning. Couples who are successful arm themselves with as much information as possible so they can feel confident, make informed decisions, and converse fruitfully with their physicians.

Even acquiring just some basic infertility information can put you on the road to further discovery. The audience at a recent regional infertility conference sponsored by the education- and advocacy-oriented RESOLVE Inc., for example, was well educated about infertility. Members of the audience were not shy about asking the speaker, Dr. Jonathan Scher, author of *Preventing Miscarriage*,[1] many complex and detailed questions during his address, titled "Pregnancy After Infertility." Dr. Scher was delighted by his audience's familiarity with his subject matter, and it gave him the impetus to include important details about advanced treatments for infertility and miscarriage—giving those present a very medically oriented and cutting-edge talk.

Like Dr. Scher's audience, you, too, can gain the respect of doctors and acquire state-of-the-art information. Your physician is apt to share more sophisticated insights with you if you are able to demonstrate a deeper-than-average understanding of infertility. Your infertility knowledge can help you regain the sense of control you lost when you learned that you couldn't get pregnant when you wanted to. This knowledge also can dispel some myths and provide you with answers you need about the medical options that have become widely available only in the last decade.

We encourage you to be a voracious reader. Read *everything* written about infertility in books, magazines, and newspapers. Watch for talk shows and news programs with infertility segments. You'll probably be surprised at the huge volume of information out there. Add to your rapidly expanding knowledge by focusing on the chapters in this book that explain and describe diagnosis and treatment. Remember, you don't have to go to medical school to understand what's happening to you.

Others can help you, too. Talk to everybody you know who has experienced infertility. One way to meet these individuals is to join RESOLVE Inc., founded by Barbara Eck Menning in 1973.[2] Through RESOLVE, you can join a support group in your area or call a hot line. RESOLVE meetings, besides providing emotional support, give members opportunities to trade medical information (how should you prepare for an endometrial biopsy?), practical information (where do you stick the needle in a Pergonal injection so that it hurts less?), and even financial information (what's the best way to submit an insurance claim to receive the optimum reimbursement?). By educating yourself, you'll not only feel calmer, but you'll also increase your chances of getting pregnant when you thought you couldn't.

2. Get in Touch with Your Feelings

The most overwhelming characteristic of infertility is how stressful it is. It's stressful because you never know how long it will last. It's stressful because it's unexpected. It's stressful because it makes you feel different and because treatments are physically demanding and often very expensive.

Different people respond differently to infertility-related stress. In her book *In Pursuit of Pregnancy,* Joan Liebmann-Smith weaves together three different but equally painful stories of how three couples coped with their infertility.[3] Researcher Margarete Sandelowski, a professor in the School of Nursing at the University of North Carolina at Chapel Hill, has investigated the emotional responses of infertile women, and reports that some infertile women describe the central experience of infertility to be one of ambiguity.[4] They are not sure why they are infertile. They aren't clear if they should try a different treatment or change doctors. They don't know when or even if they will ever have a baby. They are *confused*.

Our client Phyllis fits that profile perfectly. The thoughts that wind through her mind reflect her confusion: "Every month I can't stand the wait. Maybe this insemination will work. Should I have a laparoscopy? Should we just go on vacation? Should I forget about having my own baby and adopt?"

Nobody knows why Phyllis can't conceive. She just wishes that some doctor would tell her that she'll never get pregnant. Then she thinks she would know what to do next. But maybe not.

Other infertile women focus on the alienation of their experience.[5] They feel different from all the other women who get pregnant and have babies. They feel singled out and stigmatized by the infertility label. They can't talk to women with children; they can't talk to single women; they can't talk to voluntarily childless women. They feel like they just don't fit in. They feel *isolated and alone*.

Arlene is one of those who feel "desperately different." Everyone around her seems to be pregnant or wheeling a baby carriage. Every weekend at her synagogue there's another baby-naming. Arlene feels left out. "I am not like my sisters," she says. "They both got pregnant. I'm not like anyone in the whole world."

Time is the overwhelming aspect of other women's infertility experiences. They feel that their biological clock is running out. They respond by rushing through treatments or by changing doctors. They dwell on the past and are anxiety-ridden about the future. They think about themselves only as "ovulators" and "menstruators." Nothing else counts for them. All they can focus on is that they better get pregnant soon because time is slipping away.

Debby can't seem to think of anything else but the fact that she is forty-one and not yet pregnant. She laments her five-year relationship with Freddie. "I wasted so much time," she says. "I don't have many months left." She explains that she is going to two different doctors this week to get their opinions. She is overwhelmed by her sense of impending doom—menopause and the end of the road. Time is her primary stressor.

Infertile people say they feel anger, jealousy, repulsion, or disgust. You may feel this way, too. In fact, you may feel grief, depression, loss, confusion—many kinds of negative and potentially debilitating emotions. Despite the difficulty, *you must face your emotions and acknowledge them.*

Often the shock of infertility can make people report that they are disconnected from themselves, or completely unaware of their feelings. Find and acknowledge your innermost emotions, for these feelings may be preventing you from getting beyond the obvious sadness and grief of infertility. Remember, in terms of infertility, *all emotions are valid,* even though you may never have experienced feelings like these before. At one time or other, everyone experiences emotions that surprise them.

You might feel *angry.* At whom are you angry? There may be no clear target. Religious people may feel angry at God. Others focus their anger on abusive or neglectful parents or on women who choose to abort their pregnancies. Others prefer not to focus their anger on an external target. Instead, they turn their anger inward. They get angry at their bodies for failing to make babies.

You might feel *jealous.* Some people say they feel jealous of parents or pregnant women. They envy the ease with which friends get pregnant. They are even jealous of their previously infertile friends, even though they truly want their friend to have a baby. Your feelings may confuse you. You may feel *repulsed* when your friend asks you to hold her baby. You wonder, "How can I, who so much loves babies and wants one, feel repulsed by this innocent little creature in my arms?"

You may feel *disgusted* with yourself because you feel so inadequate. Month after month, you fail to get pregnant. Looking in the mirror, you notice how the fertility drugs make you appear pregnant. What a shame. You have a body that looks pregnant but isn't.

All, or at least some, of these and other emotions will be part of your life. Getting in touch with these feelings ultimately will help you become a happier person despite your infertility. You can begin to combat negative feelings by learning to relax. The progressive relaxation and breathing exercises in the Getting Pregnant Workout in Chapter 2 are designed to help you feel calmer. The Workout's guided imagery exercises can help you "go away" from your problem and give your mind time to heal itself.

After you get in touch with your negative emotions, realize there comes a time to move beyond them and eventually replace them with positive feelings. Emotions that are perfectly valid at one time may hinder you from exploring options at another time. Of course, there is no rule about how long you can expect to feel overwhelming sadness or anger or jealousy (and these emotions will probably never leave you entirely), but at a certain point in your infertility diagnosis and treatment you must allow yourself to get past what you are feeling so you can move on.

Some clients who come to us are already in touch with their emotions, so much so that their awareness backfires and prevents them from seeking proper, productive treatment. They are grieving and feel helpless about their loss. "This isn't my fault," they say to themselves. "I'm not responsible for what is happening to me." While it's true that the fault is not theirs nor that they are responsible for their condition, they nevertheless feel trapped by their debilitating emotions. They are fixated on negative thoughts, and their nonaction triggers a form of guilt for failing to become more involved in their treatment. This, in turn, makes their negative feelings more intense.

Either case—failing to acknowledge your feelings or feeling your emotions too much—has a strong effect on whether you will allow yourself to try to conquer your infertility and get pregnant when you thought (and felt) you couldn't. Getting in touch with your feelings, giving yourself time to experience them, and then moving past your pain into a new, more empowered phase of infertility-coping is the goal of the Get in Touch with Your Feelings Pointer.

3. Change Your Thinking

Infertility puts a strain on so many parts of your life: marriage, career, family, friendships, as well as your own identity and self-worth. We hear so many statements like, "I am a failure because I will not carry on my family line," or, "I'm defective because I have a body that doesn't work right," or, "I deserve this infertility because I wanted too much. I have a husband and a house and a job. I'm too greedy."

Dispute your irrational beliefs. You are *not a failure* because you may not carry on the family line. It's not your fault. You are doing more than most people do to have a baby. Instead of berating yourself, pat yourself on the back for the effort you are making. You are *not defective* because your body can't get pregnant. Your body works well in other areas of life; you may be a terrific tennis player or a good cook, for example. Your mind works extremely well. And your soul is gentle and kind. You are *not greedy* because you want your life to go as planned. And, as you know, babies don't always go to the ones who want or deserve them most.

The rational/emotive approach is a form of psychotherapy that focuses on restructuring thoughts and feelings to foster adaptive behavior.[6] This approach, modified for use with infertility, can provide you with the ABCs of getting pregnant when you thought you couldn't. The A (the *a*ctivating experience) refers to some real external event to which you are exposed. Your A is called infertility. The B (*b*elief) refers to the chain of thoughts about A. Your B might be, "I'm defective." C symbolizes the *c*onsequences, which are those emotions that result from B. For example, you may want to stay home and not see your friends. The D stands for *d*isputing these beliefs—which is what you must do to get out of this rut. If you do this, then E will follow—you will function more *e*ffectively.

The best way to get in touch with your irrational beliefs is to listen to what you say to yourself. The words you say to yourself and their meaning create and maintain your view of the situation. Ask yourself these questions: What's causing me the most stress? What specifically am I telling myself about my infertility? What you tell yourself gives it the meaning that it has for you.

Mary Alice and her husband, Henry, are childless. When Mary Alice asks herself, "What's worrying me about not having a baby?" she answers, "It means not being able to pass on my genes and my husband's for all posterity." When Henry asks himself, "What's upsetting me about not having a baby?" his response is different. He says, "Without a baby I can never be a Little League coach." Although different, such thoughts produce profound feelings of loss for both these people.

As you go about your daily routine, take time out to monitor your thoughts. Stop putting yourself down for feeling jealous of your friends who have babies. Accept your humanity. Stop thinking poorly of yourself because you don't want to hold your friend's baby. Would you want to work in a pastry shop if you were dieting? The urge to steer clear of situations that would be unpleasant for you is perfectly natural. It doesn't mean you're a cruel or thoughtless person.

You can also change your thinking so that you react differently in stressful situations. You can learn to use a technique called *self-talk,* which involves disputing your destructive inner dialogue. We call our version of the technique Getting Pregnant Self-Talk (described fully in Chapter 2). You can choose to say, "I'm not pregnant now. But I'm hopeful that I will get pregnant. I know the odds are tough, but I prefer to think that I'll succeed. If I don't, I'll deal with that when the time comes." Viewing your problem from that perspective, you may be able to allow yourself to hold your friend's baby after all. More importantly, instead of thinking you are a failure, you will think about how nice it will be when your time comes—for you and your partner.

4. Work as a Team

One of the most important aspects of living with infertility is working in concert with your partner. Under normal circumstances, it takes two people to make a baby. For the infertile couple, the quest seems to employ a cast of thousands. By focusing on your own emotions or the treatment you are undergoing it's easy to forget your partner. Don't! Remember that in unity, there is strength. And no matter how many doctors, nurses, technicians, friends, and family are involved, you and your spouse—the mother and father of this desperately wanted child—are the central players.

You need teamwork to survive infertility. But sometimes it's difficult to stay united. Many couples that start with similar goals part company along the seemingly endless road. Infertility requires a reordering of priorities and a change in lifestyle. When partners differ in their priorities, trouble looms. When treatment fails and a new course of action must be charted, conflict and disharmony may arise. These differences can strain a marriage that already may be taxed by physical discomfort, sexual deprivation, career disruption, financial woes, problems with relatives, and isolation from friends.

One of the most important tools for building a united front is developing excellent communication skills. Communication is the most important factor in determining the quality of your marriage. Therefore, the most important place to start communicating is in your marriage.

Like every human being, you and your partner each live in a private world of experience, and neither of you are mind readers. Unfortunately, couples make the mistake of believing that because they are married they ought to be able to understand each other—to know what the other is feeling or thinking, and especially to understand the reasons behind their spouse's actions. But in fact they don't have access to the reasons, only to the actions.

Henry sees Mary Alice's sad face. He guesses she is upset because today is their anniversary and they still don't have a baby. Indeed, the anniversary has something to do with it. Mary Alice tells him that she is sad because she ruined the special anniversary cake she was baking. Henry laughs at her for getting so upset over such a trivial thing. Henry was jumping to unwarranted conclusions which subsequently led to a rift with his wife. Had Henry questioned her, Mary Alice might have helped by being more specific to begin with.

Good communication involves Active Listening and Leveling. Eventually, Mary Alice explained to her husband that her sadness was not just about the cake but about other things as well. It was about trying to make their day special. It was about showing Henry that they had a stable, romantic marriage even though they lacked a baby. Their anniversary dinner was salvaged because they listened and leveled with each other.

So many aspects of infertility diagnosis can be less stressful and less emotionally devastating if you work as a team. Simple actions, such as accompanying each other to medical procedures or scheduling the receipt of test results when you can be together, can make life much more bearable. And being up front about fears concerning anesthesia, injections, and pain during necessary procedures helps you realize that you are in this together, despite your trepidations. Couples report that when they communicate with each other, using the Getting Pregnant Active Listening and Leveling approach, detailed in the next chapter, they feel closer and more emotionally equipped to cope with all the problems that arise from infertility.

Even after bridging communication gaps with each other, many couples find they still have difficulty discussing their ordeal with outsiders. Bear in mind that other people often can provide additional support, which brings us to our next pointer.

5. Manage Your Social Life

Rose, twenty-eight, teaches fourth grade. She's been trying to have a baby for two years. Recently, she began taking Pergonal injections and undergoing intrauterine inseminations—procedures in which timing is crucial. As a result, she is late to school three or four mornings a month. Rose also has gained weight and appears bloated. Fellow teachers whisper behind her back, wondering, "What's the matter with Rose?"

Martin is an attorney. Last year, everyone thought that this year he would be made a partner. But Martin seems different. Unbeknown to his colleagues, Martin is preoccupied with his wife's infertility treatments and test results. He's frequently on the phone, but not with clients. Everyone at work thinks something's up. Is he getting a divorce? Is he having a breakdown? Is there another woman? Whatever the problem is, his superiors surmise, Martin no longer seems to be partner material.

These stories demonstrate what can occur if you keep your fertility problems secret. Like Rose and Martin, you and your partner may have refrained from telling friends and co-workers about your problems. As a result of your new behavior or mood changes, colleagues might conclude that you're losing your edge or having a midlife crisis. Just when you need the understanding of your colleagues, family, and friends more than ever, you've alienated them.

Social psychologist Sheldon Cohen has conducted numerous studies demonstrating that social support is critical for getting through stressful situations.[7] You may feel uncomfortable discussing the intimate details with friends and co-workers, and, in fact, there may be situations in which it is inappropriate to share this information.

Ultimately, Rose and Martin told their co-workers that they were involved in fertility treatment. Rose's principal gave her time off and assigned other teachers to fill in. The whole school seemed to rally around her. Now she can go to work without feeling as though she's failing as a teacher. Martin was a little less fortunate. He opted out of the partner track temporarily. He took the pressure off himself, and his colleagues respected him for it. Martin knows that he will be able to return to a partner track once the infertility issues are resolved. But Martin is able to be present at all of his wife's important procedures and surgeries. His main concern for now is to do everything possible to have a baby.

Disclosing the secret of your infertility sometimes frees you to interact normally with the people you care about. Psychologist Sidney Jourard, a researcher of self-disclosure, suggests that distancing yourself from everyone else estranges you from yourself.[8] On the other hand, it is inappropriate to tell everyone about your problem. Use good judgment. Think carefully about whom you should tell and under what circumstances. Maybe you will feel most comfortable by telling your mother. On the other hand, you may feel better talking to a longtime friend. Whom you tell first is not important—it's the telling part that is critical. The support and encouragement you can get from your confidants is often surprising. And you'll feel better, too. It's difficult at first, but you and your partner must share what's happening, if only to unburden yourselves from feeling so isolated.

It also helps to have ready answers to embarrassing questions. Peggy took the direct approach to questions about when she planned to have children. Her answer was well rehearsed and always the same: "We want children, but we're having trouble. We're seeing the best doctor in town, and I'm hopeful all will go well. But I have trouble talking about this at happy occasions, so I hope we can change the subject." Gwen also had a prepared answer—one more risque than Peggy's: "Maybe nine months from this morning." We're not suggesting that you use either of these answers, merely that you have statements ready that let you off the hook when you feel uncomfortable. What you tell casual acquaintances and how you talk about your infertility to people who really matter will differ drastically.

Another aspect of this Pointer concerns choosing which social occasions to attend. Bear in mind that baby-related events may be difficult for many infertile women. Avoiding baby showers and baby-namings or christenings protects you from directly having to experience a recent birth. Decide whether you can tolerate such events. If attending will upset you, then you are entirely justified in steering clear.[9]

Young children's birthday parties and other family-oriented events also may be painful. Halloween, Christmas, Hanukkah, Thanksgiving, and other holidays may similarly depress you. You may decide to avoid family gatherings completely, perhaps using the occasion to get away with your partner for a few days. Or you may choose to attend the gathering only briefly and talk with individual family members prior to the event so they understand how you feel. Whatever you decide, make sure you have given these child-centered events careful consideration. Your job is to make your own life easier, not to be a dutiful daughter/ sister/friend when you are not feeling strong.

6. Be a Partner in Your Treatment

Arthur Greil in *Not Yet Pregnant* makes an excellent point when he says that "infertility . . . is in the process of becoming *medicalized*."[10] He further asserts that this medicalization puts the infertile person into a passive role with her physician, who dominates all face-to-face interactions.

How do you view your role as the patient? Do you remain passive and let your doctor run the show? Or do you educate yourself (Pointer 1) and view yourself as a partner in your own treatment?

As a partner in treatment, you will feel more able to discuss the medical options, ask questions, and voice your opinions. Of course, your doctor has a deeper knowledge of infertility diagnosis and treatment, but you know, for example, your own psychological responses to medication and your medical history better than anyone else. Failing to assert yourself with your doctor can make you feel frustrated and resentful of medical treatment that fails to meet your needs. Believe it or not, most doctors will welcome you as a partner.

By assertive, we certainly don't mean you should be obnoxious or constantly challenging your doctor's every word and action. Assertiveness, as one of the key aspects of this Pointer, means stating what you want and making every reasonable effort to get it. Being assertive means believing that it's your perfect right to want certain things.[11] Being assertive also means behaving in a way that is honest and relatively straightforward in terms of how you think and feel.

By being assertive, Marsha, one of our clients, avoided an unnecessary treatment with Clomid, a drug that she had tolerated poorly in the past. Marsha took Clomid for six months and had suffered physical and emotional side effects such as hot flashes, vaginal dryness, mood swings, and uncontrollable crying fits. She vowed never to take Clomid again. When she began treatment at a local clinic, the doctor described a particular test that involved taking Clomid. Marsha was very upset and spent several sleepless nights. She talked to her husband, who urged her to talk assertively with her doctor.

The next day, Marsha telephoned the doctor and asked him for more information about the test. Then she described her previous response to Clomid. The doctor explained that the test was important but not critical and that if she preferred not to take the drug, she didn't have to. He told her they could use other tests instead. Marsha learned a valuable lesson about asserting her needs.

You are in touch with your emotional needs and your body better than anyone else ever could be. And your instincts are, more likely than not, valid. Remember that the treatment of infertility is an inexact science. Your input can influence many aspects of your treatment. Don't underestimate your intelligence just because you don't have a medical degree, and don't be intimidated by your doctors just because they do.

7. Get Organized

Making an appointment schedule, keeping tabs on where you are in your menstrual cycle, and staying on top of mounting bills and insurance payments can seem as demanding as a full-time job. And most people must maintain a full-time job in order to secure the means to pay medical bills or obtain health insurance coverage. But we have found that couples who have a system for paying bills, recording information, following up on insurance claims, and keeping a detailed appointment calendar report less stress surrounding their infertility than do couples who have no organized system.

Recently we saw a perfect example of a disorganized couple who came for their entry interview at the in vitro fertilization (IVF) clinic where we prepare patients for the emotional aspects of infertility treatment. As they walked in, we could tell at a glance the couple had been arguing and were very angry with each other. The wife, Gina, explained that she had scheduled this interview about six weeks ago and had told Vincent, her husband, that she had done so. Vincent denied that he had been informed and was furious over having to take an unexpected afternoon off from work during a particularly busy time. Gina countered that she even heard him (through the telephone) make a note of the appointment. After about five minutes of bickering, the couple calmed down enough to participate in the interview. As the interview progressed, not unexpectedly, they were unable to answer questions about the whats and whens of their treatment history. The interview concluded when Vincent rose and stomped out of the room. Gina stayed with us, crying and saying, "I wish I could get it together."

One reason for Gina's distress was that infertility, as you know, can never be fully under the patient's control. But the major reason for her being upset—a reason that *was* under her control—was her lack of organizational skills. Losing track of what was happening alienated the couple from each another and augmented their stress of being unable to conceive a child.

The energy and time you spend staying organized is extremely valuable because it helps you gain a sense of control over your treatment. Women typically think they will remember the exact day of their post-coital test and its results. You probably think that you will never forget your endometrial biopsy and exactly what the doctor told you afterward. But with time, multiple treatments and doctor's reports can merge into a big, terrible blur. So after every treatment, we encourage you to keep a record of it—a medical one for your doctor and a psychological one for yourself.

In addition, we encourage you to keep logs of each and every menstrual cycle, master and utilize the insurance payment system we've developed (only after we lost track of a few major claims of our own), and purchase (and fill in) an appointment calendar for all future tests, treatments, and procedures so you and your partner can better anticipate what's to come in the days and weeks ahead.

8. Make a Plan

Couples battling infertility must make a myriad of decisions and judgments: what tests to have, what treatment options to explore, how many times to repeat them, how much money to spend, what doctor to select, and what procedures are most likely to bring success. Infertility decisions rank right up there with other important choices such as what college to attend and even what person to marry. While you should stay flexible to allow for medical breakthroughs, for new information about your condition, for a changing insurance policy, or even a surprise pregnancy, it's still important to construct an overall plan so you know where you are and where you're headed at any given moment.

Forging a plan forces you to think about how much money you want to spend, how long you want to keep trying, how much physical and emotional trauma you believe you can withstand, what kinds of odds you are looking for, and other critical factors. As you make a plan, you need to ask yourself some tough questions, questions that focus on your physical, emotional, and financial wherewithal. Your inner monologue may go something like this: "I want a baby. What am I willing to do to make it happen? Am I willing to endure physical pain? Am I willing to spend my money on infertility treatments instead of a vacation? Am I willing to put my social life on hold? Can I put my career on the back burner?" Answers to these questions do not come easily. As one woman we talked to put it, "Infertility hurts my brain." What are you willing to sacrifice to achieve your goal?

Once you learn about all the available treatments and how they'll affect your life and pocketbook, you're ready to develop your plan. We recommend devising a six-month plan. By keeping things finite, you can determine your monetary and emotional limits without overwhelming yourself. If pregnancy remains elusive after six months, then reevaluate and devise another plan for the next six months. Six months is a reasonable amount of time, since infertility treatment options are changing rapidly.

Once you develop your plan, stick with it unless new information warrants a change. Here's an example of a plan that was well organized and thoughtful, but not carved in stone.

In their plan, Susan and Michael decided to try three in vitro procedures. If these three procedures failed, then they would begin to take steps toward adoption. Unfortunately, the three operations were unsuccessful. But then they learned about the recent great success of a procedure in which a donor gives her eggs to the couple to be fertilized with the husband's sperm, and then the embryo is transferred to the wife's uterus. Susan and Michael decided to try three of these ovum donor attempts before adopting. First, however, some psychological issues arose that they needed to confront before they could begin their attempts. (Susan and Michael's story is told in detail in Chapter 10.)

Susan and Michael are unconventional and flexible. They represent one category of planners. Many couples we talk to proceed differently.

Some entertain several mini-plans simultaneously; they try a variety of treatment options in rapid succession, as well as pursue adoption at the same time. Others may tend to stay with one treatment for several years. There are many pathways through infertility. The case stories provided throughout the book can help you clarify what kind of planning style is most comfortable for you. Later in the book, we provide you with a framework for decision-making and some skills and exercises that can help you make a plan that gives you the greatest sense of control.

9. Don't Give Up

Overall statistics suggest that about one out of two infertile couples will eventually produce a baby. But we believe that for some couples whose problems are not too complex or who are willing to go the limit—using repeated trials with donor eggs, donor sperm, or even both—the success rate can approach 90 percent. Of course, this 90 percent figure represents what's *medically* possible. Tragically, medical possibilities require economic resources. Many of the 90 percent of people whose infertility problems could be medically remedied may be unable to afford the cost of treatment. It is truly a tragedy that family-planning decisions are so strongly affected by finances.

Naturally, some infertility treatments are more successful than others. The cutting-edge treatments that offer possibilities when nothing else would ever work get the most publicity. But their odds of success are still limited. Even the top-notch programs have a take-home baby rate of only 30 percent at best with IVF and its related assisted technologies. Simpler procedures, such as artificial insemination, can also offer you reasonable success rates. Even though we encourage you to optimistically try all possible avenues, we also encourage you to *be realistic about your odds of getting pregnant.*

To fully appreciate the odds of succeeding with a single therapy, imagine that you are sitting in your doctor's office with nine other women. Each of you has dysfunctional ovaries and is about to start Pergonal therapy. At the end of six attempts, four of you will be pregnant.

No human being could sit in that waiting room and undergo treatment unless she believed she will be one of those four. Doctors encourage that optimism. Yet they walk a tightrope between encouraging you and tempering that encouragement with a realistic perspective. When a procedure fails, they urge you to try again.

And remember, technology is evolving all the time. Today's insurmountable problem may be fixable next year. For example, since we began researching this book in 1990, embryo-freezing technology has improved dramatically. Eggs harvested from a single retrieval can be frozen in multiple "six-packs." If an initial embryo transfer fails, a new cycle can be attempted with a frozen "six-pack." So one egg retrieval can be parlayed into multiple implantation attempts.

It is important to continue when many attempts have failed. The important key is to find ways to persevere despite these repeated failures. The temptation to give up increases if you withdraw from daily activities or let the specter of infertility color everything you do. Later in the book, we will introduce motivational techniques borrowed from athletes, actors, artists, and other successful individuals who manage to keep going in the face of adversity.[12] The skills, modified for use with infertility, focus on helping you help yourself through all the various situations you must confront. You can choose those that work for you or adapt them to fit your circumstances. Armed with these tactics, you will be able to continue infertility treatment as long as it continues to hold out a realistic chance of success.

We must make one important clarification here. By telling you not to give up, we encourage you to stay focused on your goal of getting pregnant *so long as it continues to be your goal.* But you must be open to new information—medical, emotional, and financial. Sometimes this new information may lead you to change your goal. At some point, it may make sense to set a new goal: adopting, or restructuring your life to live childfree. Your goal, then, becomes to stop treatment and change direction. So, by encouraging you not to give up, we don't mean you should continue treatment endlessly when it no longer makes sense to do so.

Putting It All Together: How the Nine Pointers Combine to Help You Start Living Again

Taken individually, each Pointer probably won't seem like a major life change. But once you start putting all Nine Pointers into practice, we expect you will begin to view your infertility in a new, positive light you previously thought was impossible. Practicing the Nine Pointers can help you resume a normal, happy life even though your infertility is not yet resolved.

It's important for you to live in the present in order to make rational decisions, cope with treatment, and live a rich and rewarding life despite your infertility. It is counterproductive to regret any past actions as the real or imagined cause of your current problem. It is tempting to talk about what might have been or what you should have done. Leeanne, for example, still weeps over the abortion she had when she was eighteen, even though it seemed to be the only proper course of action at the time. "I should have had the baby," Leeanne laments. "Now my tubes are blocked, and I'll never get pregnant."

Ed, meanwhile, berates himself about the vasectomy he had during his marriage to Valerie. Little did he know back then that he'd one day divorce Valerie and marry another woman who wants children. "Who would have thought it? Me with new kids at my age, but it sounds nice," says Ed, whose children from his first marriage are grown. "When Valerie suggested a vasectomy, it seemed like a good idea. But I never should have listened to her."

Leeanne and Ed are each mired in what we call "pastspeak." They dwell obsessively on their past. What they did years ago made sense at that time. They need to live in the present. You probably have some of your own should haves and what ifs. Everybody does. But infertile people may seem to dwell on these past occurrences, perhaps to avoid the frustrations of their current dilemma. Living in the past robs you of the pleasures of today. If you live in the past, you are more likely to give up your quest to get pregnant. You must find a way to build happiness into your everyday life even as you pursue your goal of getting pregnant. Focusing on the present is more productive and healthier than dwelling on the past.

Through the Nine Pointers, Leeanne and Ed each are working to let go of their past. They are lucky to live in the 1990s. Their infertility problems can be treated—with surprisingly good results. In vitro fertilization can bypass Leeanne's bad tubes. And Ed has a better chance of successfully reversing his vasectomy than reducing his alimony payments to Valerie. Our advice to you is the same as it is to Leeanne and Ed. Don't look back. Plant yourself firmly in the present. Make a plan. Find a doctor who can help, and become an active, informed partner in treatment.

The Nine Pointers can help you avoid another common pitfall of infertility: pining for the future. Spending all your time on "futurethought" can make your precious todays melt together. Instead of living in the here-and-now, infertile couples often calculate the days until ovulation, the weeks until the pregnancy test, or the months until the next IVF procedure. This hurry-up-and-wait phenomenon is one of the most difficult problems infertile people need to overcome. There is so much to wait for: the doctor, a procedure, a drug to take effect, an operation, and, of course, the pregnancy itself. Dwelling on all you have to wait for can put your life on hold.

Dorothy lived her life nine months ahead. If she got pregnant in January, her baby would be born in October; if she got pregnant in February, it would be born in November. Each month, she got out her astrology book and read what sign her baby would be born under if she got pregnant that month. When she wasn't pregnant that month, she'd start reading the next chapter.

Dorothy is an extreme example of somebody who was unable to live in the present. Each failure seemed to pull her further from her immediate goals. Through the Nine Pointers, Dorothy reframed her thinking, got in touch with her feelings, developed a system to organize her bills and appointments, and made a plan. She scheduled some pleasant activities with her husband and with her friends. Dorothy is now working hard to live in the present.

We're not suggesting that it's going to be easy to live in the today world, but we believe that the wait for conception will be more tolerable if you train yourself to experience each day fully. But with all these worries on your mind, how can you possibly live in the present? The answer is to force yourself. Make a conscious effort to purge futurethought and pastspeak from your consciousness. Dispute any self-pitying or self-loathing sentiments you might harbor. To your negative statements like, "What's the use of buying a bigger house if I can't have a baby," for instance, prepare a convincing retort, such as, "My husband and I will feel more comfortable with more space." And be patient. Allow time to dig yourself out of the rut you have been in.

We provide some digging-out tools in the Getting Pregnant Workout, a set of skills described in the next chapter. The Workout, like the Nine Pointers, will help you start living again, even if your infertility seems far from being resolved.

CHAPTER TWO

HELPING YOURSELF THROUGH INFERTILITY: THE GETTING PREGNANT WORKOUT

As WE WENT through the diagnosis and treatment of our own infertility, we felt the same disappointment and heartache that other infertile couples feel. We learned that infertility can prevent people from living normal lives, since our own lives were incapacitated by our failures to conceive. As therapists experienced in helping others cope with emotionally charged issues, we searched for ways to adapt our counseling methods to help us through our own ordeal. Our search led us to develop our Getting Pregnant Workout.

The Getting Pregnant Workout is a series of activities that put the Nine Pointers discussed in Chapter 1 into action. The Workout blends elements used by clinical psychologists of various schools of psychotherapy—all modified to meet the unique needs of people with fertility problems. Among the traditions we draw from are cognitive and family therapy, mental imagery, communications theory, behavior modification, and Gestalt psychotherapy.

As broad as the above list seems, it was not sufficient for our program. So we included elements from the performing and visual arts, Eastern philosophy, and substance abuse recovery.

As a way to start living normally again, we began counseling infertile couples in our psychotherapy practice. These sessions provided us with new perspectives and additional psychological information, which we also incorporated into the Getting Pregnant Workout. We field-tested these techniques with our clients and presented the Workout at a meeting of the infertility support group RESOLVE Inc. Feedback from people who tried the Workout has been extremely positive. These techniques make good *clinical* sense. But the field of Assisted Reproductive Technology is so new that mental health practitioners have not yet developed or adapted a myriad of techniques to help infertile individuals cope. Many of the techniques we describe in this book are at the cutting edge. We have created them to fill an unmet need of our clients. But because the techniques are so new, they have not yet been subjected to rigorous scientific evaluation to determine precisely what percentage of people who use them benefit from them and exactly how much they benefit. We have begun to conduct this needed research and plan to report our findings as soon as they are available.

We chose the word ''workout'' deliberately. We have found that you cannot cope successfully with infertility on a casual basis. It takes psychological work to equip yourself with the tools you need to handle the tough situations that lie ahead. With practice, healthy responses to awkward or upsetting situations can become second nature.

Linda Salzer, an infertility counselor and author of the widely acclaimed book *Surviving Infertility,* tells audiences how she and her husband devised and actually rehearsed a set of signals they used to escape uneasy social encounters.[1] At one dinner dance, Linda recounts, she grew extremely anxious as several women at her table began exchanging pictures of their babies. Linda signaled her husband with a subtle hand gesture. In response, he whisked her from the table and swiftly waltzed her across the dance floor and out of the room so she could cry in private instead of embarrassing herself in front of her friends.

Like Linda, you can prepare yourself for any situation: social, medical, job-related, or financial. The Getting Pregnant Workout is most effective when practiced for several brief periods every day. The more you practice, the better you'll get at the Getting Pregnant Workout skills: relaxation, self-talk, interpersonal communication, assertiveness, decision-making, record-keeping, goal-setting, and using your imagination.

Later in the book, we'll provide further details to help you cope with specific situations—such as using the decision-making technique to choose your doctor. Throughout, we will refer to the Getting Pregnant Workout as a means toward getting pregnant when you thought you couldn't.

INFERTILITY IS STRESSFUL

The stress of infertility is inescapable. No matter what you do, you cannot entirely avoid it. Although you may be aware of your stress, you probably don't know yet how to cope with it.

The stress of infertility is both long- and short-term. Like other long-term, or chronic, stressful situations, such as poverty or cancer, there may be little you can do to change your predicament. You may feel as though you are running on a treadmill and keep failing in your attempts to jump off.

Then there are short-term, or acute, stresses that last from a few minutes to a few days. Waiting for the results of a test. Receiving a medical bill you can't afford to pay. Getting invited to a baby shower.

The Physical Effects of Stress

In times of stress, what are known as fight-or-flight hormones kick in. It happened when your cave-dwelling ancestors confronted a lightning storm. And it happens when you confront your pregnant sister-in-law. Eventually, the fight-or-flight response can exhaust you mentally and physically. It can even make you sick or more prone to physical pain. The adrenaline flowing through your body makes you tense up during an endometrial biopsy, for example. Unlike your prehistoric ancestors, however, you can acquire the knowledge to analyze, evaluate, and even challenge erroneous assumptions about your infertility. You can learn to employ a variety of adaptive techniques that can reshape your responses, lower pain, and keep your self-esteem intact.

Figure 2.1 shows how the stress of infertility can affect your body.

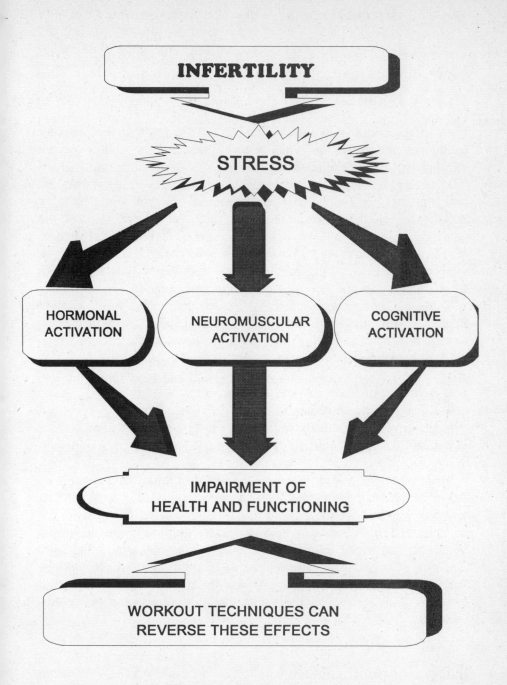

Figure 2.1.
How Infertility Stress Affects Your Body

Combating Stress: Changing Your Thoughts to Take Positive Action

Look at the bottom section of figure 2.1. It shows that the Workout techniques can reverse the impairments of infertility stress. *How* you are affected by stress depends on how you *view* your situation. Richard Lazarus, a psychologist and an eminent stress researcher, has shown that how you *appraise* a situation often determines how you are affected by it.[2] If you view the situation as a *threat* and you believe you *lack the resources to cope* with it, you will become stressed. The critical element here is your outlook. And your outlook can be changed. If you learn to view the experience differently, you can modify how you respond to what's happening and how you behave in that situation.

Recasting your view of infertility is a key component to the Getting Pregnant Workout. The techniques we present have strong theoretical underpinnings in the field of behavioral medicine, at the core of which are four principles important to people confronting infertility:

- Be aware of what you are thinking;
- Change your erroneous beliefs;
- Learn various methods and techniques to assist you; and
- Carry out these skills in daily life.

You can begin by exerting some control over what happens to you. When we talk of control, we don't mean the ability to control whether you get pregnant. We mean you can develop the belief that you are not helpless and that you can take an active role in your diagnosis, treatment, and social interactions. Figure 2.2, a model modified from the work of two Canadians, psychiatrist Eldon Tunks and psychologist Anthony Bellissimo, graphically depicts the relationship between your thoughts, your view of yourself and your capabilities, and the actions you take.[3]

The Mind-Body Connection

Thinking optimistic thoughts won't unblock your tubes or make your husband's low sperm count suddenly become normal. Nor will reducing

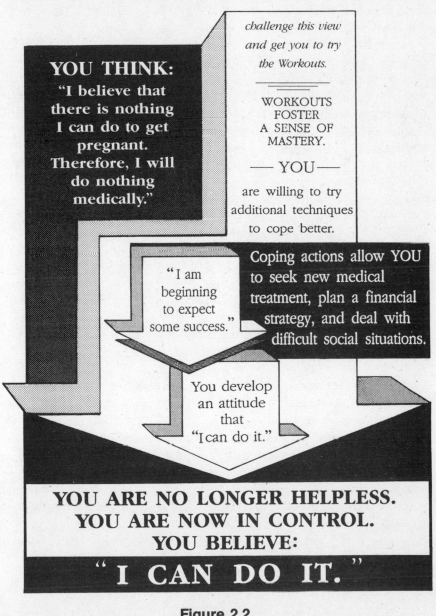

YOU THINK:
"I believe that there is nothing I can do to get pregnant. Therefore, I will do nothing medically."

challenge this view and get you to try the Workouts.

WORKOUTS FOSTER A SENSE OF MASTERY.

—— YOU ——

are willing to try additional techniques to cope better.

" I am beginning to expect some success."

Coping actions allow YOU to seek new medical treatment, plan a financial strategy, and deal with difficult social situations.

You develop an attitude that "I can do it."

YOU ARE NO LONGER HELPLESS. YOU ARE NOW IN CONTROL. YOU BELIEVE:

" I CAN DO IT. "

Figure 2.2.
The Relationship of Your Thoughts and Your Actions

your stress level. But studies suggest that relaxation has many other beneficial effects. Researcher Candace Pert, cancer surgeon Bernie Siegel, and Norman Cousins, among many others, have written about nontraditional, intellectual/emotional methods of healing.[4] These methods acknowledge that we all have a body-mind connection.

Immunologist George Solomon discusses studies suggesting that depression, a condition often associated with infertility, leads to suppression of the body's ability to provide immunity against certain diseases. "Behavioral interventions (such as psychotherapy, relaxation techniques, imagery, biofeedback, and hypnosis) should be able to enhance or optimize immune function," he believes.[5] And he predicts that eventually research will directly support his contention.

First and foremost, then, the Getting Pregnant Workout will help you relax and feel less stress. We are unable to offer any scientific evidence that the Workout will combat the *physical* aspects of your infertility. But we do know that if you perform the Workout as recommended, you will be able to manage your medical treatment more effectively.

RELAXATION: A GOOD WAY TO CONFRONT STRESS HEAD ON

Most of the infertile couples we counsel talk about loss, pain, and grief. They speak of feeling overwhelmed. And they worry about what infertility is doing to their marriage, their careers, and their view of themselves and others. To help them, we recommend techniques such as progressive relaxation, controlled breathing, and positive imagery to break the cycle of debilitating negative emotions. By using these relaxation methods, our clients have slowly replaced their negative thoughts with a sense of peace. Gradually, they find the inner strength to take the steps necessary to increase their odds of getting pregnant.

As clinical psychologist Thomas D'Zurilla describes it, relaxation works in this way:[6]

■ Relaxation *reduces emotional upheaval directly.* It helps calm you down so that you are not so overwhelmed by what you are feeling. Relaxation helps you reduce the level of your debilitating emotion.

- Practicing relaxation techniques helps you *learn to monitor your stress* and recognize the stress as it begins to occur. Mastering relaxation allows you to be on "automatic pilot," ready and able to reduce your stress as you begin to feel it.
- When you begin to achieve relaxation, you give yourself *direct access to your counterproductive thoughts* that may be keeping you from seeking treatment, preventing you from complying with your doctor's orders, or making you interact negatively with your spouse, family, or friends.

Progressive Relaxation

Progressive relaxation, pioneered in the 1930s by physiologist and psychologist Edmund Jacobson, is an effective way to relax and reduce anxiety.[7] Jacobson believed that if people could learn to relax their muscles through a precise method, mental relaxation would follow. Jacobson's technique involves tensing and relaxing various voluntary muscle groups throughout the body in an orderly sequence. According to psychologists Robert Woolfolk and Frank Richardson in their book *Stress, Sanity, and Survival,* "Despite the relative obscurity of this method, progressive relaxation is perhaps the most reliable and effective procedure of all [the different means of achieving relaxation]."[8] Since Jacobson developed and refined his techniques, people have used progressive relaxation to alleviate such diverse stress-related disorders as anxiety, ulcers, hypertension, and insomnia.

Progressive relaxation works because of the relationship between your muscle tension and your emotional tension. When you feel emotionally distraught, you automatically tense your muscles. Your muscle tension may be a *cause* of the headaches and backaches of infertility, as well as a *clue* about how you are responding to your infertility.

Mastering progressive relaxation in its pure form requires extensive training and more practice than people dealing with infertility generally have time to do. Research, however, has shown that abbreviated versions of progressive relaxation can be quite effective in alleviating the effects of stress.

Five features are critical:

PLACE: Find a quiet room where you can work undisturbed.
POSITION: To learn progressive relaxation, all parts of your body

CLOTHING:

TIME:

FOCUS:

must be comfortably supported. Find a bed, a couch, or a recliner.

CLOTHING: Wear loose clothing.

TIME: Designate about fifteen minutes daily. Try to schedule a fixed time every day so you won't forget to do your progressive relaxation.

FOCUS: Try to focus on the particular sensations that come from letting go of tension.

Prior to beginning your progressive relaxation routine, have someone whose voice you find pleasant tape-record the text in the box that follows. Tell that person to speak slowly and clearly, pausing to give you time to respond.

Lie or sit in a comfortable position. I'm going to ask you to tense and relax various parts of your body. When I say TENSE, I'd like you to tense that body part. When I say RELAX, I'd like you to let go of all tension. Try to focus on one body part at a time.

Get in touch with your breathing. Breathe out, breathe in. Imagine that as each body part is relaxed, all tension is gone.

TENSE your toes. RELAX. TENSE your knees. RELAX. TENSE your right leg. RELAX. You should feel your whole leg relaxing and settling into the floor. TENSE your left leg. RELAX. Now TENSE your buttocks. RELAX. Press your lower back against the floor. RELAX. TENSE your stomach. RELAX. TENSE your rib cage. RELAX. Feel the tension gone in your lower body.

Push your shoulders back. RELAX. Pull your shoulders forward. RELAX. Now work on your arms. Make a fist with one hand. RELAX. TENSE that upper arm. RELAX. TENSE that whole arm. RELAX. Make a fist with the other hand. RELAX. TENSE that upper arm. RELAX. TENSE that whole arm. RELAX.

Now let's work on your face and head. Clench your jaw. RELAX. Open your mouth wide. RELAX. Grimace. RELAX. Scrunch up your whole face. RELAX. Eyes closed. RELAX. Eyes wide. RELAX.

Now feel all the tension gone from everywhere in your whole body. Keep breathing. Breathe out. Breathe in. Feel completely relaxed.

Learning to Breathe

Voluntary breath control is probably the oldest known stress reduction technique. It is a major component of yoga, the ancient Indian self-help system of health care and spiritual development; T'ai Chi, a Chinese movement art form; and the Lamaze method of natural childbirth. These and other methods share a focus on the four distinct phases of the breathing cycle: inhalation, pause, exhalation, and pause. Becoming aware of these four phases is an essential step in obtaining control of your breathing pattern. Once you gain control of your breathing in a nonstressful environment, you can more readily call up your relaxation breathing during times of stress.

Your thoughts and your internal responses are closely linked. If you think anxious thoughts, your breathing becomes shallow and rapid. Conversely, shallow, rapid breathing can make it difficult for you to think calmly and rationally. If you are caught in this vicious cycle, you can either change your thoughts or change your breathing—and the other will follow. You can use controlled breathing to implement an important Pointer: changing how you think about your infertility. Also, by learning to breathe properly, you can begin to feel less fatigued, less overwhelmed by your thoughts, and more able to cope with each new procedure and treatment. As you cope better, you may become more optimistic. While not a panacea, the Getting Pregnant Breathing described above is perhaps the easiest new technique you'll master.

Again, tape-record the directions in the box. Play them back when you have a few minutes to learn to practice Getting Pregnant Breathing.

Lie on your back on a rug. Get comfortable.

Place one hand on your chest and the other on your abdomen. Without trying to change your breathing, notice which hand is rising and falling with each breath. If your belly rises as you breathe in, you are breathing from your diaphragm. If not, you are breathing from your chest.

Shift your breathing from chest to diaphragm. Inhale slowly and deeply through your nose into your abdomen to push up your hand as much as it feels comfortable. Smile slightly, inhale through your nose, and exhale through your mouth. Make a relaxed soft sound like the wind as you exhale. It should sound like "whoosh."

Continue taking slow deep breaths. Inhale. Exhale . . . whoosh. Inhale. Exhale . . . whoosh. Think of each whoosh as a sigh of relief.

- Practice this activity for five minutes at a time once or twice a day.
- At the end of each breathing time, focus on your body and its tension. By the end of a week, you should experience a noticeable difference in your tension, particularly in your neck and shoulders, and in the muscles around your jaw.
- After one week's practice, try this activity while sitting or standing.
- After one month of practicing, try this activity during a doctor's visit.

Once you've mastered controlled breathing, you can use it while driving to your doctor's office, sitting in the waiting room, or during a medical test or procedure. You can even use it while waiting to hear the results of a test. Use controlled breathing anytime you start to feel tension.

GETTING PREGNANT SELF-TALK (GPST)

Almost all infertile couples we have encountered entertain negative thoughts. One of our clients, Gloria, was trying to decide whether she should change doctors. We asked her to voice her inner thoughts. "What difference does it make," she responded. "Nobody will be able to find out what's wrong with me. I'm not pregnant with this doctor. The next one will just cost more but won't do me any good." With thoughts like these, how could Gloria ever make positive decisions? We taught her to listen to her thoughts and to say them aloud when no one was in the room. From that point, we told her to replace the negativity with positive thoughts. This self-talk method eventually motivated her to take appropriate action.

If you stop and say your inner thoughts aloud, your monologue probably sounds like this: "I'll never get pregnant. I'm sure this will go on forever. I will never be a parent." Bombarding yourself with negative thoughts like these impedes your ability to deal with the fertile world, undergo surgery, or make the first phone call to a doctor. Your negative inner statements stand in the way of what you want most. You need to learn to use the same *cognitive* technique we taught Gloria. We call that technique Getting Pregnant Self-Talk (GPST). Implementing all Nine Pointers, GPST is the single most powerful technique in the Getting Pregnant Workout.

Self-talk is a technique used in cognitive psychotherapy, a form of counseling that focuses on how thoughts and images contribute to stress. Psychiatrist Aaron Beck, one of the country's leading cognitive therapists, discusses the importance of *automatic thoughts*.[9] Automatic thoughts are those thoughts that occur in your stream of consciousness *automatically* and are rarely questioned. They are couched with *shoulds* and *musts*, and are difficult to turn off. People erroneously treat their automatic thoughts as foregone conclusions rather than hypotheses to be questioned. Your automatic infertility thoughts make you believe your situation is hopeless. These thoughts may prevent you from taking steps to help yourself.

Donald Meichenbaum, who developed the method of *stress inoculation*, believes that all people engage in an internal dialogue.[10] Your internal dialogue incorporates your expectations and evaluation of yourself and your behavior. The psychic pain you experience from inner statements such as, "I'll never get pregnant," can paralyze you. Meichenbaum teaches his clients to use self-talk to create a productive inner dialogue that replaces these defeatist ideas.

GPST, then, aims to boost your self-esteem and motivate you to act. GPST is *not* the vague, imprecise feelings you have regarding a situation, but rather the actual words you say to yourself in your mind's ear. Because self-talk requires that you say each word in your monologue (not just think it), we encourage you to try GPST by first writing down and then rehearsing your new inner monologue. Then, when you feel ready, use GPST during an actual situation. It may be helpful to think of GPST in the following steps:

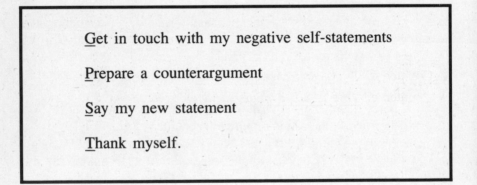

<u>G</u>et in touch with my negative self-statements

<u>P</u>repare a counterargument

<u>S</u>ay my new statement

<u>T</u>hank myself.

We'll help you get started by asking you to follow the steps and fill in the following incomplete statements. Try to be as specific as possible when writing your statements. We'll illustrate each step with responses from some of our clients.

1. Get in touch with negative statements by filling in the following blanks:
   a. I don't think I can _____.
   b. I'm afraid I will _____.
   c. I don't want to _____.
   d. I think that _____ will happen again.
   e. (Create your own phrase): _____.

Our clients said:

a. I don't think I can *take my temperature one more time.*

b. I'm afraid I will *never carry a baby to term.*

c. I don't want to *get my hopes up just to have them dashed.*

d. I think that *a miscarriage* will happen again.

e. (Create your own phrase): *This can't be happening.*

2. Prepare a counterargument for each of these negative statements. First read how our clients prepared their counterarguments.

Counter **a:** *By taking my temperature I'm upping my odds of getting pregnant.*

Counter **b:** *I know I'll find an answer to this puzzle of miscarriage.*

Counter **c:** *Perhaps getting my hopes up will get me through the next procedure.*

Counter **d:** *I'm strong enough to deal with another disappointment.*

Counter **e:** *This is not a punishment or a curse but a fact of life.*

Now prepare *your* counterarguments:

Counter **a:** _____.

Counter **b:** _____.

Counter **c:** _____.

Counter **d:** _____.

Counter **e:** _____.

3. Say your counterarguments out loud in a place where no one else can hear you. Once you've said them out loud, repeat them silently to yourself several times.

4. Thank yourself for trying to cope. We'll give you the first few thank-yous; you create several more:

a. Thanks for taking control.

b. I like myself for helping myself.

c. I'm proud of myself for working to change.

d. (Your own thank-yous go here.) _____.

Here is one more GPST memory tool to help you understand the four types of GPST statements. Examples are included with each.

Guiding yourself: *Let's figure out what this test result means.*

Psyching yourself up: *By calling the doctor I'm upping my odds.*

Soothing talk: *It's okay. This procedure will be over soon.*

Taking charge. *Come on now. Pull yourself together.*

Guiding statements help you through taxing procedures. They also assist you when you feel confused or overwhelmed. If you get a medical report that you cannot understand, don't panic. Instead, calmly guide yourself. Say, "Let's figure out what this test result means." Psyching-up statements use positive and optimistic language to motivate you. Don't let that inner voice defeat you with phrases like, "What's the use of trying?" Fight back with a psyching counterargument such as, "By calling the doctor, I'm upping my odds." Soothing talk is like your inner parent calming you down when you are scared. When you panic during an unpleasant procedure, use soothing words like, "It'll be over soon." Finally, taking-charge statements spur you into action or quiet you down if you find yourself obsessing.

LEARNING EFFECTIVE COMMUNICATION SKILLS

Study after study has found that men and women react differently to infertility. In his thoughtful research book, *Not Yet Pregnant,* sociologist Arthur Greil reports, "Husbands were not only less likely than their wives to see infertility as a threat to identity, but they were also less likely to see themselves as living in a world where painful reminders of infertility were inescapable."[11] In infertility, as in other stressful situations, women tend to focus on the emotions of the situation. Even though they often are good at taking action, they also feel compelled to talk things out. Most men, on the other hand, are less comfortable dealing with feelings. They are socialized to be task-oriented. When they face a crisis, they want to do something about it rather than talk.

Our female clients, many of whom are career women, lament that their husbands have lost interest in the pregnancy quest. The women complain that their husbands don't listen to them as they did in the beginning of their crisis. Husbands are upset when they see their previously competent wives fall apart. They find it equally difficult to participate in "endless" discussions, particularly when they are not sure what their role is or should be.

Women in our society have a mandate to become mothers. Until they fulfill that mandate, everything else gets placed on hold. The only topic worthy of discussion is getting pregnant. But as Greil notes, "There is, in American society, no 'fatherhood mandate' with the same force and intensity as the 'motherhood mandate.' "[12] The bottom line, however, is that when one member of a couple has a problem, the *couple* has a problem. In order to Work as a Team, the couple must find a way to pull together.

Greil notes that despite the gender differences in motivation to have a baby, many couples report that infertility actually strengthened their marriage. Husbands and wives felt closer because of their shared experience. Admittedly, they argued more, but these intense interactions fostered greater rapport and an increased sense of empathy. Greil concludes that infertility becomes a threat to a marriage when the husband resists his wife's demands for greater communication. But if the husband accepts infertility as a problem for the marital team and is willing to talk about it with his wife, the crisis is likely to unite them.

Facing infertility as a team makes the struggle less stressful. But when stress is high, some couples have great difficulty speaking to each other productively and rationally. A few basic communication skills, mastered today and called up when communication breaks down, can help you get back on track.

Two important communication techniques are *active listening* and *leveling*. Active listening is more than just listening attentively and quietly. Active listening means trying to understand your partner's inner world. Leveling is sharing your inner world with your partner.

Listening and leveling go hand in hand. As you listen, you participate actively. As you share your reactions, you help your partner to understand your world while he is explaining his world to you. By leveling, you help your partner to listen. When you tell him about your innermost thoughts, he begins to better understand you. Also when you level, you drop your guard. Seeing that, your partner reciprocates. By leveling, you encourage him to listen; by listening, you encourage him to level. The outcome of this productive dialogue is a mutual sense of *legitimation*. Each member of the team feels that his or her partner treats his or her concerns as legitimate and valid.

The Getting Pregnant Active Listening and Leveling approach fosters productive dialogue. The approach has three facets:

- Trying to understand your partner's world of experience;
- Conveying information about your own world of experience; and, as a by-product of the first two processes,
- Commenting on the relationship.

We've developed a checklist that can help you and your partner evaluate the nature of your communication in terms of listening and leveling:

Getting Pregnant Listening focuses on trying to understand your partner's world by:

☐ asking your partner for further clarification and expansion
☐ asking about your partner's intentions and preferences
☐ trying to probe for your partner's feelings about what's happening and about your actions
☐ testing to see whether your understanding corresponds to what your partner means

In contrast, *Not* Listening communication is characterized by:

☐ cutting off your partner before he finishes
☐ telling your partner how he feels or what he wants rather than asking him
☐ responding literally to your partner's words instead of to the meaning of what is said
☐ arguing about whether your partner said something rather than whether he meant it
☐ treating your inferences as facts not hypotheses to be tested

Getting Pregnant Leveling contains interactions that focus on:

☐ explaining your concerns
☐ showing how your concerns fit into your partner's concerns
☐ disclosing your feelings related to your partner's actions
☐ demonstrating how present experience relates to past experiences

In contrast, *Not* Leveling includes these interactions:

☐ taking action without explaining the basis for the action
☐ not sharing information indicating whether you agree or
     disagree with the position your partner is taking
☐ not acknowledging your feelings
☐ not sharing the basis for your feelings
☐ attempting to persuade

Here are some sample conversations. Use the checklist to evaluate them. Then read our evaluation.

MARY: I just got this invitation to Beth's baby shower. I—
JOHN: I know. She should know better than to invite you to these things.
MARY: No. She is a really good friend. She's so excited about being pregnant. It's just—
JOHN: That you feel so bad that she's pregnant and you're not.
MARY: No. That's not it. I wish you'd let me say what I'm feeling instead of assuming you know how I feel. It's just that I feel so bad that I can't share her happiness. I love Beth. We're best friends. And I know she'd never want to hurt me.

Here's how we evaluated this dialogue:

Not Listening:

JOHN: cutting off his partner before she finishes
JOHN: telling his partner how she feels or what she wants rather than asking her
JOHN: treating his inferences as facts, not hypotheses to be tested

Leveling:

MARY: explaining her concerns
MARY: disclosing her feelings related to her partner's actions

Not Leveling:

JOHN: attempting to persuade

How did your evaluation compare with ours? Now try this one.

DENNIS: I'm worried that I won't be able to produce a sperm sample
           for your insemination tomorrow.
PAULA: Don't be silly. You can do it. You're so sexy.
DENNIS: I'm not worried about my manliness. Did you think that's
           what was bothering me?
PAULA: Sure. You mean that's not what's really worrying you?
DENNIS: No. I'm upset because I think you'll be so disappointed in
           me. Here you've taken all these shots and spent all this
           money on medicine. And then I won't produce the sample
           and you won't get inseminated. I just think you'll feel angry
           with me. Won't you?
PAULA: No. I'd know you tried.
DENNIS: I just find that hard to believe. Wouldn't you feel let down
           after getting your hopes up so much?
PAULA: You're right. I would.
DENNIS: So why did you say it wouldn't bother you?
PAULA: Well, I just thought if I said I wasn't worried it would take
           the pressure off you.

This interaction is more complicated than the last one. Let's analyze
the dialogue in greater detail.

When Dennis says, "I'm worried that I won't be able to produce a
sperm sample," he is leveling by *explaining his concerns*. When Paula
says, "Don't be silly. You can do it. You're so sexy," she is not
leveling. She is *attempting to convince* him that he can feel sexy. She is
also not listening. She *infers* that he is upset about a problem of
manliness. She treats this inference as a fact rather than checking it out.
Dennis levels by *explaining his concerns* when he counters, "I'm not
worried about my manliness." Then he *tests his understanding* of
Paula's comment by asking, "Did you think that's what was bothering
me?"

Paula *asks for further clarification* when she says, "You mean that's
not what's really worrying you?" Dennis responds by *showing how his
concerns fit Paula's concerns* when he says, "I'm upset because I think
you'll be so disappointed in me..." He concludes by *testing his
inference* when he asks, "Won't you?"

Paula *does not acknowledge her feelings* at first. She says, "No. I'd
know you tried." But Dennis finds that hard to believe. So he further

probes to *test Paula's preferences*. He asks, "Wouldn't you feel let down?" Paula then *discloses her feelings in relation to Dennis's actions*. She admits, "You're right." Then Dennis *asks for further clarification* by saying, "So why did you say it wouldn't bother you?" Then Paula explains *how her concerns fit Dennis's concerns* by saying, ". . . if I said I wasn't worried it would take the pressure off you."

How did you evaluate the dialogue? Did you score it similarly? Perhaps you categorized a few statements differently than we did. That's okay. Several of the statements can be placed in more than one category. What's important here is learning to monitor your own communication to avoid making statements that you'll regret. Remember:

- You and your partner are two different people with different ideas about infertility. Keep the following question foremost in your mind: *How do my partner's beliefs make sense to* him, *not to me?* No matter how silly or unreasonable his beliefs seem to you, *they make sense to him.* Your task is to investigate how they make sense to your spouse. Your partner has the same task with respect to your statements.
- Whenever your partner says something about infertility that you find unreasonable, ask him to tell you more until you get to the point where you can understand how he views the situation. And of course, he must try to understand your view.
- Try to avoid the natural tendency to think you are more right than the other person. Instead, tell yourself that you and your spouse are two different people with two different views about infertility.

When you feel you've mastered these communication skills, you're ready to use them in the situations described in future chapters, and in real-life ones, too.

LEARNING TO BEHAVE ASSERTIVELY

Because you are not yet pregnant, you may consider yourself deficient or unworthy because you cannot do what fertile people can do. You may believe: "I have no right to make any demands."

Such an attitude is unproductive. Often, it manifests itself in the way you behave with the medical staff during your diagnostic workup. Many of the couples we counsel relinquish control to the medical team. They allow the doctor or technician to call the shots. Of course, doctors have a great deal of expertise, but you also have a great deal of information and experience, particularly concerning your own body. It's important to learn when and how to share this information, as well as how to ask for what you want. Only then can you Become a Partner in Your Treatment.

Start learning about assertiveness by looking at another memory device: the word ASSERT. These six statements can help you begin:

Acknowledge your rights.

Specify your goal (to yourself).

State your view of the problem.

Express and explain your feelings.

Request what you want from the other person.

Thank the other person for considering your needs.

First, you must believe that you have rights that deserve to be acknowledged. Then, you must decide what you really want, such as a doctor's appointment or a copy of your medical records. After you have clarified your needs, you must state your desire clearly when making your request. Be ready to respond to the other person's viewpoint as well.

Jane, one of our clients, started her infertility workup feeling particularly unassertive. She faithfully tried to master assertiveness training but never truly believed that she would need to use her new skills. Then something happened that convinced Jane of the importance of being assertive. Two weeks earlier, she had written a letter to Dr. A requesting that her records be sent to Dr. B, an infertility specialist very much in demand and recommended to her by Dr. A. His waiting list was three months long, and Jane had been placed at the end of the queue. On the day she phoned us, Jane had received a call from Dr. B's office explaining that the busy physician had a cancellation and could see her and her husband immediately.

Jane was ecstatic. She called Dr. A's office and explained that she needed her records that day. Dr. A's staff refused, stating that records were sent out in the order they had been requested and that Jane's records would not be ready for at least a month. Initially, Jane related,

"I saw red. All I wanted to do was scream. I felt like saying, 'Your patients must be exiting en masse if you're backed up six weeks,' but I took a few deep breaths, said a little GPST [Getting Pregnant Self-Talk], and calmly told them that the records belonged to me, that I could come over and copy them myself, and that I was unable to accept no for an answer since I needed to see Dr. B as soon as possible."

The staff continued to balk. Even Dr. A, whom Jane asked to speak with personally (a very assertive stance in itself), called her approach highly unorthodox and refused to comply. Jane calmly stated, firmly but quietly, that she would do anything to facilitate getting her records immediately. She acknowledged that Dr. A had done the best he could and thanked him for referring her to Dr. B, but she stressed that she could not wait. Even though Dr. A set up his practice in this rigid way and was cold and unemotional, he finally backed down and gave Jane her records. She didn't get a smile, but Jane knew that friendly behavior was not critical to her getting pregnant.

Jane got her meeting with Dr. B and was excited by what she learned. She told us, "Dr. B said that a new procedure might help us. We can do it next month, and maybe then I'll get pregnant. Thanks for helping me learn to ask for what I want. I always felt I deserved things but never knew how to ask."

Like Jane, you may find it difficult to ask for what you want. Yet your diagnosis and treatment has short- and long-term implications for your body and your life. Express your opinions. Clarify what you want. Make demands. Don't be afraid to make simple requests such as a sheet in a cold examining room or an appointment at 9:00 A.M. instead of 3:30 P.M. Your comfort and convenience are important. And be bold when asking for more complicated and critical considerations, even if a doctor implies that your opinions are not important. You're paying for your treatment, not asking for a handout. Insist on the best possible treatment. But be diplomatic. Avoid being obnoxious or overly aggressive in making these requests.

DECISION-MAKING

More often than not, the clients we see have no plan for their treatment. They have fallen into what Kassie Schwan has called "the infertility maze."[13] They flounder here and there with no clear direction. Having no plan makes you feel helpless, and helplessness fosters feelings of depression, so common in infertility. The way out of the infertility maze is to formulate a plan and take responsibility for making important decisions. You will have to decide whether to see an infertility specialist or an OB-GYN who does not specialize in infertility. You may have to decide how to best spend the money you have on treatment—whether to try many repeated cycles of a less-expensive low-tech treatment, or to go with fewer but more expensive high-tech treatments. The volume of information you must consider when drafting your plan of action can be daunting.

There is no simple way to make these choices. But there is a method that can help. The method we present is based on one model of decision-making discussed by psychologist Ward Edwards and on another model of choice discussed by psychologists Amos Tversky and Daniel Kahneman.[14]

First a scenario. Your mother is planning a visit during the Christmas vacation. You can't decide whether to pursue treatment while she visits or take a month's rest.

Begin your decision-making process by gathering information about the factors you must weigh. Talk to friends and acquaintances who have experienced a similar dilemma. Read books and magazine articles that discuss the problem. And then with your spouse develop a list of those factors. At the end of this phase, prioritize. A list (which we have deliberately simplified for illustrative purposes) includes these factors:

- Preventing stress to your body;
- Getting closer to your goal of having a baby; and
- Avoiding family friction.

These are just a few of the many considerations that you would list. Your next step is assigning a grade to each factor. The grade, which is a number from 1 (worst) to 10 (best), indicates the effect of each choice on that factor. So you might assign the following grades:

Factor	Choosing Treatment	Choosing Rest
1. How much will this choice prevent stress to my body?	2	8
2. How much closer will this choice bring me to my goal of having a baby?	7	1
3. How much will this choice prevent friction in the family?	1	10

Next, assign a weight from 1 (least) to 10 (most) to the importance of each factor. You need to weigh the benefit of treatment at a distant clinic against the cost of family friction that would result if your travel prevented you from spending relaxed time with your mother during her visit. You then multiply the weight by the rating to get a factor score. Finally, you add the total factor scores for each choice. Here's what your chart might look like:

Factor	Weight for this factor	Grade for treatment	Factor score for treatment (weight × grade)	Grade for resting	Factor score for resting (weight × grade)
Prevent stress to body	2	2	4	8	16
Closeness to goal	10	7	70	1	10
Avoid family friction	9	1	9	10	90
Total score			83		116

Looking at the table, you can see that your best choice would be to rest for the month. In later chapters, we will apply this technique to important decisions such as choosing a doctor. When we do, we will guide you through a more thorough examination of the various factors to take into account.

RECORD-KEEPING

Once your diagnosis begins, you'll be swamped with papers: receipts, test results, insurance forms—the sheer volume is enough to make you stuff it into a drawer and forget about it or, worse yet, leave the materials scattered around the house. Instead of becoming preoccupied with how difficult getting pregnant is, channel some of your energy into getting and staying organized. Put copies of your medical records, as well as your own logs of monthly cycles, in a convenient file or loose-leaf notebook. Getting Organized is probably the most effective way to reduce your feelings of being overwhelmed. Following the organization Pointer also can help you develop your Getting Pregnant Plan.

The Cycle Log

The first section of your notebook or portfolio will contain your Cycle Log, which will help you chart your menstrual cycle. On pages 52–53, you will find a Cycle Log form to photocopy and put into your portfolio. This log can help you record every aspect of your cycle: how you feel, whether you had intercourse, what medications you took, what your blood levels were, or what tests were done on any given day. Although you may think you'll remember that you had unusual cramps on Day 21 or that your temperature fell on Day 25, you probably won't. Daily events, even those that seem momentous at the time, often blend together or fade from memory. Detailed records of each cycle allow you and your doctor to compare one treatment or one cycle to another or begin to see patterns suggesting why you are not getting pregnant.

GOAL-SETTING

Coping with infertility is like coping with any chronic illness. Our clients often feel that their condition is entirely out of their control. While they cannot control whether they get pregnant, they *can* choose their physician, their treatment, and how long they will remain in treatment. Goal-setting is a skill that can help you enact many of the Getting Pregnant Pointers: getting organized, making a plan, managing your social life, and being a partner in treatment.

In setting your Getting Pregnant Goals, follow these do's:

- Do set realistic goals. When you set goals, consider time, travel, work and family commitments, financial resources, and all the other real-life situations that can get in the way of accomplishing these goals.
- Do make specific concrete goals. Think in terms of both short- and long-range objectives. A long-range objective might be to undergo all the tests your doctor recommends by a particular date. That particular long-range objective can require short-range objectives such as having one test during each cycle.
- Do divide the goals into discrete manageable steps. These steps are what you actually have to do to meet your goal, such as checking your temperature, making a doctor's appointment, or arranging time off from work.
- Do set verifiable milestones to check your progress toward your goals. Write—and follow—reminders such as these on your calendar: when to call for test results, fill a prescription, and mail insurance claims. You are your own best monitor, so don't cheat.

And also remember the don'ts:

- Don't set yourself up for failure. Sometimes when you are pessimistic, you expect failure before you even start. Then you might set unrealistic goals that you can never accomplish and say, "See, I knew it was impossible."
- Don't retreat into passivity. By becoming passive, you ensure that nothing good happens and thus confirm your prediction that "nothing good will happen."

CYCLE LOG

Use this log to enter important information about your cycle. The days of the cycles are listed at the left of the page. Next to the day of the cycle, write the date. Then record essential information to the right. In your notes keep track of the following (and anything else that may be important to you):

- Symptoms: any important symptoms you experienced
- Estradiol information (E2)
- Progesterone levels (P)
- Sonogram results (number of follicles and follicle size for left and right ovaries)
- Medication taken
- Questions to ask your doctor

Day of cycle	Date	Symptoms or comments	E2	P	Left ovary: size of each follicle	Right ovary: size of each follicle	Medications taken: Lupron (L); progesterone (PR); Pergonal (PG); Metrodin (ME); hCG (H); other (O)						Questions?
							L	PR	PG	ME	H	O	
1													
2													
3													
4													
5													
6													
7													
8													

Day of cycle	Date	Symptoms or comments	E2	P	Left ovary: size of each follicle	Right ovary: size of each follicle	Medications taken: Lupron (L); progesterone (PR); Pergonal (PG); Metrodin (ME); hCG (H); other (O)						Questions?
							L	PR	PG	ME	H	O	
9													
10													
11													
12													
13													
14													
15													
16													
17													
18													
19													
20													
21													
22													
23													
24													
25													
26													
27													
28													

- ■ <u>Don't</u> become exhausted. Pace yourself. Budget your energy.
- ■ <u>Don't</u> catastrophize. See the situation for what it really is and hold on to hope.

The Getting Pregnant Monthly Plan

On the next page you will see a model of the Getting Pregnant Monthly Plan. Photocopy it, punch holes in it, and insert it into the second section of your notebook. Together with your spouse, set a short-term goal—one you can envision reaching this month. *Do not make your goal, "I will get pregnant this month." Do make your goal, "This month, I will schedule and undergo the test my doctor recommended."*

The monthly plan suggests a number of possible goals for the coming month. Your first step is to decide upon a goal, either from the examples given or one that seems right for you. Once you've established what your goal is, write it on the form.

Next, use GPST (Getting Pregnant Self-Talk) to motivate yourself to accomplish your goal. Make a GPST statement that you find particularly motivating. For example, if you hate calling doctors, try psyching yourself up by saying, "By calling the doctor, I'm upping my odds." Keep your GPST statement in mind if you find yourself procrastinating.

Now you are ready to formulate an action plan. The action plan is critical and easy to put off. Make your spouse your consultant. Ask him to review the plan and add any important steps you might have omitted.

Your task for this month is to put your plan into action. At the end of this month, assess how your plan worked out. If your plan worked, congratulate yourself. If it didn't, figure out why and modify the plan for the next month.

THE GETTING PREGNANT MONTHLY PLAN

MAKE THIS MONTH COUNT. Now is the time to make sure you accomplish something important this month.

Even if you will not be able to try to conceive during this month, you must view this cycle as a chance to get closer to your goal. It's important to think of a month during which only tests occur as providing you with information that confirms or rules out causes for infertility. Cycles that fail also can provide new knowledge. You can't control whether you get pregnant this month. But you *can* do something to up the odds. This planning sheet will help you do so.

First list your goal for this month. Make it something manageable—something you can definitely accomplish. This month you can:

- Find out new information
- Get the results of an important test
- Strengthen your body and your mind
- Try a treatment
- Do something else (supply your own goal)

MY GOAL FOR THIS MONTH IS:

Now you must psych yourself up to accomplish this goal. Do this by making a *motivating GPST*. For example, a person who hates having tests might say, "By having the test, I may learn what's wrong." Write your motivating GPST below.

MY MOTIVATING GPST STATEMENT FOR THIS MONTH IS:

Now that you have a goal and you've psyched yourself up, it's time to formulate your action steps. For example, suppose you set the goal of finding out whether your tubes are blocked. You might formulate the following plan:

1. I'll contact my doctor to set up the test.
2. I'll read the section in the diagnosis chapter describing the test.
3. We'll work as a team; I'll ask my partner to read about the test and discuss it with me.
4. I'll mentally rehearse experiencing the test so I'm ready for it.
5. As a partner in treatment, I'll call the doctor to clear up any questions I might have.
6. I'll ask my partner to take time off from work to accompany me to the test.
7. I'll get the insurance material ready in advance.

MY ACTION PLAN FOR THIS MONTH IS:

In the next part of this form, write down how it worked out.

HERE IS HOW MY PLAN WORKED OUT:

Now that you took the steps to carry out your plan, congratulate yourself for taking a positive action.

CONGRATULATE YOURSELF!

USING YOUR IMAGINATION

When we tell our clients that we are going to ask them to use their imagination in helping them through their infertility, they initially reject the idea. They mistakenly fear we're going to have them imagine that they are pregnant, and they find that thought too painful. Or, worse yet, they think that we're going to ask them to imagine a sperm fertilizing an egg, and they find this scenario too weird or off-putting. Unfortunately, most of the infertile couples we see have lost so many dreams that their imagination is dulled. They are almost ready to give up. They fear entertaining any new dreams. Yet once they have learned to use imagery techniques and incorporate them into real-life situations, couples report that they feel much more able to cope with their experiences. And some even tell us that they also allow themselves to dream again.

Before you begin your imagery work, we want to clarify that we are *not* introducing imagery as a way for you to explore your complex unconscious mind. Such personal introspection takes intensive one-on-one work with a qualified therapist. What we want you to do is to gain access to your inner world of ideas, modify those images that hinder you, and expand and detail those images that help you—all for the purpose of harnessing the power of your mind to help you through infertility.

For this imagery section of the Workout, we've collected a wide range of imagery procedures, modified them, and tested them with infertile couples. The result is a series of techniques that possess amazing power. These are not mystical exercises, but straightforward techniques and scenarios that help relax, inspire, motivate, and prepare you for what you must do to enhance your chances of getting pregnant.

What Are Mental Images?

Mental images are those pictures that you see in your mind's eye when the object is no longer present or the situation is in the past. Your mental image may be visual (recorded through seeing), olfactory (recorded through smelling), auditory (recorded through hearing), gustatory (recorded through tasting), tactile (recorded through touch), or kinesthetic (recorded through moving). Your images may be spontaneous, like a daydream, or they may need some prodding and shaping.

In the Workout, we focus on developing your ability to imagine procedures and interactions that you've yet to experience. You will use these images together with breathing or progressive relaxation to reduce your stress. And you will employ these images in conjunction with GPST to help you reframe unproductive experiences and to assist you in cultivating a sense of optimism.

Mental Rehearsal

Experts believe that having a mental picture of an upcoming event can help you cope better when it happens. For example, having a mental picture of how to react in an awkward social situation—the words you'll say or the things you'll do—can be very reassuring. Likewise, the more familiar a medical procedure is, the less likely you are to panic or experience extreme discomfort during the procedure. In subsequent chapters, we describe many of the tests and treatments used to help infertile couples. If you use these descriptions to help you form a movie in your mind and then rehearse what will occur, you can prepare yourself for what will happen.

Once you develop a clear and detailed picture in your mind's eye, add some GPST. For example, while imagining that you are having one of the tests that many find unpleasant—the endometrial biopsy—you might add a soothing statement to your mental rehearsal like, "This test is almost over. I've passed the worst." Just as we encourage you to actually imagine yourself experiencing the test step by step, we also encourage you to hear yourself saying your GPSTs.

Rehearsing for a Diagnostic Test or a Medical Treatment

Jennifer Wilson-Barnett has investigated the stress of diagnostic testing. She writes that "one of the most common fears expressed by those scheduled for tests is the 'fear of the unknown.' For those experiencing a procedure for the first time, in particular, anticipation may be tainted by various fantasies."[15]

To overcome that fear, follow these steps:

- Read the description of the procedure with your spouse. Together, use the information to write a brief script of the procedure, which includes all of the relevant details (a sample script follows).
- Sit in a comfortable position. Close your eyes.
- Have your spouse actually read the script to you or tape-record it for playback at a later time. Make sure your spouse gives you sufficient time to really picture the scene. You may have to coach him to read or record at a slow enough pace.
- Mentally rehearse the scene in as much detail as possible. Allow yourself to feel the anxiety. Also picture yourself coping with the worst-case scenario, knowing that once you've dealt with your ultimate fears, you are ready for anything.

Here is a bare-bones script that you can use to structure your mental rehearsal of tests and procedures:

I'm going to read you a description of the _____ (name of test). I want you to see yourself coping with your anxiety by using the deep-breathing technique you've been practicing. I'm going to help. I'll be your coach and cheerleader. Whenever you feel anxious just raise your little finger. I'll help you relax. Take slow deep breaths. INHALE, EXHALE . . . WHOOSH. GOOD. Again. INHALE. EXHALE . . . WHOOSH. Okay. Here we go. I'm with you so you don't have to be afraid. C'mon. You can do it! Good. You're doing it. As you see yourself exhaling, get in touch with the feeling of relaxation and control the air you are bringing forth. GREAT. Add your GPST. Tell yourself, "I can do it! I've done tougher things before." GOOD. Keep breathing slowly and deeply. GREAT. Now stop that image and relax. GOOD WORK!

Following is an example of a script, based on the model above, that you and your spouse might write to mentally visualize and rehearse yourself going through a hysterosalpingogram (HSG) procedure. (You can find a detailed description of this procedure in Chapter 4.)

You've arrived at the radiologist's suite. You are signing in. The receptionist is giving you a consent slip to read and sign. It says that you will release the doctors from any responsibility for any problem that might happen as a result of the procedure. Now you're signing it. Now you're going into a dressing room, taking off your clothes, and putting on a dressing gown. The nurse is escorting you to the examination room. You are lying on the table. It feels cold. You look around and see an X-ray camera and an X-ray screen. The room is dark. Here comes the radiologist. She's putting a tube into your uterus. Now she's squeezing dye into the tube. Now you can feel the dye traveling through your tubes. You feel pressure and maybe some pain. The doctor is going behind a screen. Now she's telling you to turn to the right so she can get a picture of that side. Now she's telling you to turn to the left. Now she's finished. She's telling you to get dressed.

Mental imagery also can help you prepare for difficult or awkward situations that can arise socially or on the job. In her pamphlet *Getting Around the Boulder in the Road: Using Imagery to Cope with Fertility Problems*, psychologist Aline P. Zoldbrod encourages readers to "try working with your imagery during demanding periods in your treatment regimen, when your life feels out of control, or when you feel distant from your spouse . . . to make you feel more comfortable during social situations, or to control pain during surgical procedures."[16]

Guided Fantasies

An entirely different approach to mental imagery is called *creative visualizations* or *guided fantasies*. These activities, which deal almost exclusively with your sense of sight, focus on using images to help you relax, get motivated, or even inspire you to develop a more upbeat attitude toward fighting infertility. An important benefit of guided fantasies is that they often are accompanied by physiological changes, such as relaxation.

Guided fantasies, or mind journeys as they are sometimes called, are a set of guiding phrases, read or tape-recorded. While in a relaxed state, you are encouraged to visualize the picture or experience suggested by the reader. Generally, infertility guided fantasies require that you the listener experience the journey firsthand, with such sentences as, "Together we are going to develop a circle of friends who are your supporters," which is the beginning of a guided fantasy called Circle of Friends that appears in Chapter 6. There are just a few simple rules to remember:

- Find a calm and quiet place to practice your imagery.
- Set a regular time each day to do imagery activities. Just like physical activity, you need to practice mental activity on a regular basis.
- Sit in a chair or lie on the floor, whatever position seems to be easier.
- Start with controlled breathing, as described earlier in this chapter.
- Try to direct your focus inward, instead of on the chaos around you.
- At the beginning of each exercise, always state your goal to yourself, using GPST.
- For the time you are imaging, allow yourself to go with the images.

ONE FINAL THOUGHT

In the first chapter, we gave you Nine Pointers. In this chapter, we have given you a set of skills that will allow you to enact the Pointers. Some skills, such as Getting Pregnant Self-Talk, are so useful that they can help with all of the Pointers. Other skills, such as controlled breathing, are more limited in what they can do for you. In each of the succeeding chapters, we will describe pitfalls and obstacles to getting pregnant. Then we will show you how to apply the skills learned from the Getting Pregnant Workout to help you avoid them.

Practice the Getting Pregnant Workout on a regular basis. The Workout could very well contain the tools you need to help you get pregnant when you thought you couldn't.

CHAPTER THREE

THE MIRACLE
OF LIFE

GETTING PREGNANT WHEN THINGS
WORK RIGHT

FOR MANY who have been trying for a long time to have a baby, the thought of actually conceiving a new life seems like a miracle. Yet in truth, conception itself—even for the most fertile people—is surely miraculous. A myriad of events must occur at exactly the right time and in the proper place for pregnancy to happen.

Broadly speaking, there are four milestones to conception, some involving both partners, others involving the woman only. The first milestone is *production of a gamete,* or reproductive cell: the man's sperm and the woman's egg. Next, the *sperm meets the egg and fertilizes it* to produce an embryo. Third, the *embryo implants* itself in the uterus. Finally, the *implanted embryo divides, flourishes, and fully develops*. Each milestone is controlled by a cascade of chemical and hormonal reactions. Through feedback mechanisms, hormone production is turned on and off, just like a thermostat senses temperature changes in your house to control whether your furnace turns on or off.

Gamete Production in the Woman

A female is born with all the eggs she will ever produce—about 1 to 2 million.[1] As she gets older her supply of eggs decreases. From the onset of puberty when she has about 400,000 eggs until menopause, a woman normally has a menstrual cycle culminating in the release of one or more of those eggs. This menstrual cycle is spawned at the base of the brain, right above the *pituitary gland,* in an area called the *hypothalamus.* The hypothalamus produces a hormone called *gonadotropin releasing hormone* (GnRH). About every ninety minutes, for about one minute, the hypothalamus pumps out a small dose of GnRH.[2] This periodic pumping is necessary to set things in motion for ovulation to occur. If the hypothalamus pumps out a steady stream of GnRH, for example, the entire pregnancy process will be pushed off balance.

When the hypothalamus works properly, the GnRH stimulates the pituitary gland to release two more hormones—*follicle stimulating hormone* (FSH) and *luteinizing hormone* (LH). As its name implies, FSH stimulates the ovaries to start developing one of many *potential* follicles that are available. A *follicle* is a sac that may contain an egg. Why a particular follicle is selected over another one is a mystery. Some follicles contain healthy eggs; others contain poor-quality eggs that are unable to develop into an embryo. Ideally, FSH stimulates the follicle to grow an egg large enough to be *ovulated,* or ejected.

As the sac grows, the egg is being genetically prepared to become susceptible to fertilization. Again, timing and hormone levels are critical. FSH production must start and stop at the proper times. The ovary must secrete increasing amounts of *estradiol,* a form of the female hormone, *estrogen,* which performs many functions. It's important to note that most women rotate ovulation: They ovulate one month from the left ovary and the next month from the right.[3] Other women ovulate almost consistently from only one ovary. When one ovary is surgically removed, the other generally takes over the monthly job.

The estrogen first stimulates the development of the lining in the uterus. This lining, or *endometrium,* must grow thick enough to allow an embryo to implant and grow. Secondly, the estrogen rise increases the quantity and consistency of *cervical mucus.* You may notice this extra mucus midway through your menstrual cycle. The mucus serves as a vehicle for sperm as it journeys to the egg.

Third, high levels of estrogen in the bloodstream enlarge the opening of the *cervix*. Estrogen's fourth function is to signal the pituitary gland to stop producing FSH and to send a tremendous surge of LH instead. The LH surge signals the ovary to ovulate an egg.

In addition to stimulating ovulation, meanwhile, the LH surge also initiates a series of genetic events inside the egg. Like every cell in the human body, the egg cell contains forty-six chromosomes—strands of genetic material. When an egg gets fertilized, it combines with a sperm, which has twenty-three chromosomes of its own. (Sperm shed their other twenty-three chromosomes sometime prior to ejaculation.) If the fertilized egg retains all forty-six female chromosomes as well as the male chromosomes, the resulting cell could not grow into a healthy baby. So the LH surge prepares the egg cell to expel half of its chromosomes.

After the egg is ovulated, the leftover sac develops into a yellow structure called the *corpus luteum* (literally "yellow body"). The corpus luteum produces a second important hormone called *progesterone*. For most women there is a sharp increase in progesterone secretion at the beginning of the second half of the menstrual cycle. This part of the cycle is known as the *luteal phase*. As estrogen makes the uterine lining grow thick, progesterone makes the lining soft and spongy—a good environment for embryo implantation. If a pregnancy occurs, progesterone will continue to be secreted throughout the pregnancy. However, if there is no pregnancy, progesterone secretion stops at the end of the luteal phase. The decrease in progesterone and estrogen levels sends a signal to the hypothalamus to trigger a new stream of FSH. Then the ovulation cycle begins anew.

Gamete Production in the Man

Unlike women, men are not born with all the sperm cells they will ever have. Sperm are born, grow, mature, and eventually die (save for the ones that ultimately fertilize eggs).

Men are like women in that they also have a GnRH pump that pulses periodically, stimulating the production of FSH and LH. In men, however, LH causes the production of *testosterone*, not estrogen.

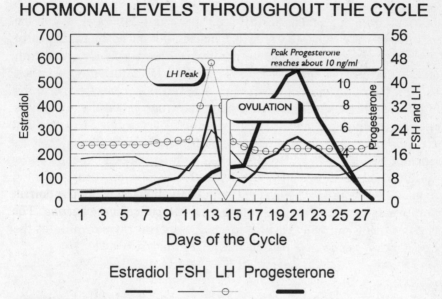

HORMONAL LEVELS THROUGHOUT THE CYCLE

Days of the Cycle

Estradiol FSH LH Progesterone

FSH and LH are in miU/ml

Estradiol is in pg/ml

Progesterone is in ng/ml

Figure 3.1

Testosterone is the male hormone that increases sex drive and stimulates development of secondary sex characteristics, such as beard growth, at puberty. FSH, on the other hand, regulates the production of immature or primitive sperm cells known as *sperm precursors*. These precursors are *not* the same as the mature sperm used to fertilize an egg. As with females, there is a feedback mechanism in males that regulates FSH and

LH levels. When testosterone levels increase, LH production decreases, and vice versa. Likewise, when sperm precursor levels are low, FSH levels rise to increase their production.

It's important to keep in mind that so-called manliness is not related to the ability to make sperm. A high sex drive can be present in a man totally lacking in sperm, just as a man with a very high sperm count can have a low sex drive.

There are other similarities between the sexes. Just as an egg begins with forty-six chromosomes, which must be reduced to twenty-three, sperm precursors have twice the number of chromosomes needed to be able to fertilize an egg. FSH plays a role in triggering this process of halving the number of chromosomes and producing mature sperm.

Mature sperm travel through a long, thin tube called the *epididymis,* where they improve their swimming ability. Eventually, they move into the *vas deferens,* then to the *seminal vesicle,* and finally into the *ejaculatory duct,* where they are mixed with semen and expelled during orgasm.

It takes about ninety days to make a fully functioning sperm. Surprisingly, a relatively high proportion of sperm are defective.[4] That is why men normally make so many sperm—many millions per ejaculation—to increase the chances of fertilization.

Journey and Rendezvous—Sperm and Egg Meet

Again, timing is crucial during this stage. First, the sperm must travel from the penis and through the vagina, cervix, uterus, and fallopian tubes to get to an egg. To optimize pregnancy, intercourse should occur just before ovulation. One reason is because the life of the egg is very short; estimates run from twelve to twenty-four hours. If intercourse does not take place at the right time (around the time of the LH surge), the sperm can travel to the right site, but fail to meet its target. If the sperm does encounter the egg, it must be able to penetrate and fertilize the egg. As you are beginning to see, both the egg and the sperm must survive an arduous journey before getting a chance at conception.

As the sperm prepares for the journey, the ovaries are getting ready to ovulate an egg or eggs. The ovaries lie just outside the end of the *fallopian tubes.* The fallopian tubes are extremely narrow, the narrowest point having an outer diameter about as wide as angel-hair spaghetti where it hooks up with the uterus. Inside the tube is a canal lined with

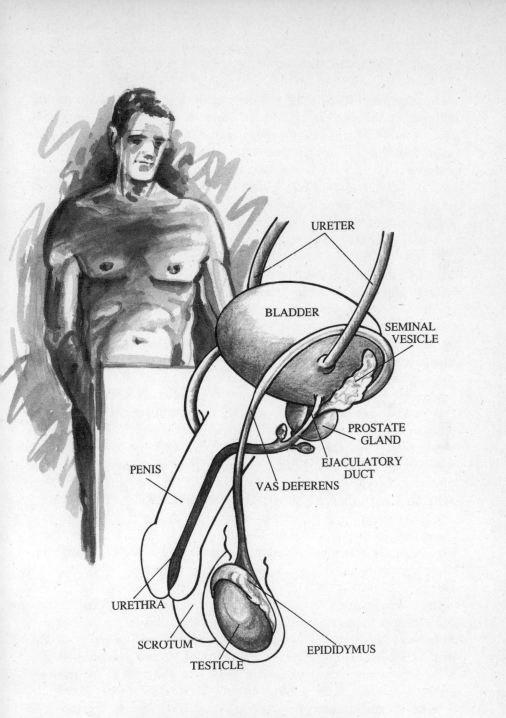

URETER

BLADDER

SEMINAL
VESICLE

PROSTATE
GLAND

EJACULATORY
DUCT

PENIS

VAS DEFERENS

URETHRA

SCROTUM

EPIDIDYMUS

TESTICLE

THE MALE REPRODUCTIVE SYSTEM

Figure 3.2

millions of tiny hairs called *cilia*. It also contains special cells that secrete a fluid that plays a critical role in fertilization. The narrow portion of the tube that joins the uterus is called the *isthmus*. The isthmus is barely wide enough to allow a fertilized egg to pass through. However, as you proceed down the tube, the tube widens into a bell-shaped structure called the *ampulla*. At the end of the ampulla are fingerlike structures called *fimbria,* which contain little petals of tissue. The ampulla is hinged to the ovary in such a way that it is able to swing over to catch the ovulated egg.

Just before the egg is ovulated, the fimbria are positioned above the dominant egg follicle. When it leaves its follicle, the egg is covered with a sticky substance that helps it adhere to a petal of the fimbria and get trapped. Once the egg is trapped, the cilia on the lining of the fimbria beat rapidly and push the sticky egg mass into the crevices of the lining of the ampulla. Here, the fluid of the lining dissolves the sticky coating and nourishes the egg. As the fluid dissolves the egg's coating, it also softens the egg's shell so that the egg will be more susceptible to penetration by a sperm.

Assuming that the man and woman have just engaged in intercourse, the man will ejaculate semen into the woman's vagina. The semen is an alkaline fluid, which protects the sperm from the vagina's acidic environment. Typically, a single ejaculate contains many millions of sperm, most of which are spewed forth during the first ejaculatory pulse. A significant percentage of these sperm are poor swimmers. They have only about thirty minutes to swim through the vagina to reach the cervix before they are destroyed by the vagina's acidity. Fewer than 1 percent of the sperm ejaculated will make it to the site of fertilization. Some sperm, however, can live up to three or four days in the cervical mucus.

Once sperm reach the cervix, they encounter the cervical mucus, which, under the influence of estrogen, has built up during the first half of the woman's cycle. The estrogen has created an abundance of thin, stretchy mucus that, under normal conditions, serves as an ideal sperm transport system. First, one sperm begins to nudge at the mucus and eventually succeeds in poking a hole in it. That sperm enters the cervical mucus, and other sperm follow it through this opening. The cervical mucus holds the sperm at the opening of the cervix, releasing only a few at a time.

When the sperm reach the cervix, they are freed from the seminal fluid, which enables them to wiggle their tails more readily and swim

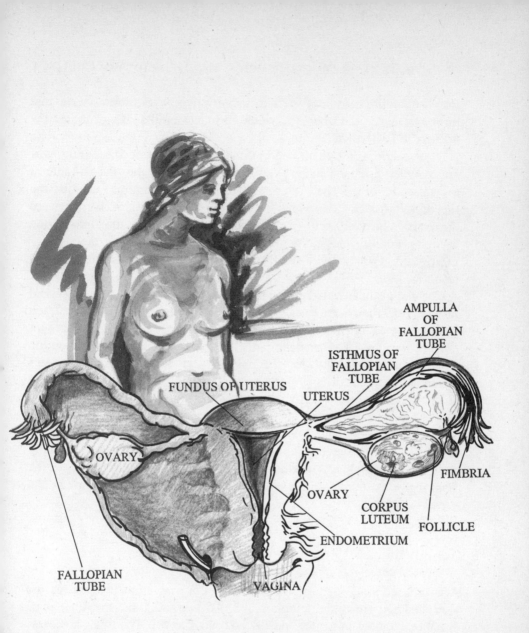

THE FEMALE REPRODUCTIVE SYSTEM

Figure 3.3

faster. Over the next forty-eight to seventy-two hours, a few sperm pass through the cervix to begin a journey to the ampulla, where the egg is waiting to be fertilized.

Most sperm don't swim straight and thus never find the egg. A few are expert swimmers, though, and make their way into the isthmus of the fallopian tube. There they find themselves swimming against the tide created by the cilia, which are propelling the egg downward, toward the uterus. In addition to pushing some sperm back, the fluid in the fallopian tube enables the strongest sperm to further hone their swimming skills. Eventually, a small group of these strong-swimming sperm reach the egg.

The pointy heads of the sperm are covered by a cap, which is shed just prior to their attempt at penetration. After shedding the cap, each sperm secretes an enzyme called *acrosin,* which further softens the outer shell of the egg. Like battering rams, these top-of-the-line sperm butt up against the *zona pellucida,* the hardest part of the shell, with their arrowlike head. If all goes well, one sperm will soon break through the shell and penetrate, wiggling its tail wildly to give it momentum. As soon as it enters the egg, the shell closes up again to prevent any other sperm from coming in. The egg literally swallows the sperm, and the two cells combine their chromosomes. The now-fertilized egg, called a *zygote*—the first stage in embryo development—is ready to begin the final leg of its journey to the uterus, where it will attempt to implant and grow.

Womb with a View

The cilia continue to beat rapidly, propelling the fluid that carries the fertilized egg down the fallopian tube. At the same time, the muscles of the tube contract to further aid the embryo's travel. The tube, however, retains the embryo for about three days until the uterine lining is ready to receive it. If the embryo is released too soon, it will be unable to grow into a fetus.

When it enters the uterus, the embryo has developed to the point where it contains many cells surrounded by a hard outer shell. It is now called a *blastocyst.* The blastocyst floats around searching for a place to implant. Soon a portion of the shell dissolves. The fertilized egg hatches and implants in the endometrium, which, as you recall, has thickened under the influence of estrogen and softened under the influence of progesterone. The embryonic cells secrete yet another hormone, called *human chorionic gonadotropin* (hCG), which stimulates the corpus luteum (vacated egg sac) to continue secreting progesterone. In this favorable environment, the implanted embryo grows and develops over the next nine months.

NOT GETTING PREGNANT WHEN YOU THOUGHT YOU COULD

Given the complexities of conception, it is no wonder that fertile couples have only a one-in-five chance of conceiving during any given month. Yet, even with those odds, 90 percent of couples without fertility problems will achieve pregnancy within one year.

If you are not one of those lucky ones, you may be tempted to believe simply that the odds have worked against you. But it is that line of reasoning that will not be to your benefit if you delay seeking a medical evaluation at this point. Postponing diagnosis can waste precious time, especially if your problem is easily correctable. It's our belief that the sooner you find out what, if anything, is wrong, the sooner you can cradle your baby in your arms.

Here we examine what can go wrong at each stage of the process. Later in the book we will discuss the various procedures and drugs available to correct many of these problems.

The Woman Fails to Ovulate

As we pointed out previously, you are born with a crop of about 1 to 2 million eggs and will produce no more. Each month, your ovaries grow about 1,000 follicles, of which one will become the dominant egg sac. The remaining 999 follicles will wither and die. If 1,000 of the 400,000 eggs are used up each month, the entire supply of eggs will be exhausted in about thirty-three years. So for a forty-year-old woman who began ovulating at age fourteen, the countdown to egg depletion is only about seven years. For this woman, the biological clock begins to take on awesome dimensions.

One reason older women have trouble conceiving is ovarian failure—

they simply used up their supply of eggs or the few remaining ones are of very poor quality. But for younger women, the failure to ovulate probably lies elsewhere.

The ovulation process is controlled by numerous hormones whose levels must attain a proper balance. The GnRH pump must be pulsing properly every ninety minutes or so. Adequate amounts of FSH must be secreted by the pituitary during the first half of the month, and the ovaries must respond by producing sufficient amounts of estrogen. The estrogen levels must rise during the first half of the cycle (the follicular phase) and reach sufficient levels to trigger an LH surge, which will eject the egg from its follicle.

If your hormonal levels are off balance, you will not ovulate, or you will ovulate eggs before they are ripened. Other problems that can affect ovulation include polycystic ovaries, high prolactin levels, and other less-common conditions that are discussed in Chapters 4 and 5.

The Man Fails to Produce Sperm

Just as with ovulation, hormones regulate sperm production. Therefore, indirect evidence of whether a man is producing sperm can be gathered through hormonal testing. As we noted earlier, FSH controls the production of sperm precursors (immature sperm). If a blood test shows an adequate FSH level, it means the man is making these precursors. However, in order to have sperm that can fertilize eggs, these sperm cells must mature and lose half their chromosomes. Cases where this does not happen are exceedingly rare.

By obtaining a semen sample, a laboratory technician can check the number of sperm, their shape, and their ability to swim. All three factors give doctors enough data to diagnose whether the man has a problem.

The Egg Does Not Get Fertilized

If the woman is ovulating and the man is making sperm, infertility may result from a problem in the rendezvous stage. These problems may involve *travel, timing,* or *penetration.*

TRAVEL

The sperm that are ejaculated must travel from the vagina to the fallopian tubes where they can attempt to penetrate the egg. Sperm can be blocked, lost, or killed before they reach their destination. The acid in the vagina may kill all the sperm. The cervical mucus may be too thick to allow penetration, or the mucus may contain antibodies that are lethal to sperm. Ironically, the sperm itself may have antibodies that cause it to self-destruct. Also, sperm may be poor swimmers. Instead of swimming straight to the tube, they may swim off course or in circles and never reach their destination. Or they may be straight swimmers but too weak to buck the tide in the female's reproductive tract.

Like the sperm, the egg also can encounter travel problems. Although a fine egg may have developed and been ejected from the ovary, it may never be caught by the fimbria. To catch the egg, the tube must have rotated into the proper position. But an adhesion or scar tissue might have interfered with the structure's ability to move and turn. If this is the case, the egg gets lost in the abdomen instead of making its way down the tube.

TIMING

Mature eggs can only live in the body for twelve to twenty-four hours. If sperm aren't available during this window of opportunity, fertilization cannot occur. Sperm can live in the woman's body longer than eggs, up to four days in some cases, in fact. A supply of sperm must be released to get to the tube several hours before the egg's estimated time of arrival. Sperm that died waiting should be replaced by fresh arrivals.

PENETRATION

The third main cause for a lack of fertilization stems from a sperm's inability to penetrate the egg. The shell of the egg is hard. It needs to be softened by enzymes secreted in the fallopian tube. The sperm also secretes enzymes that further soften the shell. Nearby sperm actually help to break the shell and assist the chosen sperm to penetrate. Once the sperm breaks the shell, it has to flap its tail powerfully to gain the momentum to drill in. The point of its head must be sharp enough to cut through the protective covering until the sperm is safely inside the egg. If any of these factors are problems, fertilization will not occur.

Fertilized Egg Fails to Implant

Generally, three types of problems can thwart success during the implantation stage. These involve *travel, roadblocks,* and *lodging*.

TRAVEL

The fertilized egg must be swept through the fallopian tube on a current of fluid. It must pass through a narrow opening linking the tube and the uterus. Then it must land upon a soft spongy endometrium where it takes up residence. Problems with the fallopian tube muscles or the cilia may impair movement of the fertilized egg.

ROADBLOCKS

The narrow passage leading from the tube to the uterus may be blocked by inflammation, thereby preventing the fertilized egg from leaving the fallopian tube. If this happens, the fertilized egg can die, or worse, it can implant and begin to grow in the tube. This *ectopic,* or tubal, pregnancy can be life-threatening if not treated promptly.

LODGING

Finally, if the fertilized egg enters the uterus, it must land on the soft spongy endometrium and implant there. Throughout the early stages of pregnancy, the endometrium is nourished by a constant supply of progesterone. This lushness will not occur if there is insufficient progesterone being produced either naturally or through drug therapy. Scar tissue, adhesions, or fibroid tumors inside the uterus also can prevent implantation.

The Implanted Embryo Divides for a Time but Fails to Flourish

If things have gone well at each of the previous stages, a pregnancy test will be positive. From this point on, the embryo must continue to be nourished or it will die and miscarriage will occur, sometimes before the woman even realized she was pregnant. Researchers estimate that a large percentage of pregnancies end this way.[5] Since infertile couples tend to take pregnancy tests at the earliest possible moment, they are often painfully aware of early miscarriages. Even when an embryo begins to grow, many problems—with both the developing fetus and with the mother—can contribute to a miscarriage.

Nature has a way of fostering preservation. Some embryos were not meant to develop because the resulting fetus would be deformed. Some eggs, particularly very old ones, are genetically nonviable. Even if they are fertilized, they may contain genes that could contribute to a genetically defective baby. To prevent these defects, nature causes a spontaneous abortion—a miscarriage.

THE DISORDERS OF FERTILITY

Various factors—male, female, or unexplained—can prevent you from getting pregnant. Male problems almost always are associated with sperm production, sperm transport, or the health of the sperm itself. The root of female problems, on the other hand, can lie in the ovaries, fallopian tubes, uterus, cervix, or any combination thereof. As you see from Figure 3.4 showing the distribution of infertility causes in the United States doctors are unable to pinpoint the cause of infertility in almost one fifth of cases.[6]

Ovulatory Disturbances

Ovulation is the key to conception. More than one quarter of all infertile couples have ovulatory disturbances. Some disturbances are:

- A woman may not ovulate;
- A woman may fail to ovulate consistently;
- A woman may produce eggs that are too ripe;
- A woman may produce eggs that are not mature enough;
- A woman may produce many tiny egg follicles that fail to ovulate.

CAUSES OF INFERTILITY

Percentage Distribution of Each Cause

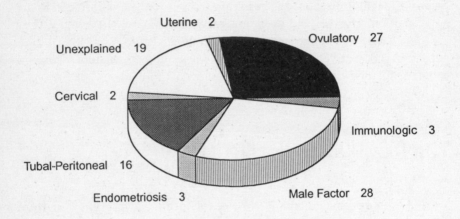

Figure 3.4

For ovulation to occur, a woman's body must produce various hormones in proper sequence in the right amount and at the right time. Chapter 4 covers ways to detect whether you have an ovulatory problem.

Tubal Problems

Blockages or adhesions involving the fallopian tubes are another major cause of infertility. A common cause of blockages and adhesions is *pelvic inflammatory disease* (PID), which usually stems from sexually transmitted infections such as gonorrhea, chlamydia, or mycoplasma.

Some women are born with damaged fallopian tubes. A major cause of this damage is the fetus's exposure to diethylstilbestrol (DES), a drug prescribed to pregnant women to prevent miscarriages in the early 1950s.

Damaged fallopian tubes also can result from an ectopic, or tubal, pregnancy. The ectopic pregnancy can not only cause adhesions or blockages, it can literally rupture the tube. Damaged tubes may be unable to transport the embryo into the uterus, increasing the risk of another ectopic pregnancy. Chapter 4 covers the tests doctors use to discover these problems, some of which can be corrected surgically.

Endometriosis

Endometriosis is a condition in which the lining of the uterus, the endometrium, grows outside the uterus causing scarring, pain, or heavy bleeding each month. It affects an estimated 8 percent of the female population. For unknown reasons, a small amount of endometrium backs up into the fallopian tubes and into the abdominal cavity instead of flowing out of the body through the vagina. This wayward tissue catches hold in the reproductive system and continues to respond to hormonal changes, behaving as though it is still inside the uterus even though it's not.

Endometriosis sufferers describe pain—during menstruation or other times in the cycle—as the primary symptom. Pain may or may not signal endometriosis, however. And women with endometriosis may not necessarily feel pain. Endometriosis can mimic many other disorders including colitis and PID. Moreover, the severity of the symptoms don't always match the severity of the disorder. Very few disorders associated with infertility have so many unanswered questions. And doctors aren't sure exactly how endometriosis prevents pregnancy.

Cervical Problems

Cervical problems can involve the mucus in the cervix or the structure of the cervix itself. Mucus problems usually hinder conception, while structural deformities can make staying pregnant difficult. Mucus can be too scant, too thick, too acidic, or otherwise hostile to sperm. Mucus problems can shorten the life of the sperm or prevent it from swimming to the egg.

In addition to hostile mucus, bacteria in the cervix can kill sperm. The responsible microorganism, which is sometimes hard to identify, is studied by means of a cervical culture test. When the cervix is infected by one of these microorganisms, it becomes inflamed. Inflammation of the cervix is referred to as *cervicitis*.

Uterine Problems

Three types of uterine disorders can impair fertility and sometimes be corrected surgically. Women can have congenital uterine abnormalities such as *bicornuate uterus:* one that is divided by a wall of tissue. While structural abnormalities don't necessarily prevent conception, they can be a source of repeated miscarriages.

A second uterine disorder is fibroid tissue within the smooth muscle of the uterus. *Fibroids* do not always cause infertility, but when they do, they usually result in a miscarriage rather than in a failure to conceive. A fibroid is most likely to interfere with conception if it grows near the entrance to the tubes, obstructing the embryo's way into the uterus.

A final type of uterine disorder involves infections. One such infection can result from a *dilation and curettage* (D&C) and can cause Asherman's syndrome—adhesions between the opposing walls of the uterus and destruction of the endometrial cavity.

Male Problems

By all accounts, a significant proportion of infertility problems are attributable to a male factor, such as:

- Making no sperm, called *azoospermia;*
- Making sperm that fail to reach the ejaculate (because of a blocked duct, for example);
- A low sperm count, called *oligospermia;* or
- Ejaculating enough sperm, but some aspect (their ability to move or their shape, for example) prohibits them from fertilizing the egg.

Rapid weight gain, weight loss, or malnourishment also can hurt sperm quality or quantity. DES exposure in the womb is another factor that can create fertility problems in males.

Radiation treatment or chemotherapy also can cause sperm problems. Also, chronic alcoholism can create impotence and contribute to male infertility. Exposure to high heat from Jacuzzis, long-distance driving, or the wearing of tight underwear also can contribute to male infertility, as can infection of the genitourinary tract. The primary diagnostic tool for detecting male fertility problems is a *semen analysis,* discussed in detail in the next chapter.

YOUR ROAD TO PREGNANCY

Once you have become pregnant, you can look back at this chapter and marvel at the miracle of conception. For now, though, we urge you to Educate Yourself About Infertility—our first Pointer. Educating yourself is critical to Becoming a Partner in Your Treatment, another Pointer. Consider the knowledge you gained through this chapter your first step toward getting pregnant when you thought you couldn't.

CHAPTER FOUR

DIAGNOSTIC TESTING: FINDING OUT WHAT IS WRONG

WHEN YOU are having trouble getting pregnant, time is a precious commodity. Each month that passes without a pregnancy is likely to increase your level of stress. It therefore is in your best interest to find the source of the problem and correct it as quickly as possible. Having accurate information about your menstrual cycle helps your gynecologist determine which diagnostic tests to order or whether you need to see a specialist.

Diagnostic tests help figure out why you are not yet pregnant. Most of these tests are performed by physicians. However, you can also collect information on your own that can save time and be helpful in aiding your diagnosis. We begin with what you can do on your own to Become a Partner in Your Treatment.

DETECTING OVULATION

Infertility problems can be detected either directly or indirectly. The only *direct* evidence of ovulation is pregnancy. Indirect evidence can be provided through an endometrial biopsy, through an analysis of your hormonal levels during specific days of your menstrual cycle, through a cervical mucus check, basal body temperature charts, and home ovulation predictor kits. These charts and tests look at clues that arise from the hormonal events associated with ovulation. Try to keep your information organized so that you can readily share it with your doctor. The Cycle Log in Chapter 2 should help.

Cervical Mucus

As your estrogen levels change, so does the quantity and quality of the cervical mucus. Around the time of ovulation, mucus production increases, and it becomes clear and stretchy almost like raw egg white. One test you can do yourself is to examine your cervical mucus during your cycle. Try to discern when it changes from scant to copious and from thickish to thin and stretchy. After ovulation, it changes again from the consistency of egg whites back to a small amount of thick mucus.

Basal Body Temperature

Another hormonal event you can monitor indirectly is the level of progesterone in your bloodstream. At the beginning of the cycle, the progesterone level is low and your body temperature is correspondingly low. Just before ovulating, there is an LH surge, associated with a drop in basal body temperature. Following the surge, the egg is ovulated from the follicle, and the remaining sac becomes the corpus luteum, which secretes high amounts of progesterone. When this happens, body temperature jumps one half a degree to a whole degree.

You can chart these temperature changes using a basal body temperature (BBT) thermometer. Most basal body thermometers come with temperature charts. These charts also are produced by pharmaceutical companies. Your doctor should have an ample supply of temperature charts to give you. All charts contain spaces in which to date each day of your cycle. The first day of your menstrual period is Day 1. In addition to graphically showing any temperature changes, the chart also helps you determine exactly how long your cycle is and how regular you are. Here is a sample chart:

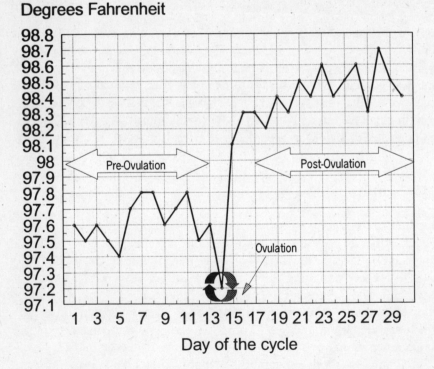

Figure 4.1

For charting to be of value, you *must* heed the following precautions:

- Take your temperature *as soon as you wake up*.
- Do *not* move around before taking your temperature.
- Record the temperature on the chart right after you take it. Do not rely on your memory.
- Record your temperature every morning.

Your BBT changes constantly according to activity levels and time of day. Readings taken anytime other than the moment you wake up are useless. Keep your thermometer, chart, and a pencil at your bedside. Shake the thermometer down immediately after recording your temperature so it is ready for the next morning's reading.

Keeping track of your temperature can be nerve-racking. A reading that is not what you hoped for may tempt you to fudge or to take a second reading. Resist this impulse because inaccurate data can mislead a doctor into thinking you are ovulating when you really aren't.

Ovulation Predictor Kits

In addition to monitoring your BBT and cervical mucus, you also can test your urine for an LH surge, which generally occurs thirty-four to thirty-six hours before ovulation, the time of peak fertility.[1] There are some half dozen brands of ovulation predictor kits on the market, and all are available without a prescription. They vary in complexity as well as in price (the average is about $40 for a five-day supply of testers). All of the kits require that you either collect your urine and mix it with chemicals or put the urine in contact with a chemically treated surface. A color indicator will tell you whether you are having an LH surge.

Most kit manufacturers claim that ovulation will occur twenty-four to forty hours after the change in color on the indicator stick.[2] The tests are reliable if used effectively. Test your urine for three or four consecutive days, beginning about four days before the time you usually ovulate as shown by previous BBT charts. For most women this will be between Days 9 and 13 of their cycle.

Once you have a positive test, stop testing and be sure to have intercourse within the window of time recommended on the kit's instruction leaflet. Note on your BBT chart when the LH surge occurred.

When you first run a series of ovulation-predictor tests, you may feel like a mad chemist. But rest assured, you soon will be able to perform the tests in a more matter-of-fact way once you get accustomed to the procedure. Knowing when to time intercourse is a definite help in getting pregnant.

COLLECTING MEDICAL HISTORY INFORMATION

Another way to aid your gynecologist is to gather critical medical history in a systematic and organized way. To help, we provide you with separate forms for both you and your partner to photocopy, fill out and give, along with your temperature charts and a list of questions, to your gynecologist during your consultation.

WOMAN'S MEDICAL HISTORY FORM

Name: _____

Age: _____ Years married: _____ ☐ 1st marriage ☐ 2nd marriage

Height _____   Weight _____

Menstrual History Information:

Age at first period: _____

Characteristics of early periods:

☐ cramps   ☐ light flow   ☐ heavy flow

☐ erratic period

How long did it take for your periods to become regular? _____

Do you remember anything unusual about your early menstrual history? _____

Current Menstrual Information:

When was your last period? _____

How long is your typical menstrual cycle (from the beginning of one period to the
    beginning of the next period)? _____

How many days do you bleed? _____

Do you have:

☐ cramps   ☐ clotting   ☐ heavy flow

☐ light flow   ☐ irregular flow

Is your period usually regular? _____

Have you had any missed periods lately? _____

Has it been some time since you had a period? _____

Can you tell when you are ovulating? _____

What are the signs:

☐ pain in your ovaries   ☐ pain in your lower back

☐ heavy watery cervical mucus   ☐ other

History of Birth Control:

Have you ever used birth control? _____

Have you used:

☐ birth control pills   name _____ date of use _____ duration _____
☐ diaphragm   date of use _____ duration _____
☐ IUD   kind _____ date of use _____ duration _____

Woman's Medical History Form (*cont'd.*)

☐ condom
☐ sponge/foam
☐ rhythm method
☐ coitus interruptus

If you used an IUD or birth control pills, describe your cycles while using either of them:

What were your cycles like after you stopped using them?

How long has it been since you stopped using birth control?

Pregnancy History:
Have you ever been pregnant? _____

Pregnancy History

Year	Spontaneous abortion? Yes/No	Therapeutic abortion? Yes/No	Ectopic pregnancy? Yes/No	Any infertility treatment for this pregnancy?	How much time did it take to conceive?	Did this pregnancy result in a live baby?	Was the current husband the father?

General Medical Information:
What was the age of first intercourse? _____
Have you had any sexually transmitted diseases? _____
☐ gonorrhea   ☐ syphilis   ☐ chlamydia
☐ venereal warts   ☐ herpes   ☐ pelvic inflammatory disease (PID)
☐ other

When did you have them? _____
How were they discovered and treated?

Have you ever had:
☐ vaginal infections   ☐ abnormal pap smears

Did your mother take the drug DES while she was pregnant with you? _____
    If yes, how did you find out?

    Has any doctor commented on your DES exposure?

Have you had any surgeries or illnesses that required hospitalization?

Name of illness or surgical procedure	Date	Reason for hospitalization	Findings	Complications

Have you had any chronic illness now or in childhood? _____

Have you ever been on medication for a long time? _____

Are you taking any medication now? _____

Are there any chronic diseases or conditions in your family? _____

Lifestyle History:

Name of exercise	How often do you do this exercise?	How much time do you spend on this exercise?

Does your weight fluctuate much? _____
Do you diet? _____
Have you ever had an eating disorder? _____
Do you drink alcohol? _____
        How often? _____
        How much? _____

Woman's Medical History Form (*cont'd.*)

Do you smoke cigarettes?
    How often? _____
    How much? _____
Are you exposed to any chemicals or radiation on your job? _____
_____
_____

Do you consider yourself to be under a lot of stress at home or at work? _____

History of Infertility:

How long have you been trying to get pregnant? _____
When did you discontinue contraceptives? _____
Intercourse:

Frequency (times/week)	Position	Lubricant? Yes/No	Douche? Yes/No	Pain? Yes/No

MEDICAL HISTORY: MALE

Name: _____

Age: _____ Years married: _____ ☐ 1st marriage ☐ 2nd marriage

Height _____ Weight _____

Childhood Information:

Were you an: ☐ only child ☐ middle child ☐ last child

Were you born
 prematurely? ☐ yes ☐ no

Were you
 circumcised? ☐ yes ☐ no

Did you ever have
 mumps? ☐ yes ☐ no At what age? _____

Did you ever have
 surgery for a
 hernia? ☐ yes ☐ no At what age? _____

Sexual Information:

What was the age of first intercourse? _____

Have you ever
 fathered a
 child? ☐ yes ☐ no

Have you
 ever had
 gonorrhea? ☐ yes ☐ no

Have you ever
 had syphilis? ☐ yes ☐ no

Is intercourse
 painful? ☐ yes ☐ no

Do you have
 trouble
 maintaining an
 erection? ☐ yes ☐ no

On a scale from 1 (low) to 5 (high), how would you characterize your current sex
 drive? _____

Do you ejaculate in the vagina without difficulty? ☐ yes ☐ no

Medical History: Male (*cont'd.*)

Genitourinary Information:

Have you ever been treated for an infection of the testicles: ☐ yes   ☐ no

Is urination
   painful?   ☐ yes   ☐ no

Did you ever
   have
   undescended
   testes?   ☐ yes   ☐ no

Was the problem
   corrected?   ☐ yes   ☐ no

Did you ever
   have any injury
   to your testes? ☐ yes   ☐ no

Have you ever
   had a
   vasectomy?   ☐ yes   ☐ no

Have you ever
   had varicocele
   surgery?   ☐ yes   ☐ no

Other Information:

Do you use hot
   tubs regularly? ☐ yes   ☐ no

Are you exposed
   to high
   temperatures
   at work?   ☐ yes   ☐ no

Are you exposed
   to radiation at
   work?   ☐ yes   ☐ no

Were you ever
   exposed to
   Agent Orange
   in the military? ☐ yes   ☐ no

What type of
   underwear do
   you use?   ☐ boxer shorts   ☐ jockey shorts

Do you drive long
   distances on a
   regular basis? ☐ yes   ☐ no

Have you had any surgeries or illnesses that required hospitalization?

Name of illness or surgical procedure	Date	Reason for hospitalization	Findings	Complications

Have you had any chronic illness now or in childhood? _____
Have you ever been on medication for a long time? _____
Are you taking any medication now? _____
Are there any chronic diseases or conditions in your family?

Lifestyle History:

Name of exercise	How often do you do this exercise?	How much time do you spend on this exercise?

Does your weight fluctuate much? _____
Do you diet? _____
Have you ever had an eating disorder? _____
Do you drink alcohol? _____
    How often? _____
    How much? _____
Do you smoke cigarettes?
    How often? _____
    How many? _____

This information probably will have to be supplemented with data gathered through laboratory tests and medical examinations. Knowledge of the tests and procedures described in this chapter should prepare you for whatever your diagnosis might be. Finding out that you have a problem is discouraging news. But remember that many fertility problems can be fixed or circumvented and that advances in this area of medicine are happening all the time.

BEGINNING THE PARTNERSHIP

Prior to testing, your doctor will probably request a consultation session with you. Try to have your partner accompany you to this visit to help you Work as a Team. During this initial visit, your doctor will review your medical histories and probably schedule some diagnostic tests, technically known as an *infertility workup*. Be on alert that this workup is physically taxing, emotionally draining, and can deplete your finances quickly if you have no health insurance. The diagnostic process may span many months.

Life during diagnosis is extremely stressful. You may feel bombarded by disturbing and possibly conflicting thoughts. It's quite normal to want several things at the same time. You want to learn what the problem is. You want to hear there is no problem. You want to know whether the problem is fixable. The bottom line is you want to know whether you will ever be pregnant.

If you are feeling scared or overwhelmed at this point, realize that just knowing the names of the tests, what problems they might uncover, and what you can expect to happen during your workup will provide some relief and may give you a sense of control.[3]

When you schedule your doctor's appointment, make sure you tell the nurse or secretary the purpose of the visit: to begin diagnosing why you are not yet pregnant. When you see the doctor, request that you have a Pap smear, cultures of your cervix, and some basic hormonal tests and blood work.

Many of the hormonal tests must be conducted on a particular day of your cycle, for example Day 3 for FSH. So try to schedule your visit to correspond with the early days or the midpoint of your cycle. Don't worry if your cycle is irregular. You can have your entire physical during that day and then return on another day to have blood drawn.

This initial visit is your first opportunity to Become a Partner in Your Treatment. As a partner, you should take the responsibility of setting an agenda for the visit. The agenda should be:

- What do we know?
- What do we need to find out?
- What do we do next?

When talking to your gynecologist, explain clearly that you have been trying to get pregnant for X months and would like to begin testing as soon as possible. When you leave the office, you should have a clear-cut Getting Pregnant Plan for the next several months, fulfilling yet another Pointer.

Dealing with Experts Other Than Your Primary Care Physician

Unfortunately, the key to getting the diagnosis and treatment you want can mean seeing a battalion of specialists. Many of the tests described in this chapter can and should only be done by experts who perform them regularly. Although your gynecologist can orchestrate the general plan of action, you most likely also will require the services of radiologists and laboratory technicians, as well as urologists who specialize in male infertility.

Unlike your own doctor, who is familiar with your personality and probably has a good bedside manner, doctors in these specialties may see patients only once or for short periods of time. They may be gruff or cold. Their relationship is not with you but with your personal physician to whom they will submit the results of your test. Prepare yourself for this detachment by realizing that the doctor's expertise and competence—not charm—are the only important factors. You want to get pregnant, not find a new friend, so seek emotional support outside the specialist's office.

THE TESTS THEMSELVES

The simplest tests are generally performed first, either in your doctor's office or in a laboratory.

Hormonal Analysis for Women

Even if your BBT shows the appropriate rise and fall in temperature and your LH surge kit reveals a color change, your doctor may order a hormonal analysis to confirm that your ovaries are functioning normally. These tests are almost always covered by health insurance. You need only have a few vials of blood drawn, a relatively painless procedure. Having the test done does not prohibit you from trying to get pregnant during that month, although you may experience some stress awaiting the test results.

Here is a list of the hormonal tests your doctor might order and when in your cycle these tests are generally done:

- FSH (Follicle Stimulating Hormone) level, monitored between Days 3 and 6 of your cycle. The normal base level is between 5 and 20 mlU/ml on Day 3. The peak FSH level at mid-cycle is two times higher than the base level.[4]
- LH (Luteinizing Hormone) level, monitored when Day 3 FSH is taken and again around mid-cycle. A normal base level is between 5 and 20 mlU/ml. During the mid-cycle peak the level is about three times as high as the base level value.
- Estradiol level, monitored at various times. During the follicular phase it can normally range between 25 and 75 pg/ml. During the mid-cycle peak it can range between 200 and 600 pg/ml, and during the luteal phase it will be between 100 and 300 pg/ml.
- Progesterone level, monitored at mid-cycle and seven days after; the level at mid-cycle is typically under 2 ng/ml on the day of the LH surge and rises to between 10 and 15 a week later.[5]
- Prolactin level (too much prolactin can inhibit ovulation), monitored at any time during the cycle. It is normally less than 25 ng/ml.

Semen Analysis for Men

While you undergo ovulation tests, your husband's sperm quality and quantity can be analyzed through a test known as a *semen analysis*. To obtain a semen sample, the man must ejaculate through masturbation into a sterile cup. Lab technicians have told us that some couples have brought in samples in Tupperware salt shakers. This is not advisable. For best results, obtain a sterile specimen cup from your doctor or pharmacist.

The sample can be collected at home, in a doctor's locked examination room, or in a lab that has a private room for this purpose. (If religious practices conflict with masturbation, other methods of obtaining semen can be used. Consult a clergyperson.)

If the specimen is to be obtained at home, be sure to keep the semen at room or body temperature en route to the lab. The sample should be provided thirty-six to ninety-six hours after the man last had intercourse and should be brought to the lab within one to two hours of leaving the man's body. The test is usually repeated at least once to increase reliability.

Specifically, the lab technician will measure:

- *semen volume:* how much liquid is produced (normal value is 2 to 6 milliliters);[6]
- *semen density:* how many sperm per milliliter of semen? (at least 20 million sperm per milliliter is considered sufficient to conceive);
- *pH:* acidity or alkalinity (7-8);
- *sperm morphology:* shape of the sperm (at least 50 percent should be of normal, oval shape);
- *sperm motility:* swimming ability (graded on 5-point scale):
    0: sperm are not moving,
    1: sperm are staying in place and vibrating,
    2: sperm are moving slowly,
    3: sperm are moving forward in a straight line at a good pace,
    4: sperm are racing forward in a straight line
    (the total percentage of motile sperm should be at least 75 percent);
- *semen viscosity:* how thick or watery (good semen is not too thick); and
- *sperm agglutination:* how much clumping (good semen has no significant clumping).

Results are usually available within one week. The lab sends results to the referring physician, who will pass the information along to you.

While there are no ill effects associated with providing a semen sample for analysis, there could be some emotional upheaval should the specimen prove to be less than ideal. It is important to emphasize to your husband that the quality of a man's sperm has nothing to do with his masculinity or sexual attractiveness. If the semen analysis reveals a problem the doctor may order one or more of these additional tests: a *fructose test,* a *testicular biopsy,* and *hormonal analysis.*

Fructose Test

This test is done *only* if the semen analysis reveals a complete absence of sperm. Its purpose is to determine whether an obstruction is preventing sperm from getting into the ejaculate.

Sperm cells and the seminal fluid are produced in separate areas of the testes. They flow through separate tubes, which merge into a single tube, the vas deferens, which carries the semen out of the penis during ejaculation. The seminal fluid contains a sugar called fructose. If no fructose is detected in the semen, the doctor knows there must be a blockage somewhere before the epididymis. Results should be available within one week.

Testicular Biopsy

If a fructose test reveals no sugar, the doctor may order a testicular biopsy to determine whether the man is making sperm. The biopsy examines the entire sperm production line—the area where sperm precursors are made, whether precursor sperm cells are changing into mature sperm, and whether sperm tails are being formed. It seems remarkable that so much information can be gathered by examining a tiny snip of tissue, but it helps to remember that all these things happen on a microscopic level.

The biopsy is taken under local anesthesia, usually in the doctor's office. The doctor, preferably a urologist, makes a one-quarter-inch incision in the scrotum and snips a small piece of tissue from the testes. The tissue is sent to a lab and examined under a microscope. The actual removal of tissue takes about ten minutes, and results are available in a week or two. Taking Tylenol prior to the test can reduce pain.

While physical discomfort is minimal and temporary, most men who undergo a testicular biopsy experience anxiety. They are concerned about both their masculinity and their potential ability to father a child. Again, it is important to be emotionally supportive of your husband as he waits for the results of this test.

Hormonal Analysis for Men

Analyzing the levels of hormones in the man's blood is another method of finding out possible causes of a low sperm count. The man's pituitary gland may not be secreting enough FSH to stimulate the testes to make sperm, for instance.

DOES THE COUPLE HAVE A PROBLEM?

Once the doctor has established that the woman is making eggs and the man is producing sperm, the next logical question is: "Can the sperm get to the eggs to try to fertilize them?" There are several barriers that can keep this from happening.

During the initial consultation, the physician should determine whether the couple are using a proper intercourse technique. Although there is no special technique or position that will assure a pregnancy, there are some improper ones that can prevent sperm and eggs from meeting. If the doctor discovers that you are using one of these, he will advise you of an appropriate change.

Post-Coital Test (PCT)

In perhaps 2 percent of infertile women, the cervical mucus is hostile to sperm and kills them long before they can swim to the egg. Hostile mucus can be diagnosed through a *post-coital test,* or PCT. This test also is known as the Huhner test and is performed two to twelve hours after intercourse.[7] However, there is no need to feel pressured to rush in immediately with your sample.

A PCT also can be performed twenty-four hours after intercourse to determine the sperm's long-term survival in the vagina. A negative finding may stem from poor-quality mucus, acidity, inadequate sperm, lack of estrogen, or from sperm-killing antibodies in the woman's vagina. It is not always clear which is to blame.

Prior to the PCT, you will use your basal body temperature chart and LH test kit to determine when you are ovulating. Just before ovulation, you will be instructed to have intercourse. When you arrive at the doctor's office, the gynecologist extracts a small sample of cervical mucus and examines it under a microscope to see how many sperm are alive and swimming. The procedure takes a few minutes, and some doctors allow you to view the sample under the microscope. While the PCT is relatively painless, it can cause emotional upset due to the sex-on-demand pressures.

Testing for Bacterial Infections

One of the earliest tests that should be done is a genital tract culture to look for bacterial infections. Many different strains of bacteria can live in the male and female genital tract and can cause a variety of problems at many different stages of the pregnancy process. Some of these bacteria are transmitted in Ping-Pong fashion from one partner to the other during sexual intercourse. Certain bacteria may create problems, which interfere with ovulation. Bacteria may contribute to a low sperm count or to sluggish sperm swimming. Bacteria also can advance the formation of scar tissue, which can block sperm transmission or damage the sperm production apparatus in the testes.

For women, certain bacterial infections can be a factor in pelvic inflammatory disease. These bacteria include chlamydia, T-mycoplasma, streptococcus, and enterococcus, among others. The cervical mucus and the semen should be tested for the presence of a bacterial infection. These infections are, in most cases, easily treatable with antibiotics.

As benign as this testing seems, it can spur emotional distress because a chlamydia infection can bring up discussions of past sexual activity.

Immunobead Test for Antisperm Antibodies

The body has an immune system designed to prevent attack by foreign bodies. The husband's sperm cells normally are treated as friendly foreigners by the woman's body. But some women's bodies mistakenly treat sperm as an enemy and send antibodies to destroy them. The woman can have antibodies that attack the head, the tail, or the midpiece of the sperm. Antibodies to the head can make the sperm incapable of penetrating the egg. Antibodies to the tail can impair the sperm's ability to swim properly.

Sometimes, too, a man can produce antibodies that actually attack his own sperm. This is a serious problem. Fortunately, the incidence of these antisperm antibodies is low for both the male and female populations.

To find out whether either or both members of the couple are producing antibodies, the doctor orders an Immunobead Test. A blood sample is drawn and a mucus sample obtained from the female, and a blood and semen sample is obtained from the male. Results, available in a few weeks, are given in terms of percentage of antibodies attacking the head, midpiece, or tail of the sperm.

The doctor will discuss the specific proportions of the various types of antibodies found. In those instances in which significant immunological problems are encountered, the doctor may discuss using one of the Assisted Reproductive Techniques described in Chapter 7.

DOES THE WOMAN HAVE A PROBLEM THAT IS PREVENTING FERTILIZATION?

If the tests for ovulation suggest that you are ovulating, the doctor needs to find out whether the ovulated egg is getting into the fallopian tube. Some women have adhesions, or scar tissue, that impede the ability of the tube to rotate into position to catch the egg. Even if the tube is in position, the egg may not be picked up because the fimbria at the upper end of the tube may be damaged.

If the egg does get into the tube, it may get stuck in one spot, unable to travel to the location of the sperm. The tube itself may contain internal adhesions, or fibroids, which act like roadblocks preventing movement of an egg.

There are several diagnostic procedures that provide information about the internal and the external condition of the fallopian tubes. These tests differ in terms of their cost, physical discomfort, risks, and the amount of information they provide. Understanding these tests can give you an idea of which ones should be done before others and whether the costs and risks are worth it.

The Hysterosalpingogram (HSG)

Useful information about the internal condition of the fallopian tubes is provided by a *hysterosalpingogram,* or HSG. The HSG does not allow the doctor to *directly* see the actual inside of the tube. Instead, it only shows the *outlines* of the tube. Only a new experimental procedure called *falloscopy* allows the doctor to *directly* observe the inside of the tube.[8] Not only can the doctor see it, he or she can perform minor surgery to correct some problems.

A hysterosalpingogram is an X-ray picture showing the shape of the uterus and the fallopian tubes and whether the tubes are open. The X ray also can reveal scarring in the reproductive tract.

To obtain the X ray, a tube is inserted into your uterus and dye injected into the tube. As soon as the dye begins to travel through your tubes, you will feel mild to moderate discomfort. Performed in a radiologist's office or hospital, the procedure takes about thirty minutes and is done early in the menstrual cycle prior to ovulation.

It is not unusual to feel emotionally distraught over the HSG procedure. You may be worried, and rightly so, that the test will reveal blocked tubes. You may be upset about having to sign a waiver releasing the doctor from responsibility should anything go wrong. You may feel uncomfortable about having to get undressed in front of an unfamiliar doctor. And finally, since your doctor may have prescribed antibiotics, you may be worried about a bacterial infection resulting from the procedure. To cope, we recommend that you:

- Work as a Team. Have your partner read the description of this procedure and write a script to help you mentally rehearse it. In addition, have your partner accompany you to the test.
- Make a Plan. Use the Getting Pregnant Workout techniques to rehearse the procedure, and relax using controlled breathing before and during the HSG. Part of your plan should be taking three or four ibuprofen tablets several hours before the test to reduce discomfort. Your doctor also may prescribe antibiotics prior to the test to minimize the possibility of infection.

Hysteroscopy

As useful as the HSG is, it does not allow the doctor to directly examine the tubes and the uterus. It also does not allow the physician to determine if there are adhesions on the outside of the tube. If the physician must examine the outside of the tube for scarring, a laparoscopy will be ordered.

Like the HSG, a hysteroscopy is looking for blockage problems that may be preventing fertilization and implantation. Unlike the HSG, a hysteroscopy can include procedures to correct some of these problems through surgery.

The hysteroscopy looks for problems such as adhesions, polyps, fibroids, or the formation of a wall in the uterus called a *septum*. For example, the results of a hysteroscopy may indicate excessive scarring, which can prevent an embryo from implanting properly in the uterus.

The hysteroscopy takes thirty minutes to two hours and is generally done near the end of the cycle, a few days before menstruation is due. Under some circumstances, a hysteroscopy can be performed in a doctor's office using a combination of local anesthesia and a sedative. More commonly, the hysteroscopy is performed on an outpatient basis in a hospital operating room under local or general anesthesia. Sometimes the hysteroscopy can be combined with a diagnostic laparoscopy. It is generally performed by a surgeon who may also be your infertility specialist.

Before the procedure, you must disrobe, put on a hospital gown and lie on an operating table, which may feel cold and uncomfortable. During the procedure, the uterine cavity is inflated with carbon dioxide or a sterile water solution. The doctor inserts a telescopic instrument called a *hysteroscope* through the cervix. Using a scalpel or a laser attached to the end of the hysteroscope, the doctor can cut away adhesions or polyps he might see. While the doctor is examining the inside of the uterus, he can also obtain tissue for an endometrial biopsy.

The operation itself is not very painful. You may feel nauseated afterward from the anesthesia. Some patients vomit and many are groggy after the procedure. Patients sometimes feel a temporary pain in the shoulders and the neck from carbon dioxide bubbles rising from the abdominal cavity. Do not be alarmed by these symptoms. The body will absorb the bubbles within the next twenty-four hours, and the pain will disappear. Lying down prevents the bubbles from rising and also relieves pain.

To cope with the anxiety over the surgery, use the same Pointers described for the HSG. Ask your doctor if he plans to do a laparoscopy or endometrial biopsy, and if so, discuss with him the pros and cons of scheduling the two procedures simultaneously.

Diagnostic Laparoscopy

While the hysteroscopy concentrates on the inside of the uterus, the *laparoscopy* provides much valuable information about the *outside* of the tube as well as what's going on in the abdominal cavity. Laparoscopy is usually recommended for women who used IUDs in the past, have had a previous tubal pregnancy or painful periods, or have failed to become pregnant after a year of trying.

A laparoscopy is performed in a hospital or outpatient operating room under general anesthesia. Be aware that you will be wearing a hospital gown and be wheeled into the operating room while you are still conscious. After you are unconscious, a needle will be inserted through your belly button. Carbon dioxide gas will be introduced to inflate the abdominal cavity and make it easier for the surgeon to view the internal organs. As incision will be made in the belly button and a laparoscope inserted.

Through the laparoscope, the surgeon inspects the uterus, tubes, and ovaries for evidence of adhesions, endometriosis (uterine lining outside the uterus), or other problems, and fixes what can be corrected. Occasionally, another instrument is inserted through an incision elsewhere in the patient's abdomen. After the operation is completed, the incision or incisions are closed with one or two stitches and covered with a Band-Aid. The patient is taken to the recovery room. A few hours later, she is discharged.

The surgery takes a minimum of thirty minutes and a maximum of several hours if the surgeon needs to correct many problems. It is advisable to have a surgeon who specializes in this procedure perform the laparoscopy. Although the surgery is quite safe, complications such as perforated blood vessels, bowels, or stomach have occurred in a small minority of cases.

The side effects, both physical and emotional, are similar to those of the hysteroscopy.

To cope:

- Work as a Team. Have your partner read the description of this procedure and write a script to help you mentally rehearse it. Have him accompany you to the operation.
- Be a Partner in Your Treatment. Assertively discuss your concerns about anesthesia with the anesthesiologist and insist on a protocol that will minimize the likelihood of discomfort.

CAN THE SPERM FERTILIZE THE EGG?

Once the aforementioned tests and surgeries confirm that the man is making sperm and that there are no blockages in the woman's reproductive tract, the next logical question is: "Are the man's sperm capable of fertilizing the woman's eggs?"

The ultimate test to answer this question is *in vitro fertilization*. When the doctor retrieves a woman's eggs and places them together with her husband's sperm in a petri dish, the doctor can actually see whether the sperm successfully penetrates and fertilizes the egg. Short of that, there is no direct measure.

Hamster Penetration Test

Since there is no easily obtained measure of fertilizing ability, some doctors have tried to get an indirect indicator of the sperm's ability to fertilize an egg using a *hamster penetration test*. The idea is that if a man's sperm can penetrate a hamster's egg then it probably can penetrate a human egg as well. There is controversy, however, regarding the value of this test. Some doctors believe the information gleaned from this test is useful. Others believe that the conditions of the test are so unlike those in nature that the test does not provide valuable information.

DOES THE FERTILIZED EGG IMPLANT IN THE ENDOMETRIUM?

The next step is ensuring that the embryo can implant successfully in the endometrium. The endometrium is the lining that grows inside the uterus and is shed each month during menstruation when pregnancy does not occur. When the endometrium is too thin or not soft enough due to a lack of estrogen or progesterone, respectively, successful embryo implantation is less likely. When things work properly, the LH surge ovulates an egg, and the leftover corpus luteum secretes progesterone, which makes the endometrium soft and lush. If the woman has what is called a *luteal phase defect,* the endometrium is not ready to receive the embryo when it arrives in the uterus.

Endometrial Biopsy

To determine the receptivity of the endometrium, the doctor performs an *endometrial biopsy,* a procedure in which a tiny piece of lining is extracted and examined. The biopsy is performed in the doctor's office before the expected onset of the next menses. By studying the tissue sample, it is possible to date the age of the endometrial tissue. Endometrial tissue is dated on the basis of an idealized twenty-eight-day menstrual cycle. Careful laboratory investigations of endometrial development have revealed how endometrial tissue should look at different ages. Using these standards, the age of the biopsied tissue is determined.

The observed age is interpreted relative to the *start* of the menstrual period *following* the biopsy. Then the doctor counts backward from the first new cycle day until he reaches the day on which the biopsy was performed. So if the biopsy was performed three days before the onset of the next menses, the laboratory tissue analysis should look like tissue that is three days prior to menstruation. If the histological (tissue) date is more than two days out of sync with the date determined by counting backward from menstruation, then a luteal phase defect is said to exist. The endometrium is not ready for the egg and may have difficulty allowing for implantation.

Extraction of the tissue sample takes about ten minutes. The biopsy is done around Day 26 or 27. You may actually be pregnant at this time. But be assured that the risk of a miscarriage due to a biopsy is less than one in one thousand. Nonetheless, you may wish to have a pregnancy test before the procedure. During the procedure, the woman lies on a table just as she would during a pelvic examination. The doctor inserts a speculum into the vagina and examines the cervix. He cleans the vagina and then grasps the cervix with a clamp. That may cause a sudden cramp, and the patient may be startled. A good physician will alert the woman ahead of time and talk her through this phase in a calm manner. Then the doctor inserts a little plastic straw and creates negative suction to extract a bit of the lining. The effect of this action sometimes produces a sensation similar to a menstrual cramp. The woman may feel discomfort for several minutes following the procedure. Some women bleed and should use a sanitary napkin.

Women typically are frightened by the endometrial biopsy, but that fear can be lessened by the realization that the information gained through the procedure can be vital to getting them pregnant. To cope:

- Work as a Team. Have your partner read the description of this procedure and write a script to help you mentally rehearse it. Also have him accompany you to the test.
- Make a Plan. Use the Getting Pregnant Workout techniques to relax. Use GPST. Tell yourself, ''It's going to be easy; the pain is minor and will subside shortly.'' Before the procedure, take a mild pain medication such as Motrin.
- Be a Partner in Your Treatment. Ask your doctor to prescribe Valium, which you can also take before the biopsy. A half tablet can help you relax during the procedure. The more relaxed you are, the less discomfort you will experience. Also, ask your doctor whether lidocaine can be used.

BEYOND IMPLANTATION

Once implantation takes place, the concern becomes making sure that the embryo continues to grow and develop into a healthy baby. For information on those stages of pregnancy, we refer you to Dr. Jonathan Scher's excellent book *Preventing Miscarriage.*[9]

Diagnosing the reason or reasons for infertility takes good detective work and skilled craftsmanship. As with any job that you contract for, you want to use only highly skilled professionals. Some doctors are jacks of all trades. They do both the detective work and the repairs. As a consumer of medical care, it is your responsibility to make sure that the doctors you are working with are experienced. And remember, the doctor who is a skilled technician may not necessarily be a skilled diagnostician. In Chapter 6 we include a Doctor Interview Guide that has important questions for you to ask when selecting the infertility specialist that is best for you.

Also keep in mind that *the ability to make an accurate diagnosis does not require the skills to perform the test*. That means your gynecologist may diagnose you solely by reading the laboratory and surgical reports. That also means that you can logically deduce that some tests are inappropriate or redundant for your case, given what you already know. For that reason, it is essential that you assert yourself in discussing your case with your doctor.

CHAPTER FIVE

THE TREATMENTS
OF INFERTILITY

As in diagnostic testing, infertility treatment runs the gamut from the simplest and cheapest to the more complicated and costly. "Simple" and "cheap" are relative terms, however. As you have already read in Chapter 3, reproduction is complicated business. The ways of correcting fertility problems are, therefore, by definition, complicated. But don't let the strange-sounding names or procedures intimidate you. None of these concepts are beyond your comprehension, especially if you try to remain objective. Once you know what to expect, you can anticipate how various procedures may affect your body, your mind, and your pocketbook.

This chapter focuses on the relatively simple, or low-tech, treatments to correct your fertility problems. These treatments include drug therapy, artificial insemination, and surgery. Artificial insemination with donor sperm also is a low-tech treatment, but we address that topic along with other third-party pregnancy approaches in Chapter 9. Once you have Educated Yourself about these low-tech ways of getting pregnant, you can go on to Chapter 6, which addresses the emotional and psychological aspects of the issues covered in this chapter.

After obtaining a diagnosis from your physician—even if the diagnosis is unexplained infertility—it's time to begin Making a Treatment Plan in earnest. Depending on your doctor and your case, you may be advised to pursue one of two conflicting strategies. One strategy suggests that you go directly to the high-tech assisted reproductive technologies, which claim higher success rates and shorter time to success.

The other strategy explores less-invasive, less-costly low-tech treatments first. Couples pursuing this strategy may try a simple low-tech treatment for several cycles. If that treatment fails, the couple graduates to a more aggressive low-tech treatment (a different fertility drug, for example) for the next several cycles. Only when they've exhausted all the appropriate low-tech treatments do they consider moving to the high-tech arena.

Remember: *Regardless of what your doctor recommends, the ultimate choice is yours*. The path you choose will reflect your finances, your timetable, the advice of your physician, and a host of other individual considerations, not the least of which is your psychological well-being.

We believe you owe it to yourself to at least consider low-tech treatments before trying high-tech measures such as in vitro fertilization. This week, as we are writing this chapter, seven women at IVF New Jersey, where we counsel couples, learned that they were pregnant—not through in vitro, but as a result of taking drugs to stimulate egg production followed by intrauterine insemination—the mainstay of low-tech treatment.

INFERTILITY TREATMENT DRUGS

Most people, when they are trying to conceive a child, stop taking all drugs—even aspirin and alcohol. So it's ironic that for many infertile couples their only chance of becoming pregnant is by using drugs—fertility drugs, that is. Listen to the conversations between patients combating infertility, and the topic is almost always centered on medications: dosage, administration, costs, effectiveness, and side effects.

Here are the pros and cons, costs, and side effects of the pharmaceutical arsenal available at this writing.[1] We urge you to ask your doctor whether newer, better drugs have hit the market since.

Clomiphene Citrate

The most commonly prescribed drug to correct ovulation problems is clomiphene citrate, sold under the brand names Clomid and Serophene. By manipulating hormonal output, this oral medication stimulates the ovaries to produce one or more eggs in women who do not otherwise ovulate, have irregular cycles, or infrequent periods. Clomiphene may also be prescribed to induce superovulation in women who have unexplained infertility in order to make more egg targets for sperm.

Clomiphene, priced at about $6 a tablet, is generally taken for five consecutive days beginning on Day 3 to Day 5 after the onset of menstruation. The standard dosage is one tablet (50 milligrams) a day. If your body responds properly to the drug, you should ovulate about a week after you have taken the last tablet. If pregnancy does not result, the doctor may increase the dosage to two or three tablets a day with the next cycle. The doctor also may prescribe the drug for more than five days. While you can safely take up to 250 milligrams daily, most women need only 150 milligrams a day or less to ovulate.

While on clomiphene, be sure to carefully record your basal body temperature (BBT) each morning, and perform ovulation predictor (LH surge) tests beginning on Day 10 of your menstrual cycle (see Chapter 4). Unless you are being artificially inseminated, your doctor will likely advise you to have intercourse every other day for at least one week starting about four days after you've taken the last tablet.

Following these guidelines, about 80 percent of women treated with clomiphene will ovulate, and 40 percent will get pregnant within six cycles.[2] Those women who do conceive have about a 10 percent chance of giving birth to twins.

Caution: Clomiphene therapy often lengthens a woman's cycle by two, three, or even more days, which can give her a false sense of being pregnant.

Researchers have found that if clomiphene treatment has not led to a pregnancy after six cycles, however, it is unlikely it ever will.[3] If you have not gotten pregnant after six clomiphene cycles, therefore, it is time to Make a New Plan.

Clomiphene creates some undesirable physical and emotional side effects in certain women. The most common physical side effect is a reduction of cervical mucus, which can be counteracted by taking estrogen. Other women report bloating, weight gain, hair loss, vision changes, and headaches while on clomiphene therapy.

Many patients we counsel report fairly substantial emotional side effects from clomiphene as well. To investigate this phenomenon, we placed an inquiry in the national RESOLVE Inc. newsletter. Within several weeks, we received about thirty letters stating that clomiphene produced an array of negative emotional effects. Norma, a social worker, described profound depression, which caught her off guard, since she generally was an upbeat person. Abby called Clomid's emotional impact "devastating." Phyllis said she was so depressed that she would sit and cry for hours. Others reported that they would suddenly burst into tears without provocation. Nanette described apparitions that haunted her. (Clomiphene sometimes changes pressure in the eye, which can cause what seem like ghostly flashes of light.)

In contrast, some women wrote that they had no significant emotional side effects. Although our survey was informal, it is clear that the response varies substantially from person to person. So if you're feeling sad and "cry at every Hallmark Card" commercial like Jean told us, or have dramatic mood swings during a clomiphene cycle, you are not going crazy; you're just having intense responses to the drug, particularly because of its anti-estrogen characteristics.

Dr. Melvin Taymor, clinical professor emeritus at Harvard Medical School, calls clomiphene "one of the most widely used medications in gynecology; unfortunately, it is also one of the most misused.

"Most infertility specialists will have had the experience of seeing many patients who at the very first interview have already been on clomiphene—sometimes up to one year or more," Dr. Taymor continues. "Many of these patients have not had a simple basal body temperature chart followed to see whether or not they are ovulating. In addition, many have had no infertility workup. This misuse has probably been fostered by the fact that clomiphene citrate has been called a 'fertility drug.'

"The fact is that if a patient is ovulating normally on her own, there is little likelihood that clomiphene will further increase the quality of that ovulation. The administration of clomiphene without a workup will, in most instances, only delay the resolution of the problem. In addition, clomiphene may have inhibiting effects upon fertility" such as diminishing the quality of the cervical mucus.[4]

Dr. Taymor's warnings are worth heeding. To avoid misuse of clomiphene or any fertility drug, you must Become a Partner in Your Treatment. Be sure your doctor has completed an adequate workup before determining whether clomiphene treatment is appropriate in your situation. If it is not, you should move on to another treatment that is right for you.

Clomiphene also can be used in men in an effort to improve sperm count. A typical male regimen is taking 25 milligrams of clomiphene daily, with interspersed five-day rest periods. The therapy is generally continued for up to nine months.

Pergonal/Metrodin

Human menopausal gonadotropin (hMG), usually referred to by its brand name Pergonal, is much more powerful than clomiphene. Unlike clomiphene, Pergonal is administered by injection only and requires much more intensive monitoring, as well as an additional drug, hCG (human chorionic gonadotropin), to trigger ovulation. Pergonal contains equal parts of the hormones FSH and LH, which are extracted from the urine of post-menopausal women, purified, and freeze-dried in glass ampules (small glass containers that keep the medicine fresh and sterile). Before injection, the white powder must be reconstituted with sterilized water. The FSH and LH in Pergonal have a direct impact on the ovaries, causing them to produce several eggs during one cycle, giving sperm more targets.

Another ovulation-induction drug, similar to Pergonal, is Metrodin, which contains almost pure FSH. Like Pergonal, Metrodin directly stimulates the ovary to make multiple follicles and requires careful monitoring. Metrodin is usually indicated for women with an elevated LH level and a low to normal FSH level. Metrodin is often administered along with Pergonal.

According to research studies, about nine out of ten women treated with Pergonal will ovulate. Most women begin Pergonal injections on Day 2 to Day 4 of their cycle. Typically, patients are injected with one, two, or three ampules (75 units per ampule) of Pergonal daily for seven to twelve days.

Pergonal injections should be administered around the same time each day, and most doctors prefer evening doses, between 7 P.M. and 9 P.M. For most women, the schedule means that their partners must give the injections. At the end of this chapter is a detailed guide to help both of you through the rigors of Pergonal therapy.

The number of Pergonal days is based on results of ongoing blood tests and ultrasound scans of the ovaries. The blood tests measure estradiol levels, and the scans enable the doctor to measure the growing egg follicles and the size of the ovaries themselves. While inconvenient, this intensive monitoring is vital to avoid overstimulating the ovaries, a condition that can lead to discomfort or pain.

Most doctors order the first blood tests and scans on Day 3, before your first injection. This initial monitoring is to ensure that you have no residual ovarian cysts or follicles left over from previous cycles. The next monitoring is generally done on Day 6, then every day or every other day, depending on the individual. When the follicles grow big enough, you will stop taking Pergonal and get an injection of hCG, which will cause your eggs to ovulate.

Since you will produce several eggs with Pergonal, the risk of having multiple births becomes higher than average, about 26 percent.[5] And there is no direct evidence that Pergonal causes birth defects.

Pergonal therapy can be used in conjunction with intercourse, artificial insemination to the cervix (intracervical insemination), or artificial insemination directly into the uterus (intrauterine insemination, or IUI). Some doctors use a combined dose of Pergonal and clomiphene with or without insemination.

Physical side effects of Pergonal may include breast tenderness, swelling or rash at injection site, abdominal pain and bloating, and enlarged ovaries. Emotional side effects may include mood swings and depression. However, some women, rather than feeling depressed, experience a sense of elation, known as a Pergonal high. Interestingly, our inquiry about Pergonal side effects in the RESOLVE Inc. newsletter solicited only one letter and one phone call describing emotional problems. This was in marked contrast to the large number of complaints about clomiphene.

One side effect from Pergonal, albeit a rare one thanks to the advent of sophisticated monitoring, is hyperstimulation syndrome, a condition in which the ovaries grow abnormally large. The condition may require hospitalization, during which a catheter may be placed in the abdomen to drain excess fluids that build up. Contrary to popular belief, Pergonal does not make ovaries explode.

Perhaps the most painful aspect of Pergonal is its damage to your pocketbook. Depending on where you live, the drug can cost $50 to $75 a dose or more (Metrodin costs about the same). If your insurance does not cover pharmaceuticals, you may find yourself canceling a vacation or foregoing that new stereo in order to pursue your pregnancy quest. Syringes, by the way, should not cost more than $2 apiece.

Lupron

In cases where the Pergonal response is poor or a woman has had a previous cycle canceled because of premature ovulation, doctors may choose to put the woman on Lupron (leuprolide acetate), which halts production of ovarian hormones, prevents ovulation, and lowers the woman's estrogen level. By shutting off the communication between the pituitary gland and the ovaries, Pergonal or Metrodin becomes the sole source of follicle stimulation. Generally speaking, the use of Lupron together with Pergonal is reserved for high-tech treatment. Lupron is injected once a day with the same tiny needle used by diabetics to administer insulin.

Lupron is a drug used for multiple purposes in treating infertility. It also is used to treat endometriosis, which is caused by excess estrogen. When Lupron is administered, ovarian follicles stop growing, a woman stops having her period (temporarily), and, as a result, stops making estrogen. This decrease in estrogen is the goal of Lupron treatment for endometriosis.

Lupron is injected daily or monthly in the treatment of endometriosis. Sometimes Lupron is used in conjunction with surgery, sometimes without. When used without surgery, treatment may last up to six months. About six to eight weeks after the drug is discontinued, periods resume. Average cost of Lupron: $220 for a 2.8 milliliter vial, which can last for approximately one month, depending on the specific daily dose. Potential side effects of Lupron include hot flashes, vaginal dryness, a diminished sex drive, depression, and breast tenderness.

Synarel

Like Lupron, Synarel (nafarelin acetate) is used to combat endometriosis. Instead of being injected into the body, however, Synarel is taken as a nasal spray, and has the same potential side effects as Lupron.

Danazol

Danazol (Danocrine) is a derivative of testosterone, a male hormone. Since endometriosis is the result of excess estrogen, danazol is designed to reduce estrogen levels. The standard dose of danazol is two 200 milligram tablets twice a day, or a total of 800 milligrams a day. The treatment is continued for six to nine months. While danazol does not *cure* endometriosis, it prevents its growth temporarily. Once a patient stops taking the medication, the endometriosis returns. While doctors advise against trying to get pregnant while on danazol, there is a six- to twelve-month window of opportunity to conceive after stopping the drug and before endometriosis potentially builds up to where it was before treatment.

Unfortunately, danazol has a number of undesirable side effects. A deepening of the voice, a decrease in breast size, weight gain, hair growth in various parts of the body, and acne occur in some patients, particularly when high doses are used. Lower doses reduce the side effects but also reduce the drug's ability to fight moderate or severe cases of endometriosis. Since the FDA approved Lupron and Synarel in the early 1990s, danazol is not prescribed as often, primarily because of its side effects.

hCG/Profasi

Human chorionic gonadotropin (hCG) is a clear liquid that is injected into the buttocks to trigger the release of the eggs after blood tests or ultrasound scans indicate that the eggs are mature. HCG is frequently given during Pergonal cycles, as well as during clomiphene cycles. In addition, hCG also is used to improve the quality of a man's sperm. Marketed as Profasi, hCG is obtained from the urine of pregnant women, refined and purified. It costs about $45 for 10,000 IU; $25 for 5,000 IU. Physical side effects of hCG may include abdominal distention, abdominal pain, and headache. Emotional side effects may include irritability, restlessness, depression, and fatigue.

Parlodel

Parlodel (bromocriptine mesylate) is prescribed for women whose pituitary produces too much prolactin, which can cause a milky discharge from the breasts, menstrual irregularity, lack of ovulation, and infertility. Parlodel can also be used in the treatment of polycystic ovarian disease. It is taken in tablet form one to three times daily until blood tests indicate prolactin levels are normal.

There is a fairly high incidence of mild adverse reactions to Parlodel, including nausea, vomiting, headaches, dizziness, fatigue, light-headedness, abdominal cramps, nasal congestion, and drowsiness. Some women are able to avoid the nausea and cramps by taking bromocriptine via vaginal suppositories. Parlodel's cost: $1.50 to $2.50 per dose.

There are several similar drugs on the market that also reduce prolactin secretion. These include Pergolide and Lisuride.

Progesterone

Progesterone is used to treat patients having a luteal phase inadequacy. Progesterone is also given to women after they are artificially inseminated to help support a possible pregnancy. Under normal circumstances, progesterone is produced by the ovary in slight amounts just before ovulation and in increasingly greater amounts by the corpus luteum during the luteal phase. Progesterone also is produced in large quantities by the placenta during pregnancy.

When the woman fails to produce enough progesterone, the hormone can be taken in vaginal or rectal suppositories, pills, or injections. Many women prefer suppositories because the injections can be painful. Make sure, however, you are taking *natural* progesterone, which does not cause birth defects. There also are *synthetic* forms of progesterone known as progestins, which can harm a fetus and therefore should be avoided when you are trying to get pregnant. Cost of progesterone is about $2 a suppository. Some women describe unwanted physical side effects, including mild acne, oily skin, oily hair, and increased hair growth.

Antibiotics

Antibiotics are used to treat bacterial infections and to prevent the possibility of infections that can impair fertilization or embryo implantation. A frequently prescribed medication for treating or preventing such infections is doxycycline. A typical regimen is two 100 milligram tablets daily for fourteen days. Side effects may include upset stomach. Antibiotics are sometimes prescribed as a preventive measure for both members of the couple in conjunction with a high-tech treatment such as IVF.

INSEMINATION AS A TREATMENT FOR INFERTILITY

Artificial insemination is a procedure that separates reproduction from sexual intercourse. The procedure involves placing the husband's sperm into the wife's vagina, cervix, or uterus so that she can become pregnant. Initially, many couples view insemination as unnatural. But after they have time to think about the procedure, they usually welcome it as a means to assist them in their pregnancy quest. Some even welcome insemination as a break from sex on demand. Doctors are often pleased to use insemination as a way to help couples feel that they are doing something to remedy their problem.

Intracervical Insemination

Intracervical insemination is the least invasive form of artificial insemination. The goal is to get the sperm, which may be poor swimmers, as close as possible to the cervical mucus so that they avoid the treacherous journey through the vagina. The cervical mucus acts as a reservoir for the sperm, releasing a few at a time during the next twenty-four to forty-eight hours. In this way, the chances are very good that some sperm will arrive in the fallopian tube at the time the ovulated egg gets there.

Since you may be artificially inseminated with sperm from your husband or from a donor, doctors draw a distinction between the two for clarity. This chapter addresses only artificial insemination by husband (AIH). AIH is performed in the doctor's office, usually the day after you detect an LH surge. Your husband provides a semen sample. The doctor draws it up into a syringe. You will lie on the examining table with your feet in stirrups. The doctor first inserts a speculum and then puts the syringe into the opening of your cervix and squeezes out the semen. The whole procedure takes less than a minute. The doctor then inserts a cap, similar to a diaphragm, over your cervix to help keep the sperm pooled in the area. You remove the cap using your fingers about twelve hours later. Cost of the insemination runs about $100.

Success rates for intracervical insemination vary depending on the nature of your fertility problem, what, if any, fertility drugs you are taking, and how many inseminations you have attempted. The pregnancy rate is higher (26 percent to 56 percent) when the problem is a low sperm count compared to a cervical problem, when the pregnancy rate is only 17.5 percent.[6] If after six trials of AIH you are not pregnant, it's probably time to try another technique or conduct more diagnostic tests.

Intrauterine Insemination

Intrauterine Insemination (IUI) consists of introducing washed semen directly into the uterus. IUI is recommended to counter a variety of male factor problems, such as low sperm count or high semen viscosity (clumpiness). IUI is also recommended in cases where the woman's cervical mucus is hostile to sperm, is not plentiful enough, or is too dense. People with unexplained infertility also may benefit from IUI. The goal of IUI is to introduce the sperm directly into the uterus and bypass the cervix, thus enabling more sperm to travel a shorter distance to the fallopian tubes and the waiting egg.

IUI may be done with or without clomiphene or Pergonal therapy. The advantage of combining IUI with fertility drugs is that you are increasing the number of targets for the sperm to reach. Superovulation, and the monitoring and hCG injection that go along with it, also help the doctor to more precisely time the IUI to coincide with when your eggs are most likely to ovulate.

IUI is similar to intracervical insemination in that the husband produces a semen sample into a sterile cup. It differs, however, in that a nurse or technician washes the sample to remove prostaglandins (hormonelike substances) that would otherwise cause cramping in the uterus. Then the technician places the sperm in a tube containing culture media. This tube is then placed into a centrifuge, which spins the sperm so that they are separated from the semen. The sperm sink to the bottom of the tube and the other material is removed. The dirty culture media is then replaced with fresh culture media.

At this time, the strongest swimming sperm swim up into the media. This procedure is referred to as swim up, which allows the doctor to use the best sperm for the insemination. It takes one to two hours to prepare a sperm sample in this manner. If your husband's sperm have poor motility, it might take a bit longer to give slower-swimming sperm more time to reach the top.

Be aware that the swim up procedure is not appropriate in some situations. Your doctor will know what techniques take best advantage of your husband's sample. Many women worry that the sperm will die unless the insemination takes place immediately after the sample has been prepared. Be assured that this is not the case. Once the sample is ready, it is placed in an incubating device until the time of the insemination.

When the IUI is about to begin, you will lie on an examining table. The doctor will insert a speculum into your vagina and introduce the washed sperm directly into your uterus with his or her choice of several possible types of catheters. Catheters vary in their rigidity, and doctors differ in how high in the uterus and how close to the tube they introduce the sample. You may feel some cramping during the insemination, but it should pass in a few minutes. We encourage you to relax and/or use mental imagery (see Circle of Friends in Chapter 6) to get you into a relaxed and peaceful state of mind. After the insemination, you will probably be told to remain lying down for about ten minutes. There is no need for a cervical cap with IUI. IUI fees run about $125 each for sperm preparation and insemination.

The reported success rate of IUI varies depending upon the nature of the problem. Dr. Nancy Allen and her colleagues, researchers at the Vanderbilt University Medical Center, reviewed published studies about the use of artificial insemination for various problems.[7] Success was reported as the percentage of couples who became pregnant after several attempts. When the major problem was male factor, the average success rate was 25 percent. When the problem stemmed from cervical factors, the average success rate was 60 percent, since IUI enables the sperm to bypass the cervix completely. And when the problem was immunological, success, on average, was 22 percent.

A more recent study done at Yale reported similar results: The overall rate of IUI success was 24 percent.[8] Our own review of published data that appeared during 1990, found overall IUI success rates averaging close to 28 percent.[9]

When you think about your own attempts to become pregnant, you probably do not think about your success rate after *many* cycles; rather, you focus on your chance of success for *that* cycle. For studies reporting success *per* cycle, the percentage is about 9 percent.

But we believe that the per-cycle success rate can be made considerably higher than 9 percent. What's needed to improve the success is careful timing. And while doctors all agree that timing is crucial, they disagree upon how long after hCG the insemination should take place. It is our *personal* belief that inseminations are most likely to succeed when they are performed thirty-six to forty-two hours after hCG. This belief is bolstered by the results of a study done at Duke University. In the Duke protocol IUIs were performed thirty-eight to forty hours after hCG. Doctors at Duke report a take-home baby rate of 14 percent *per cycle*.[10]

SURGERY

In addition to drugs and insemination, surgery is also used to remedy certain infertility problems. Sometimes it is used by itself and sometimes it is combined with drugs to optimize success.

Endometriosis Surgery

Surgery is indicated only when the endometriosis is moderate or severe.[11] The operation's objective is to remove the migrated uterine lining, which can cause tremendous pain and impair fertility. Once done with scalpels, endometriosis surgery now employs lasers to vaporize the endometriosis and adhesions. Doctors charge up to $5,000 to perform laser surgery, and that does not include anesthesiologist and hospital charges.

Surgery for Other Female Disorders

There are countless conditions for which surgery is indicated. New surgical techniques have created possibilities to repair problems that twenty years ago could not be remedied. Here are just a few of the many possibilities that can be surgically corrected: Uterine polyps and fibroids, which can prevent embryo implantation, can be removed surgically. A uterine septum can be similarly removed or reconstructed. Tubal blockages can be repaired through microsurgery.

Surgery to Correct Male Infertility

A similar situation exists in terms of surgery for male infertility. One type of male fertility surgery is a *varicocelectomy,* which is used to correct a varicocele. A varicocele is a varicose vein in the scrotum, which causes the temperature in the testis to be abnormally high. Optimally, sperm need a relatively cool environment, several points below core body temperature.

The varicocelectomy involves tying off the impaired vein and redirecting the blood flow. Doctors are divided in their opinion about whether this procedure is advisable. Just as many doctors strongly advocate performing a varicocelectomy, others have cautioned against having this operation performed. Many couples feel that despite this controversy they are willing to undergo the pain, cost, and discomfort involved just to have a chance at success. Doctors charge about $2,300 for a varicocelectomy on one side, $4,550 for both sides.

Another type of surgery involves clearing a blocked duct. Through microsurgery, surgeons may be able to clear blockages in the tiny ducts of the vas or epididymis. Because the success rate is relatively low, men with duct blockages often use other procedures to retrieve the sperm.

Another type of male fertility surgery is the vasectomy reversal. Just as in the previously described procedures, this operation does not guarantee that fertility will be restored. Moreover, if the reversal is performed more than five years after the vasectomy was done, there is a good chance the man has developed antibodies against his own sperm, which can destroy his ability to impregnate his partner.

MEASURES OF INFERTILITY

Infertility treatment requires that you interpret a myriad of numbers. Mostly, these numbers represent various levels of hormones in your blood. Doctors monitor the progression of your treatment cycle so they know how well you are responding to the drugs. It's important for you to know what they are talking about and to record the information in your Cycle Log. By doing so, you Become a Partner in Your Treatment. Here is a rundown of what some of these numbers mean.

ESTRADIOL LEVEL

Estradiol is a measure of the estrogen produced by the developing follicle or follicles. This level rises daily throughout the cycle. In natural cycles when no fertility drugs are used, the estradiol level reflects the size of the follicle. But when drugs are used and multiple follicles develop, the estradiol level by itself is not a good predictor of the size of the follicles. Generally speaking, though, doctors want to see a level of 1,000 to 2,000 picograms per milliliter (pg/ml) with *multiple* follicles. Such levels indicate that at least some follicles have matured and that it is time for an hCG injection to cause the eggs to ovulate.

DAY 3 FSH LEVEL

The Day 3 FSH level is an indicator of ovarian reserve—that is, the number and quality of eggs available to be fertilized. Studies have shown that a level greater than 25 milli-international units per milliliter (mIU/ml) predicts a very low likelihood of getting pregnant.[12] Ideally, patients respond best to infertility treatment when FSH levels are below 20 mIU/ml on Day 3.

PROGESTERONE LEVEL

The progesterone level is another important indicator of ovulation and pregnancy. In a basal body temperature chart, the average temperature during the luteal phase of the cycle is between 0.3 and 1.0 degrees

Fahrenheit higher than in the follicular phase of the cycle. This higher temperature is the result of the increased secretion of progesterone following ovulation. It takes a level of about 0.4 nanograms per milliliter (ng/ml) of blood to produce this temperature rise. In a non-drug-stimulated cycle, the average progesterone level on the day of the LH peak is about 2 ng/ml.

If a woman does not get pregnant, the progesterone rises to its highest point, about 15, during the middle of the luteal phase and then drops down to around 0 when menstruation begins. On the other hand, if a pregnancy occurs, the corpus luteum continues to secrete progesterone for about ten weeks. The level during those weeks averages around 25. After that, the placenta creates increasing progesterone levels, which can get as high as 125 ng/ml.

BETA hCG

A beta hCG test is used to determine whether a woman is pregnant. The test is extremely sensitive and can detect pregnancy as early as eight to ten days after ovulation. Usually, however, the test is done at least two weeks after ovulation or artificial insemination. HCG levels rise rapidly during the beginning of a pregnancy. Typically, during the early part of the pregnancy, the level doubles every two days, although the doubling time can range between one and a half and three and a half days.[13] Two standards are used to measure hCG: the second international standard and the international reference preparation.

PROLACTIN LEVEL

A doctor is unlikely to be interested in your prolactin level unless you have a milky discharge from your breasts, your periods are irregular, or you have a luteal insufficiency. Normally, prolactin, a hormone, is produced by the pituitary gland in large quantities only to stimulate the production of breast milk if you are pregnant or breast-feeding. High levels of prolactin also inhibit ovulation. So if you are not pregnant and your prolactin level is elevated, it could be causing your fertility problem.

FOLLICLE SIZE

With the advent of vaginal ultrasound devices, it is possible to visualize not only the uterus and ovaries, but also the egg follicles that develop in the ovaries. The follicles appear as round, dark circles on the video screen.

Ideally, follicles should grow about 1 to 2 millimeters a day. The optimal size for mature follicles is between 18 and 23 millimeters in non-drug-stimulated cycles. When a patient is taking fertility drugs, she usually produces multiple follicles, which may differ in their rate of growth. But even a follicle under 18 millimeters can release a mature egg. According to Dr. Colin McArdle, a radiologist at Harvard Medical School, "Mature ova [eggs] may be obtained from follicles between 12 and 34 millimeters."[14]

Doctors use the size of the largest follicle as their guide for follicle maturity. When the largest follicle reaches about 16 millimeters, it is usually time for an hCG injection to prompt the follicles to release the eggs. Even after the hCG injection, follicles can continue to grow another 2 to 4 millimeters before releasing the egg. So a patient whose ultrasound revealed a largest follicle of 16 millimeters and then had an hCG injection may still release an egg from an 18 to 20 millimeter follicle.

THE CLOCKS AND CALENDARS OF INFERTILITY

Properly timing fertility treatments can make a difference between getting pregnant and not getting pregnant. Infertility specialists sometimes disagree on the optimal timing of certain drugs and procedures. By being a Partner in Your Treatment, you may be able to tailor a procedure so that it is best suited for you. Here are some of the most common questions our clients ask us about timing.

HOW LONG AFTER hCG ADMINISTRATION IS AN EGG OVULATED?

Arthur Wisot, M.D., a professor at UCLA School of Medicine, and David Meldrum, M.D., past president of the Society for Assisted Reproductive Technology,[15] believe that ovulation should occur about thirty-six to forty-four hours after hCG. According to Dr. Sherman Silber, a St. Louis–based infertility specialist, the hCG triggers ovulation between thirty-six and forty-eight hours.[16]

HOW LONG DOES IT TAKE AN OVULATED EGG TO GET TO THE FALLOPIAN TUBE?

According to Dr. Silber, this trip occurs very rapidly. He says, "The process of grasping the egg and moving it into the interior of the tube requires only about fifteen to twenty seconds. Once the egg is safely within the tube, it is transported within five minutes toward, but not into, the narrowest region of the tube.[17] According to Dr. Robert Franklin, a professor of obstetrics and gynecology at Baylor College of Medicine, it then takes one to two hours for the egg to travel the length of the tube to where fertilization can occur.[18]

HOW LONG AFTER OVULATION IS AN EGG ABLE TO BE FERTILIZED?

There is some disagreement here. According to Gary S. Berger, M.D., an adjunct professor of maternal and child health at the University of North Carolina, and Marc Goldstein, M.D., director of the Male Reproduction Unit of Cornell Medical School, "There is a relatively short period in each cycle during which the egg may be fertilized—probably only about eight to twelve hours."[19] According to Dr. Stephen Corson, director of the Philadelphia Fertility Institute at Pennsylvania Hospital, the "egg maintains its fertilization potential for twelve to twenty hours *after* ovulation."[20] And according to Dr. Silber, "After the egg is released from the ovary, it is only capable of fertilization for about twelve, or possibly at most, twenty-four hours."[21]

HOW LONG CAN WASHED SPERM LIVE IN THE UTERUS?

Again, there is no definitive answer to this question. Dr. Edward Diamond, former director of the Diamond Institute for Fertility, claims that the top of the uterus is a "hostile environment" for sperm, which survive no more than six hours at this site.[22] Dr. John Kerin, a professor of obstetrics and gynecology at the UCLA School of Medicine, also believes that it is important "to inseminate within hours of ovulation as the endometrial cavity appears to be hostile to sperm longevity."[23]

HOW LONG AFTER MY hCG INJECTION WILL I BE INSEMINATED DURING AN INTRAUTERINE INSEMINATION?

Earlier in this chapter, we noted that there is a wide discrepancy in the success rates reported by different doctors who perform IUIs. Dr. Nancy Allen and her colleagues, in a paper reviewing the success of intrauterine insemination, state that "perhaps the most important variable is the timing of the insemination."[24] The egg is ovulated anywhere from thirty-six to forty-eight hours after the hCG shot. It is important, therefore, that the insemination be well timed. An insemination done at about thirty-four to forty-two hours after hCG is probably the ideal time.

HOW MANY DAYS DO I TAKE PERGONAL?

The amount of time and the dosage depends upon your response. On the average, women take Pergonal injections for seven to twelve consecutive days.

HOW SOON AFTER INSEMINATION SHOULD I HAVE A PREGNANCY TEST?

Generally speaking, you can have a meaningful pregnancy test two weeks after insemination. However, you should wait a few days longer if you've taken an additional shot or shots of hCG several days after insemination to support a possible pregnancy. The reason for waiting is to avoid the possibility of a false positive pregnancy result due to residual hCG from the injection.

DO I HAVE TO HAVE MY PERGONAL SHOTS AT THE SAME TIME EACH DAY?

No. There is some leeway, but you should try to take your shots within the same two-hour period each evening. For example, if you normally take your shot at 8:00 P.M., you could take it as early as 6:00 P.M., or as late as 10:00 P.M. Be prudent, but not overly rigid, about the timing. If you have a special occasion that will prevent you from taking your shot until 11:00 or 12 P.M., don't panic. It's okay. Just try to avoid this situation too often.

GUIDE TO GIVING INJECTIONS

Starting a program of treatment can be exciting as well as a bit scary. Most partners have never given injections before. Wives are often reluctant to be injected by their husband. That's understandable.

Despite these fears, we've found that most couples get through the injection phase just fine. After a few injections, in fact, many of our clients report the procedure becomes almost second nature. One of the things that's helped is getting clear instructions. Most infertility clinics offer injection orientation classes led by a nurse. Couples about to begin Pergonal or other injection therapy watch a demonstration and receive a slew of information, usually quite rapidly. Participants may be reluctant to ask questions in front of a group. They fail to realize that a large portion of the audience probably has the same questions.

Following are step-by-step instructions designed to supplement any orientation class or one-on-one lesson you might participate in. If, after reading our instructions, you still have questions, call your doctor's office.

Throughout your infertility treatments, you will find yourself doing many things you never imagined doing. Giving or getting injections is but one.

Remember: You Can Do It!

Materials needed:

Alcohol:	Box of alcohol pads
Syringes:	a supply of syringes; 22-gauge; 1½-inch for administering Pergonal, hCG, and progesterone injections
	a supply of syringes; 14- to 16-gauge for drawing progesterone more easily than with the 22-gauge syringe
Pergonal	a supply of ampules
Water	a supply of water solution ampules
hCG	one vial of water and one vial of hCG
	NOTE: Insist that you are given a form of hCG that comes in *two separate bottles.* Do *not* attempt to work with the form of hCG that comes in an attached double-bottle unit.
Progesterone	a supply of vials
	NOTE: Progesterone comes in two different oil bases: peanut oil or sesame oil. The typical base is peanut oil. If you experience discomfort when using the regular progesterone, ask your physician whether you should try the sesame oil variety.

Pergonal injection procedure:

1. Place alcohol pad over protrusion on ampule. This will protect you if glass splinters. Holding on to the pad, break the protrusion on the water ampule. Then repeat this procedure to break the protrusions on the remaining Pergonal ampules.
2. Peel off plastic wrapper from 22-gauge syringe.
3. Holding plastic cap that's over the needle, twist to make sure needle is secured in cylinder. Remove cap.
4. Pull out plunger of syringe and push back in to make sure that it is drawing.
5. Carefully insert needle into water ampule. *If the needle touches the outside glass of the ampule or any other object, it may become contaminated. Discard the needle and use another one!*
6. Pull up plunger of syringe to draw *entire contents* out of water ampule.
7. Insert the needle into the first Pergonal ampule. Inject *one third** (or one half if you're using two Pergonal ampules, or the whole thing if you're using one). Repeat this procedure with the remaining ampules. This mixes the Pergonal with the water, creating a clear, sometimes foamy solution.
8. Insert the needle into the first Pergonal ampule. Hold the ampule horizontally. Tilt the syringe so that it is at a 30 degree angle to the ampule. *Place your thumb on the winglike structure on the syringe and press the syringe against the ampule.* With your index and middle fingers, pull up on the plunger to extract the contents of the ampule. Repeat this procedure with the remaining ampules.
9. Tap the cylinder of the syringe of get rid of any air bubbles.
10. Holding the syringe with the needle up, gently push on the plunger until a tiny bead of liquid appears on the tip of the needle.
11. Locate a spot on the buttocks for the injection. To find the location, spread your thumb and index finger against the hip bone. Locate a spot about three inches below this location. Use this spot for injections. You will be rotating spots each day. Find the comparable spot on the other cheek for the next day's injection. On the third day, you will return to the first cheek, but locate a spot slightly away from the site of the first day's injection, and so on.
12. Insert the needle all the way in, *perpendicular* to the plane of the buttock *(not at an angle)*.
13. Hold the syringe with one hand and draw the plunger out slightly to see if any blood appears on the needle. If blood appears, it means you've hit a blood vessel and need to try again. If no blood appears, proceed.
14. Inject by pushing plunger in fairly quickly. Pull out needle fast.
15. Place an alcohol pad on the site for a few minutes.

---

*PLEASE NOTE: Each patient will be told how many ampules of Pergonal to use each day. You mix equal amounts of water with each Pergonal ampule. In our example, you mix one third of the water with each of the three ampules. But if you were taking only two ampules, you'd mix half of the water with each!

hCG injection procedure:

1. Make sure you are working with two separate vials. Wipe top of liquid vial with alcohol pad. Discard pad. Wipe top of powder vial with *a different pad* and discard pad.
2. Hold water vial upside down, and insert needle into water vial. Pull back plunger to extract *2 cc's* of water.
3. Insert needle into the hCG powder vial. Push in the plunger to inject water to mix with the powder.
4. Hold the powder vial mixture upside down. *Make sure that the needle is below the level of the liquid at all times to avoid getting air bubbles into the syringe's cylinder.* Slowly pull back the plunger a little at a time to extract the entire contents of the hCG mixture.
5. Follow the same procedure as above, beginning with Step 10.

CHAPTER SIX

USING THE GETTING PREGNANT WORKOUT TO HELP YOU THROUGH TREATMENT

Now THAT we've introduced you to the many treatment options to combat infertility, it's time to confront the emotional issues that are bound to crop up during treatment, if they haven't already. To help you through this phase, we have created a fictionalized couple—Amanda and Al Gambino—who are a composite sketch of dozens of couples we have met and counseled over the years. The Gambinos' concerns are typical of infertile couples: finding a competent infertility specialist, educating and motivating themselves to begin injecting Pergonal, reducing sexual performance anxiety, remaining optimistic in the face of failure, and putting themselves first without feeling selfish.

DECISION-MAKING: SELECTING A DOCTOR

For six months, Amanda and Al have been following the advice of Amanda's gynecologist but have not yet conceived. They have kept

129

careful temperature charts, used Clomid, monitored Amanda's LH surge, and made love every other day, just as the doctor instructed. Since their doctor can find no reason for their fertility problem, the Gambinos are faced with a tough decision: Should they change doctors, and to whom should they turn?

Like so many women, Amanda was initially reluctant to start from scratch with a new physician. She hated the idea of having to search one out, get used to him, repeat her medical history, and start treatment in unfamiliar surroundings.

But what began as a pleasurable part of their marriage has turned into a nightmare of scheduled, sometimes unemotional intercourse for three weeks followed by devastation each time Amanda's period started. Their whole world seemed on the brink of collapse. Amanda and Al knew that her gynecologist, who does not specialize in infertility, had done all that he could do even though he would not admit it. Once coming to terms with that realization, the Gambinos' next step seemed crystal-clear: find a doctor who could provide specialized fertility treatments.

They wanted a specialist who was not only knowledgeable about infertility and experienced treating it, but one who was also compassionate and exhibited confidence in his ability to diagnose and treat their particular problem.

Training of the Infertility Doctor

Unfortunately, any doctor can hang out a shingle that says "infertility specialist," and some with little or no infertility training do advertise themselves this way. The American Fertility Society, the professional association devoted to the promotion of knowledge in fertility and allied fields, says that a variety of medical specialists—OB-GYNs and reproductive endocrinologists, among others—practice as infertility specialists. But medical schools don't train doctors to be infertility specialists. These specialists are usually trained first as gynecologists or endocrinologists if they wish to specialize in female infertility. Doctors interested in male infertility first become urologists, andrologists, or endocrinologists. Once completing their primary training, doctors obtain additional training, usually in the form of a fellowship or a second residency, in the field of reproductive endocrinology, for example.

Also, many doctors who have been practicing their primary specialty—

say gynecology—for several years might take intensive infertility seminars, such as those sponsored by the American Fertility Society. Not all infertility specialists do this, however. Even though Amanda's gynecologist advertises himself in the Yellow Pages, in newspaper ads, and on his shingle as an infertility specialist, he keeps patients under his care long after their needs outdistance his experience and training.

The message here is: Buyer beware. Don't let a doctor learn infertility treatment by practicing on you. He or she may be experienced with just a few treatments, like prescribing Clomid, and that's it. As Amanda is about to do, you should consider leaving your current doctor and looking for a specialist. At the very least, this new doctor should be a member in good standing of the American Fertility Society. To help, we refer you to the Doctor Interview Guide that appears later in this chapter.

What You're Looking For

Like most women, Amanda has an image of the perfect infertility specialist. He should have excellent training, be available twenty-four hours a day, 365 days a year; stay current on all new treatments, possess the sensitivity of Marcus Welby, have an office down the street, and accept whatever insurance pays him or charge next to nothing. The chance of finding a doctor with all of these traits is nil.

After deciding on some basic requirements, Amanda begins compiling a list of available specialists from the Yellow Pages, her local RESOLVE Inc. chapter, the American Fertility Society's latest membership directory,[1] and recommendations from friends and co-workers who have used fertility specialists. It's important to consult a variety of sources, since the physician who helped your friend or sister-in-law get pregnant may or may not have the expertise to deal with your particular problem. From that list, Amanda makes a smaller list of six doctors who are within a sixty-minute driving distance from her home.

A pen and pad at hand, she calls each doctor's office and asks about the physician's philosophy, success rate, and fee structure. In some cases, she speaks with the doctor directly. Many people are intimidated by the thought of asking doctors about their training, fees, or rate of success. Don't be. If you were hiring any professional, whether an electrician, a hairdresser, or an interior decorator, you'd ask questions about fees and experience. Remember, a doctor is providing you with

DOCTOR INTERVIEW GUIDE

Medical Training/Infertility Specialty:

- In what area was your primary training?

- Are you an infertility specialist?

- What is your training in infertility?

  Did you do a residency or a fellowship in reproductive endocrinology?
  Where did you acquire your specialty?

Experience:

- Have you ever done any of the following procedures:
  diagnostic laparoscopies
  hysterosalpingograms
  intrauterine inseminations
  intracervical inseminations

Logistics of treatment:

- What percent of your practice is devoted to infertility?

- Will I see pregnant women in the waiting room?

- Can I do most of my testing/treatment in the office or do I have to go elsewhere?

  Do you do ultrasounds in your office?
  What lab work is done in your office and what information do you have sent out?
    estradiol
    progesterone

FSH
beta hCG (pregnancy tests)
semen analysis

- Where do your patients get their medication?

- Are there multiple doctors in the practice?
    Can I select a primary care doctor?
    Do you arrange for doctor coverage when you are on vacation?

Hours:

- What are your office hours?
    Do you have early-morning, late-afternoon, Saturday, Sunday hours?

- What are your callback hours?

- What kind of flexibility is there for scheduling specialized treatment?
    I work from _____ to _____ and need to have my work done early/late/lunchtime. Can you accommodate me?

- Do you see your patients promptly or should I expect to have a long wait?

Financial

- What are your fees for the following procedures:
    E2
    ultrasound
    IUI

- When does payment need to be made?

- Do you arrange to bill the insurance company directly?

Factors to Take into Consideration

Amanda and Al's notes:	Notes about each doctor
Factors Al and I consider important	
1. Doctor's level of expertise	All three are competent doctors
2. Success statistics (how many people with problems like ours got pregnant)	Como has a cult reputation. Heard that Gold inflates his success statistics.
3. Cost of this doctor's services	All are very expensive
4. Doctor's bedside manner	Como is a charmer. Murphy is sweet. Gold is cordial, but aloof.
5. Individualized treatment (e.g., will the doctor tailor treatment to my case or will he use a protocol similar to one used for all other patients?)	Gold puts everyone through the same mill. Murphy will do anything you want. Como has some flexibility but not as much as Murphy.
Factors Suggested by Friends and Acquaintances:	
1. Is the practice limited to infertility?	Murphy has pregnant people in the waiting room. Como prohibits pregnant women or babies from coming to his office. Gold's practice is limited to infertility, but he allows kids in the office.
2. Does this doctor provide seven-day-a-week coverage?	Murphy and Gold do. Como doesn't but arranges for someone else to do inseminations when he's not available.

3. Is this doctor willing to work with us in terms of insurance coverage?	All seem willing to work with patients.
4. Does this doctor have flexibility in the times when he schedules procedures?	All seem to be flexible.
5. Office appearance	Murphy keeps parenting magazines and duckies in the waiting room. Has TV blaring all the time. Como's office looks like a classy French boudoir. Gold's office has that industrial look.

Factors suggested by articles and books I read:

1. What sorts of facilities does the office have for the husband to produce a semen sample?	Como has limited facilities, prefers you to do it at home and bring it in. Gold has a special room with a VCR and dirty magazines. Murphy has a bathroom with a lock.
2. How quickly can I get an appointment?	Como has a six-month waiting list. Murphy has a two-week wait. Gold seems able to take patients on short notice.
3. How quickly does this doctor give test results to patients?	Gold gets results to you immediately. Other two take longer.
4. How easy is it for the patient to speak with this doctor?	Gold filters all calls through his staff. Murphy and Como return calls fairly quickly.
5. How much time does it take to travel to and from this doctor's office?	Murphy is ten minutes away. Gold is forty-five minutes away but has a parking lot. Como is one hour away, and you must park in a parking garage.

services that you, or your insurance company, are paying for. It is your right to ask questions.

In one case, a doctor responded to Amanda's inquiries with: "How dare you question my experience and ask me these questions." Alarm bells went off in Amanda's head, and justifiably so. That doctor might not have had the extensive training his advertisement suggests, she surmised. Even if he were well trained, the fact that he was too arrogant to answer her questions indicates he is unlikely to ever regard her as a Partner in Her Treatment.

Amanda knew that by carefully shopping for the right doctor, she was sparing herself the grief of hopping aimlessly from doctor to doctor, hoping the next one will be better than the last.

Dr. Leon Speroff, president of the American Fertility Society, suggests that the physician treating infertility should keep four goals in mind: seeking out and correcting the causes of infertility, providing accurate information and dispelling misinformation, providing emotional support, and counseling a couple concerning the proper time to discontinue treatment.[2] These goals represent the ideal. Expecting your doctor to meet at least the first two goals is certainly realistic.

Before making a final decision, Amanda and Al vowed to stick with this newly selected doctor long enough to give his prescribed treatments time to work. Clients ask us how long is long enough. It's hard to answer that question because every case is different. Our rule of thumb is to give a doctor at least six months before considering getting another opinion, especially if the doctor is attentive and responsive to your needs and is suggesting treatments that you've read about in this book.

Amanda put this decision-making activity into action. First, she and Al listed every factor important to them. To prod her thinking, Amanda talked with her friends and acquaintances who used fertility specialists and read all she could on the topic. Once her list was complete, Amanda's next step was to find a match between her ideal doctor and the ones who practiced in her area. Based on her telephone interviews, she pared her list down to three: Dr. Gold, Dr. Como, and Dr. Murphy. Amanda then scheduled consultations with all three. You may not have three fertility specialists in your area, or you may feel you need to choose between just two. Do what your circumstances, instincts, and pocketbook dictate. And check with your health insurer, since many policies will pay for at least two consultations.

(Please turn to pages 134–135 to read Amanda and Al's notes.)

Next, Amanda assigned a grade from 1 to 10, with 10 being the best, to each doctor for each factor.

FACTOR	Grade for COMO	Grade for GOLD	Grade for MURPHY
1. Doctor's level of expertise	9	8	7
2. Success statistics (how many people with problems like ours got pregnant)	10	7	7
3. Cost of this doctor's services	2	4	5
4. Doctor's bedside manner	8	5	8
5. Individualized treatment (e.g., will the doctor tailor treatment to my case or will he use a protocol similar to one used for all other patients?)	7	3	9
6. Is the practice limited to infertility?	10	9	5
7. Does this doctor provide seven-day-a-week coverage?	4	8	7
8. Is this doctor willing to work with us in terms of insurance coverage?	10	8	10
9. Does this doctor have flexibility in the times when he schedules procedures?	8	8	8
10. Office appearance	10	7	4
11. What sorts of facilities does the office have for the husband to produce a semen sample?	2	10	7
12. How quickly can I get an appointment?	1	9	8
13. How quickly does this doctor give test results to patients?	3	9	6
14. How easy is it for the patient to speak with this doctor?	7	2	8
15. How much time does it take to travel to and from this doctor's office?	2	5	9

Then Amanda assigned a weight, from 1 (not at all important to her) to 10 (crucial) to each factor. She multiplied the weight by the grade to get a *factor score* for each doctor. When she finished, she had scores on each of the fifteen factors for Como, Gold, and Murphy. Finally, she added up each factor score and got a total score for each doctor. Here is how she did it:

Based on the total scores, Amanda could plainly see that her best

Factor	Weight for this factor	Grade for Como	Factor score for Como	Grade for Gold	Factor score for Gold	Grade for Murphy	Factor score for Murphy
1. Doctor's level of expertise	10	× 9	= 90	× 8	= 80	× 7	= 70
2. Success statistics (how many people with problems like ours got pregnant)	10	× 10	= 100	× 7	= 70	× 7	= 70
3. Cost of this doctor's services	2	× 2	= 4	× 4	= 8	× 5	= 10
4. Doctor's bedside manner	4	× 8	= 32	× 5	= 20	× 8	= 32
5. Individualized treatment	9	× 7	= 63	× 3	= 27	× 9	= 81
6. Is the practice limited to infertility?	9	× 10	= 90	× 9	= 81	× 5	= 45
7. Does this doctor provide seven-day-a-week coverage?	9	× 4	= 36	× 8	= 72	× 7	= 63
8. Is this doctor willing to work with us in terms of insurance coverage?	9	× 10	= 90	× 8	= 72	× 10	= 90
9. Schedule flexibility	4	× 8	= 32	× 8	= 32	× 8	= 32
10. Office appearance	5	× 10	= 50	× 7	= 35	× 4	= 20
11. Facilities for husband to produce semen sample	2	× 2	= 4	× 10	= 20	× 7	= 14
12. How quickly I can get an appointment	9	× 1	= 9	× 9	= 81	× 8	= 72
13. How quickly this doctor gives test results to patients?	3	× 3	= 9	× 9	= 27	× 6	= 18
14. How easy it is for the patient to speak with the doctor	5	× 7	= 35	× 2	= 10	× 8	= 40
15. Travel time to office	7	× 2	= 14	× 5	= 35	× 9	= 63
Total Score			**658**		**670**		**720**

choice was Dr. Murphy. She immediately called and was able to make an appointment the following week.

On pages 140–141 there's a blank chart to help you in your doctor selection. Photocopy it. Follow the steps. Once you've made your choice, you can begin to be a Partner in Your Treatment and Make a Plan. Remember, the steps are:

- List factors;
- Gather information;
- Assign grades;
- Assign weights;
- Multiply weights by grades to get factor scores;
- Add up factor scores to get each total score; and
- Pick the choice with the highest total score.

Factor	Weight for this Factor	Grade for Dr. 1
Total Score		

Factor score for Dr. 1	Grade for Dr. 2	Factor score for Dr. 2	Grade for Dr. 3	Factor score for Dr. 3
tal Score				

LISTENING AND LEVELING: TALKING ABOUT PERGONAL

Pergonal is the drug mainstay of almost every couple engaged in infertility treatment. Every night, countless husbands are opening glass ampules, mixing powder and liquid, filling syringes, and injecting FSH/LH into their wives' buttocks. These men may not be gleeful about what they are doing, but they are certainly dutiful because they know that the drug will stimulate their wives' ovaries to produce multiple egg follicles, thus upping their odds of getting her pregnant.

Amanda found out almost immediately what a big step it is from simply swallowing Clomid pills to taking Pergonal injections. She and Al were open with each other about their hopes and trepidations. Al was afraid of killing Amanda by injecting an air bubble into her accidentally. Amanda wasn't sure if she trusted her klutzy husband, who can barely turn on the dishwasher, to act as her combination chemist and nurse. But the Gambinos couldn't afford the luxury of hiring a trained medical professional to give the injections, so they opted to Work as a Team and face their fears head on. To accomplish this, they mentally rehearsed the injection skills, and added some Getting Pregnant Listening and Leveling.

"I Trust You but I'm Scared." "So Am I."

Using the following exercise, Amanda and Al were able to get in touch with their emotions and better understand what each was going through.[3] Amanda read the italicized text to Al, who, using his mental imagery skills, would close his eyes and listen. After she finished the passage, Al would look at her and tell her what he thought about the passage. Amanda then would use the active listening skills she learned in the Getting Pregnant Workout until she truly understood how he felt.

"Close your eyes and picture the following scene. You are about to give me an injection of Pergonal. You are preparing the medication. Using an alcohol pad, you break open three vials of Pergonal and one of water. You stand the vials up carefully. You peel off the plastic wrapper from the syringe. You make sure the needle is secured in the cylinder. You pull out the plunger and push it back in to make sure that it is

drawing. You carefully insert the needle into the water ampule. You pull up the plunger of the syringe to draw up the entire contents of the vial. You insert the needle into the first Pergonal ampule and inject one third of the water into this ampule. You insert the needle into the second ampule and inject another third of the water. Now you insert the needle into the last ampule and inject the remaining water.

"You insert the needle into the first Pergonal mixture and draw it up. Now you do the same with the second ampule. You draw up the remaining solution. You tap the syringe to make sure there are no bubbles. You slowly push in on the plunger until a small bead of liquid appears on the tip of the needle.

"Now you approach me. You locate a spot on my buttock. You insert the entire needle perpendicular to the plane of my buttock. You hold the syringe with one hand and draw the plunger out to see if any blood appears on the needle. There is none. You then push the plunger in quickly to inject the Pergonal. Now you pull out the needle quickly. You cover the site of the injection with an alcohol pad."

Amanda then asks Al to make a *true statement* about what he's feeling concerning Pergonal. When he has made that statement, Amanda asks him yes-or-no questions each beginning with "Do you mean . . . ?" to further clarify what he's feeling. She continues to probe in this manner until Al responds yes a total of three times. You may have to ask as few as three questions or as many as twelve. Remember, your job is to listen to your partner, to ask good questions, to accept his responses, and to validate all his yeses.

Here is what Al and Amanda said. Remember, husbands' concerns and responses are as individual as they are, so if you try this exercise, don't feel you must mirror Amanda and Al exactly.

AL: *"This whole thing is upsetting me."*
AMANDA: *"Do you mean that you want me to give up on the Pergonal and IUI?"*
AL: *"No."*
AMANDA: *"Do you mean that you wish we could have a baby naturally?"*
AL: *"No."*
AMANDA: *"Do you mean that you're afraid that you don't have the coordination to do this?"*
AL: *"Yes."*

AMANDA: *"Do you mean that you're afraid that you'll cause me pain?"*

AL: *"Yes."*

AMANDA: *"Do you mean that you want to hire a nurse to give these injections?"*

AL: *"No."*

AMANDA: *"Do you mean that you're afraid that you'll inject me with air bubbles?"*

AL: *"Yes."*

By the end of their dialogue, Amanda has a better understanding of what's bothering Al. Now they switch places, remembering that once Amanda has made her statement, she can answer only yes or no to Al's questions.

AMANDA: *"I'm afraid of doing the Pergonal shots."*

AL: *"Do you mean you want someone else to inject you?"*

AMANDA: *"No."*

AL: *"Do you mean you think I'm totally uncoordinated?"*

AMANDA: *"No."*

AL: *"Do you mean you think that I might break the needle in your buttock?"*

AMANDA: *"Yes."*

AL: *"Do you mean you think I'll inject you in the wrong place?"*

AMANDA: *"Yes."*

AL: *"Do you mean that you think this will ruin our marriage?"*

AMANDA: *"No."*

AL: *"Do you mean you are worried that I will resent you if I can't go out with the boys if you're scheduled to have an injection?"*

AMANDA   *"Yes."*

DAYDREAMS WITH A PURPOSE: COPING WITH THE DEMANDS OF TREATMENT

Amanda and Al discovered that mental imagery could provide them with some very concrete assistance in meeting the demands of their treatment. Besides helping them mentally rehearse injections, relax their minds, and reduce stress, mental imagery also helped Al produce a semen sample on demand.

In most IUI cycles, the woman is the focus 95 percent of the time. The husband's big moment arrives when he produces a sample to be used for insemination. Although it takes only a few minutes, his contribution is pivotal. It is no wonder, then, that Al felt so pressured that he had difficulty producing a sample. The thought of failing to perform terrified him. He feared he wouldn't get aroused, that he'd lose his erection, or worse yet, that he'll miss the cup. He suffered from performance anxiety, a feeling akin to stage fright.

One way to help alleviate performance anxiety is to produce a sample well before the insemination—one that can be frozen. Even though frozen sperm has a statistically lower success rate than does fresh sperm, it can be used if all else fails. Another consideration that can reduce performance anxiety concerns where to collect the sample: at home or in the doctor's office. If you live more than an hour from the office, your husband should probably produce the sample at the office. If you live close by, let your husband make the decision. Some doctors provide rooms with erotic videotapes; other doctors just provide bathrooms or an examination room with a locking door. The very act of helping your husband Make a Plan to produce a sample will lower his anxiety.

Amanda found that Al felt less pressured when she encouraged him to create fantasies to help him become aroused on insemination day. In fact, Al and Amanda created fantasies and tried them out a week or so beforehand. Al would remember the most successful fantasy and re-create it to help him produce a sample.

Another way Amanda helped Al get aroused was by recording a fantasy audiotape, which he listened to on his Walkman. The Gambinos Worked as a Team to concoct a particularly arousing fantasy. Some wives, if they feel brazen enough, make a surprise tape for their husbands. Many find this exercise fun, a welcome relief from the rigors of infertility treatment. It is important to tell your husband that his sexual fantasy life is an important part of his participation in your pregnancy quest.

Amour

To get you started, we have developed "Amour," an imagery exercise for producing a sample. We've included a model text below, one that some men find arousing. You may wish to record it as is or personalize it.

"Imagine that you and I are making passionate love. You are feeling deeply aroused and want to heighten your pleasure. You touch your body in a place and in a way that causes waves of pleasure to engulf you. I whisper words of encouragement in your ear, telling you how much I am turned on by watching you give yourself so much pleasure. You are extraordinarily excited. My words and my touch arouse you to the heights of pleasure. These feelings mount higher and higher and explode in a burst of ecstasy."

Your husband may not respond to audio stimulation, preferring a sexy magazine instead. You should support whatever works for him.

HELPING YOURSELF STAY OPTIMISTIC: HANGING IN THROUGH REPEATED CYCLES

Treatment can only work if you faithfully follow the regimen prescribed by your doctor. But you are not a machine. You have worries, doubts, and other factors that can interfere with your ability to follow the protocol. Moreover, it's hard to sustain enthusiasm and motivation, particularly when you learn that you face yet another month of treatment.

What motivates you to get out of bed at the crack of dawn so you can make it to the doctor's office by 8:00 A.M. and be at work by 9:00? What prevents you from giving up? The obvious answer to these questions is: YOU. But sometimes you need help. Optimism and motivation can become increasingly elusive as failed attempts to conceive mount up. And at some point, you may want to stop burdening your friends and relatives with your fertility problems. But you can still allow others to help you through the trials of fertility treatment by using your imagination.

Circle of Friends: A Series of Motivational Imagery Activities

From the beginning, Amanda felt that she had no one to turn to when Al could not be by her side; all her important friends and immediate family lived far away, and her beloved grandmother, who had always been her staunchest ally, had recently died.

Her fertility specialist had suggested she try six cycles of Pergonal and intrauterine inseminations before moving to any more advanced assisted reproductive techniques. Amanda knew that course of action almost guaranteed at least one failed attempt, since the best Pergonal/IUI statistics she read about show that only 14 percent of women got pregnant each month. After six months, Amanda had a 60 percent chance of becoming pregnant.[4]

To cope with the anxiety of this reality, Amanda conjured up visions of her grandmother by her side. Seeing her grandmother's smiling face in her mind's eye gave Amanda the confidence, strength, and motivation to endure almost anything.

Here is a series of three interrelated activities to help you adapt Amanda's experience to your personal situation. To derive the greatest benefit from these activities, read the descriptions of all three before engaging in any one of them. Record, or ask your partner to record, the italicized texts onto audiotape.

CIRCLE OF FRIENDS

The first part of this activity represents the beginning of your active search for people to assist you in remaining optimistic through repeated treatments. If you have recorded the text, turn on the tape recorder now.

Together we are going to develop a circle of friends who are your supporters. This group can consist of your relatives, colleagues at work, childhood friends, neighbors, friends who belong to your church or temple, or any other friends that are meaningful to you. These people can be from your past or present life. They can be people who are living or dead, as long as their memory is strong and clear. You can select a religious figure, a person from history, or a contemporary individual you admire.

Allow yourself to think about people you know who can be your supporters in getting pregnant. Do not worry now about thinking of numbers of people; one or two or even three are fine. Picture each of those persons, one at a time. You may first find that person inside your head, or even in front of you, looking at you. That person can be whispering in your ear. Remember, that person can appear to you anywhere you want him or her to be. Get a clear picture of that person in your mind's eye.

Now imagine that that person is talking to you, coaching you in preparation for the treatment you are about to undertake. Try to hear and remember what that person is saying. Sometimes even words are not important, but rather the feeling you get when that person is with you. Allow yourself to see and hear all the people you've thought of. Take as much time as you want. (You may wish to pause the tape recorder here.) When you are finished, open your eyes, read the following directions, and fill in the forms below.

For each group of lines, fill in names of the people who came to mind when you allowed yourself to find your supporters. If you did not find someone for a particular category, go on to the next category. If someone comes to mind while you are filling in the form, you may add that person, even though he or she did not surface during the time you were concentrating on developing your circle. We will admit latecomers.

Relatives:

_____

_____

_____

Colleagues at Work:

_____

_____

_____

Childhood Friends:

_____

_____

_____

Neighbors:

_____

_____

_____

Friends from Church or Synagogue:

_____

_____

_____

Other Meaningful Friends:

_____

_____

_____

Someone You Admire, Respect, or Revere from Religion, History, or Contemporary Society:

_____

_____

_____

CREATE YOUR CIRCLE

Before you begin this part of the activity, look over your list of people. In the next part of the exercise, you will be asked to recall the people on your list. Try to remember as many people as you can, but don't worry if you feel you won't be able to remember them all. Next time you do the exercise, you may remember more or different people, or even add a new one. If you have recorded the following text on a tape recorder, turn on the tape recorder now.

Get into a relaxed frame of mind. Allow yourself to recall the people who are part of your group of supporters. Don't worry if you can only remember one or two people. Start with those. If you remember more as you go through this activity, you can add those people to your circle.

Picture each of these persons seated in a circle. Now walk into the center of the circle and take a seat. Look around. Slowly focus on the face of each friend—one by one. Picture each person smiling at you and telling you how much he or she wants what you want for yourself. Really allow yourself to look at and hear each person. As each person smiles at you and speaks to you, you feel yourself becoming stronger and more optimistic. When you feel ready, stand up and leave the circle knowing that these friends and their various strengths are with you. When you have left the circle, turn the tape recorder off. But try to keep a part of this person with you in your heart for as much of your day as possible.

INVISIBLE FRIEND

For this part of the activity, you will select one or two specific people to take with you when you need support. You may find their support helpful when you need motivation to get up early in the morning to travel to a clinic. You may need their support when you are about to undergo a procedure. And you may especially need their support and encouragement when you have to bounce back after a failed procedure. If you have taped the activity, turn on the tape recorder now.

In this first activity you will use your friend to help you with an upcoming treatment. Allow yourself to be relaxed. Select one of your friends who was sitting in the circle to prepare herself or himself to accompany you to your next treatment. In your mind's ear, have a conversation with your friend about the procedure you are about to have. This friend is extraordinarily supportive and everything he or she tells you makes you feel strong. Try to focus on several of the key sentences that your friend tells you. He or she may tell you, for example, "You can do anything you set your mind to." Or, "Remember how you worked so hard to get what you wanted. You did it then and you can do it now." Or, "Remember how you made it through that last treatment. You can do anything you set your mind to." After you have drawn strength from these phrases, allow yourself to believe that your friend can come with you and talk to you during the difficult time of your next procedure. Believe that he or she can come with you and believe that your friend can give you the strength you need to get through the treatment.

Practice imagining you and your friend conversing once or twice a day for a week or so before the treatment. Each day that you picture you and your friend talking, your friend's words will have a more powerful influence on you. On the day of your procedure, your friend will exert a powerful influence over you and the success of your treatment.

In the next part of this activity, you will use your friend to help you be strong and hang in after a procedure that failed. Allow yourself to be relaxed. Select one of your friends who was sitting in the circle to support or console you after a failed treatment. In your mind's ear, have a conversation with your friend about the procedure that failed. Your friend is extraordinarily understanding and gives you an opportunity to feel sad. But he or she also tells you things that make you feel strong. Try to focus on several of the key sentences that your friend tells you. He or she may tell you, for example, "You had setbacks before and you bounced back. You did it then and you can do it again. Every time you keep trying, the odds of success get better." After you have drawn strength from these phrases, allow yourself to believe that your friend will be there to understand your pain and support you whenever you need her or him.

Practice imagining you and your friend conversing once or twice a day for a week or so while you recover. Each day that you picture you and your friend talking, your friend's words will have a more powerful influence on you. Gradually, your friend's words will heal the hurt of the failed procedure.

TAKING CHARGE OF YOUR SOCIAL LIFE

Just when Amanda thought she was feeling strong, she received an invitation to a friend's baby shower. The invitation triggered a cascade of tears, which left Amanda shaken for hours. The mere thought of walking into an infantwear department to buy a gift made her quiver. But how could she disappoint her friend by being conspicuously absent from the shower?

Just as fertility patients must be assertive with their physicians at times, so must infertile people learn to be assertive in the social arena. Even the most well-meaning friends and relatives can pressure you without realizing it. This pressure may be real or imagined on your part, particularly when it comes to holidays and pregnancy-related events. We know of one infertile woman who became physically ill during her niece's christening and had to leave the ceremony.

To help you avoid such disasters, we've developed a series of activities to help you Manage Your Social Life and, in doing so, draw you and your partner closer to each other. These activities build on your GPST, mental imagery, and assertiveness skills.

No More Life on Hold: A Series of Socially Liberating Activities

Even though you may feel obsessed with your infertility treatments, you must still live in the real world. Pregnant women and people pushing baby carriages will cross your path almost daily. News of friends and relatives becoming pregnant and giving birth will also come your way. Infertile women have actually reported the urge to run over a baby carriage or shoot a pregnant friend. Stoic men with fertility problems have cried at the sight of a community league soccer game. Otherwise low-key couples report screaming matches over whether to visit a relative who just had a baby.

If the trials of daily life don't get to you, holidays and other special occasions can. To cope, you must first recognize and acknowledge the kinds of events that will cause stress for you or your partner. Only then can you plan your schedules to be as stress-free as possible. Careful planning is the key to taking charge of your social life.

IDENTIFYING TOUGH SITUATIONS

The following activity will help you identify situations you found difficult in the past, which helps you anticipate what might be stressful in the future. We've included three charts to get you started: one for you, one for your partner, and one for you as a couple. Take some time now to recall social and family situations you found awkward, unpleasant, or downright awful as a result of your infertility. To get you started, we begin each chart with situations that the Gambinos found unpleasant. The exercise works best if you and your partner complete your own lists separately before completing the couple list together.

Social Situations: Wife	
Easy Situations	**Difficult Situations**
1. Taking my sister's kids to the movies	1. Going to a baby shower for my friend, Connie, who conceived easily

Social Situations: Husband	
Easy Situations	**Difficult Situations**
1. Attending a christening	1. Watching a Little League game

Social Situations: Couple	
Easy Situations	**Difficult Situations**
1. Going to a RESOLVE social function	1. Going to the family Thanksgiving dinner

PROS AND CONS

Next, list the pros and cons of participating in each of the situations you listed. Here is what Amanda wrote regarding her discomfort in going to Connie's baby shower.

SITUATION: Going to Connie's Baby Shower	
Why I Should . . . (go to the shower)	**Why I Shouldn't . . . (go to the shower)**
1. Because I'm polite. My mother taught me that it's the right thing to do.	1. I'll want to cry when I think that she's having a baby and I can't have one.
2. She's my good friend. She came all the way from Cleveland to be one of my bridesmaids.	2. I'll resent her for her good fortune.
3. My friends will think that I'm rude and selfish if I don't show up for Connie's shower.	3. After I come home, I'll be in such a bad mood that I'll get into a fight with my husband.

Here's a chart for you to write pros and cons for your own situations. Before filling in the chart, photocopy it to use with your husband's list and your couple's list.

SITUATION: _____	
Why I Should... _____	Why I Shouldn't... _____

Completing these charts should help you understand the kinds of demands that you put on yourself. Sometimes people feel as though they have *no choice* about what they do—that they *must* do certain things, regardless of any emotional upheaval it might trigger. But you have more freedom than you might realize.

We are not trying to teach you to be selfish or irresponsible. We are saying: Be kind to yourself, and give your friends and relatives credit for their ability to empathize with your plight. You have very sound reasons to avoid painful social situations. By "arguing" with the part of yourself that shackles you to social conventions, those reasons will become clearer. The inner dialogue activity that we present next is taken from Gestalt psychotherapy.

Gestalt psychotherapists emphasize human *polarities*. That is, each person's psyche is made up of many parts, which have different and often opposing desires. According to Gestalt psychotherapists Erving and Miriam Polster, people should allow their various parts to make contact with one other: "This reduces the chance that one part will stay mired in its own impotence, hanging on to the status quo. Instead, [each part] is energized into making a vital statement of its own needs and wishes, asserting itself as a force, which must be considered in a new union of forces."[5]

Through the following exercise, you can give voice to your conflicting feelings through a form of debate. We use the baby shower as an example, but you can adapt the exercise to any situation you wish.

EMPTY CHAIR

You are going to participate in a debate between two parts of yourself: one part says you *should* go to the baby shower, and the other part says you *should not* go.

Sit opposite an empty chair facing you. Become the part of you that says, "I should go to the shower." Imagine that you are putting the part of you that says, "I should not go," in the empty chair. Tell yourself why you should attend. After this opening statement, go sit in the other chair. Refute your "should go" argument, telling your first part why she is wrong. Do this for a few minutes, then switch back to the other chair. In this way, you are creating a dialogue, of sorts, with yourself.

Here is a sample of what we mean:

Should Go:

You really should go to the baby shower. Your mother brought you up to be polite and do the right thing. She would be appalled if she knew that you didn't go to the shower. She would say, "What kind of daughter did I raise?" (Switch seats)

Should Not Go:

You're so bogged down in always "doing the right thing." What about your needs? Must you torture yourself? Don't you deserve to be kind to yourself? You know how upsetting it will be for you to go to that shower. You know how nasty you'll be to your husband after you get back. (Switch seats)

Should Go:

Don't keep making excuses for yourself. You can always find some justification to avoid your obligations. But you know deep down that you're being selfish. If everyone acted this way, nobody would ever do anything nice for anyone else. (Switch seats)

Should Not Go:

But you know that you're not a selfish person. You've always gone out of your way to do nice things for other people. You do grocery shopping for your mother. You give money to charity. If you weren't dealing with your infertility, there's no question that you'd go. But this just isn't the right time for you. (Switch seats)

Remember, these are not lines to memorize, they're merely an example to follow. You can use the Empty Chair activity anytime you want to argue with yourself about what you "should" or "should not" do. You might be surprised by the intensity of your feelings.

YOU CAN REDUCE YOUR STRESS

We don't expect you to follow each and every element of the Workout throughout your pregnancy quest. Pick and choose the exercises that suit you at any given moment. The daily demands of infertility treatment can be quite time-consuming, and we realize that it's not always easy to stay with the Workout program. But even if you try to do just one or two of the exercises described in this chapter, you may find that it is possible to reduce the stress that accompanies most situations.

CHAPTER SEVEN

THE "ART" OF GETTING PREGNANT: ASSISTED REPRODUCTIVE TECHNOLOGIES

In 1978, a baby girl, Louise Brown, was delivered in England. In most ways, she is a normal child. What makes Louise special is that she was conceived through fertilization that took place outside the human body—in a laboratory.

The world's first "test-tube baby," Louise Brown was born thanks to the pioneering efforts of Drs. Patrick Steptoe and Robert Edwards. Not surprisingly, Louise's birth revolutionized reproductive medicine and offered new hope to countless infertile couples. Since her birth, tens of thousands of infants have been delivered as a result of *in vitro fertilization*, more commonly known as IVF. Over the last fifteen years, IVF techniques have been refined and improved to the point where they are now considered standard fertility treatments.

IVF is one of several alphabet soup terms that will be discussed in this chapter. These terms fall under the general category of *assisted reproductive technologies*, or ART. Medically, ART is not a quantum leap from the treatment you already may be trying. But psychologically,

ART represents a major step for infertile couples: the last hope of producing a child that is theirs genetically.

Because of its complexity, ART is usually explored only after low-tech procedures have failed. And because of its costliness, ART may indeed be a couple's last shot at parenthood because of its drain on their pocketbook, as well as on their emotional life.

Medically, ART embraces many of the low-tech procedures and regimens covered in earlier chapters: Pergonal injections, blood monitoring, ultrasound scans, semen samples, and maybe even a laparoscopy. What's different is that eggs are physically removed from your body. Once removed, the eggs are mixed with sperm in a petri dish and allowed to fertilize before being transferred into your womb, or the eggs are placed back into your fallopian tube along with your husband's or donor sperm.

Psychologically, people who attempt these procedures must come to grips with the fact that ART is a further cry from lovemaking than is artificial insemination. At least during an insemination, sperm is introduced through your vagina, albeit via a tube and syringe. With ART, eggs and sperm disappear behind closed doors, often returning as pre-embryos several days later.

WHAT IS ART?

Assisted reproductive technologies make use of laboratory procedures to examine eggs and enhance their likelihood of being fertilized. Although there are several variations on ART, they tend as a group to be referred to as in vitro fertilization (IVF). *"In vitro"* means "in glass"—in reference to the glass laboratory dishes in which fertilization takes place. Like tissues that are called "Kleenex" and photocopying procedures referred to as "Xeroxing," assisted reproductive techniques are often referred to as IVF. Despite the fact that some clinics use ART procedures that do not fertilize the eggs in a laboratory dish (e.g., GIFT procedures), they still call themselves IVF clinics.

At this writing, there are close to two hundred IVF clinics operating nationwide, some free-standing, some hospital-based. (For a complete list of these facilities, contact the American Fertility Society. The address appears in the appendix.)[1] In addition to IVF, currently available

ART techniques include: GIFT (gamete intrafallopian transfer) and ZIFT (zygote intrafallopian transfer), both of which will be explained later in this chapter.[2]

THE ELEMENTS OF ART

Downregulation

The use of the drug Lupron for *downregulation* of your pituitary gland's functioning has been one of the most dramatic developments in recent IVF technology. Downregulation means that Lupron temporarily inhibits the production of the pituitary hormones FSH and LH so that the doctor can artificially regulate your menstrual cycle. It also allows the doctors to control egg development and minimize the chance that you will ovulate your eggs before they can be retrieved. In addition, Lupron helps to increase the number of eggs you produce as well as improving the quality of those eggs. In a survey conducted in 1990, 75 percent of all American IVF clinics reported using Lupron as part of their protocol.[3]

Downregulation with Lupron takes ten to twelve days. At this time, you will get your menstrual period and be ready to begin your superovulation medication. You will continue taking Lupron, while you are also taking the superovulation medication. Lupron is injected once a day into your thigh or stomach with a tiny needle.

Superovulation

Superovulation is probably the most publicized and most anxiety-provoking aspect of ART. Perhaps the anxiety stems from fears that the use of drugs will somehow cause birth defects in future offspring or diseases of your own reproductive system. There are no scientific grounds for those fears, however. The superovulation drugs Pergonal and Metrodin are *natural*, not synthetic. They are combinations of the hormones your pituitary gland normally secretes. These drugs have been used for more than twenty years with no reported adverse side effects for the mother or the baby.

Depending on the individual and how much medication they are given, these drugs help your ovaries grow up to a dozen or more mature eggs rather than the single egg, which normally develops each month. Since most women ovulate naturally, you don't need these drugs for ovulation induction. Rather, you take these drugs to enhance the doctor's ability to obtain multiple eggs for potential fertilization. Infertility specialists agree that your chances of becoming pregnant improve if you produce many eggs. Multiple eggs potentially can result in multiple embryos. And by transferring several embryos to your uterus at once, the odds of at least one of them implanting and growing into a baby increase.

The two most common superovulation drugs are Pergonal and Metrodin. Pergonal is a combination of two hormones: FSH and LH. Metrodin is almost pure FSH. These drugs are injected daily into your buttocks. Although the needle may look intimidating, the injections are virtually painless because the needle pierces fatty tissue and should not hit any nerve endings. Dosage varies depending on the IVF program and the patient. But probably you will be taking more Pergonal (or Pergonal and Metrodin) each day than you did for a Pergonal-IUI cycle. Expect to inject the fertility drug or drugs for seven to twelve days per cycle.

Taking larger doses increases the risk of *hyperstimulation syndrome*. This severe hyperstimulation of the ovaries can cause nausea, vomiting, abdominal swelling, and rapid weight gain. Severe hyperstimulation can occur if you take large amounts of Pergonal, have extremely high estradiol levels, and then use hCG to ovulate your eggs in preparation for an insemination. When the hCG shot is given, some of the many eggs may not ovulate. Instead, they may leak large quantities of estrogen into the abdominal cavity. It is this estrogen overload that produces the negative side effects.

As rare as hyperstimulation syndrome is during low-tech procedures, it is even less common with ART. The reason is that doctors physically remove, or *aspirate,* the eggs, and in the process minimize the likelihood that the corpus luteum will leak estrogen that might trigger hyperstimulation. Also, if scans and blood tests indicate the patient is at high risk for hyperstimulation, the doctor refrains from administering hCG and cancels the cycle. Through careful monitoring, then, you can safely take high doses of fertility drugs with little fear of hyperstimulation syndrome.

Monitoring: Blood and Ultrasound

Your response to the medication will be monitored via blood tests to determine your estradiol (a form of estrogen) level and ultrasound scans of your ovaries. Undergoing this monitoring is a mixed blessing. It's a relief to know that your doctor is checking how fast your eggs are growing every day or every other day. Monitoring ensures that eggs grow as large as possible, but not so large that they are overripe or so mature that they ovulate before they are ready to be retrieved. But you pay a price for your doctor's vigilance. And we don't mean only money.

Most clinics want you to arrive early in the morning to have your blood drawn. Early often means between 6:30 and 8:30 A.M. Arriving at a distant clinic may mean leaving your home before dawn. And getting there early doesn't necessarily mean avoiding the crowd. Chances are, you will be one of many women waiting to be monitored. While comparing notes with others can be a source of support, being amid so many infertile women also can make you feel depressed or overwhelmed. Also, starting your day at an IVF clinic and then going to work can make you feel nervous and preoccupied.

While you are still only half awake, a nurse will stick a needle into your vein and then an ultrasound technician will insert a probe into your vagina. The probe is used to obtain an ultrasound scan of your ovaries. Using high-frequency sound waves, the probe produces a picture of your ovaries and follicles on a video screen. To help you stay involved in your treatment, many clinics will give you a notepad and have you write down a series of numbers the technician calls out as she scans. "Twelve on the right." "Fifteen on the left." These are not football plays. They are the diameter—in millimeters—of the egg follicles that are being measured on the screen. The lead follicles must be at least 16 to 18 millimeters in diameter before they are ready to be aspirated.

Doctors need to obtain your blood early in the morning to allow sufficient time for a laboratory to analyze your hormone levels. Doctors get their lab reports early in the afternoon and use this information, together with your ultrasound results, to adjust your dosage for that evening's fertility drug injection. You will be notified of the doctor's decision by phone later in the day.

Figuring out the logistics of receiving this vital information can be stressful, especially if you don't want to be called at work where colleagues or customers might overhear your conversation. You may worry that a message left on your answering machine may be unclear. You may want to speak personally to the doctor if you have questions or concerns. Or you might elect to sit by the phone to make sure you don't miss the call.

In addition to telling you how many ampules of Pergonal to inject that evening, some doctors also will tell you your estradiol level. Getting information about estradiol levels can be troubling. It's easy to obsess over the numbers, plaguing yourself with questions such as, "Is it going up enough?" "Am I doing okay?" If your doctor routinely shares estradiol levels, we recommend Getting Organized by keeping track of them in your Cycle Log. If your levels fail to match last cycle's levels, don't worry. It is not unusual for women to respond differently to the same doses of Pergonal month to month. One woman who had two children thanks to Pergonal said she was better able to cope with the intensive monitoring by trying to stay emotionally neutral whether the news was good or bad.

Triggering Ovulation

When your doctor decides that your follicles have reached optimal development, he will prescribe an hCG (Profasi) injection. Like Pergonal, hCG is injected into your buttocks and is not particularly painful. Egg retrieval will be scheduled thirty-four to thirty-six hours after this injection.

Egg Harvest

Eggs are harvested using one of two different methods. The first, rarely used today, involves egg retrieval through *laparoscopy*. This surgical procedure requires general anesthesia. A surgeon inserts a laparoscope, a long telescopelike tube, through an incision below or in the belly button. Looking through the laparoscope, the surgeon guides a needle through the patient's abdomen into a mature ovarian follicle. When pierced, the follicle collapses and the follicular fluid and egg are aspirated. Follicles also are flushed with a special salt solution to help remove any eggs that were missed by the initial aspiration. Research has shown that flushing can collect eggs that would otherwise have been left behind and that these eggs can be fertilized and result in live births.[4] The laparoscopic retrieval generally takes about two hours.

The other, more popular, technique is called *ultrasound guided transvaginal aspiration*. This procedure requires no incisions and uses only intravenous sedation. The doctor inserts an ultrasound probe into the vagina. When a mature follicle is identified, he guides a needle through the vagina and into a follicle to be aspirated. All the eggs are aspirated and flushed. This procedure usually takes about an hour.

Whichever approach is used, the retrieved eggs are given to a specialist called an embryologist, who examines the eggs under a microscope and assigns them a grade from 1 (worst) to 5 (best).

Doctors take care to ensure that you are physically comfortable during the retrieval procedure. For most women, the outcome—whether enough healthy eggs will be harvested—is more stressful than the procedure itself. Although a pregnancy can occur even when only a single egg is harvested, more eggs means your chances of success are greater. Likewise, a harvest of eggs that are of inferior quality has a poor prognosis.

Fertilization

When you try to get pregnant on your own, you have to wait at least two weeks to learn whether your egg got fertilized. With IVF, you get important information within twenty-four to forty-eight hours after egg retrieval. This is because the site of fertilization is changed from inside the body, where it is invisible and unknown, to outside the body—a glass dish in the laboratory.

Each harvested egg is placed in its own glass dish filled with a special IVF culture medium. Your husband's or a donor's sperm cells that have been washed and specially prepared are also placed into the dish. Each dish then goes into an incubator. In about twelve hours, an egg that was fertilized will divide and become a two-celled *pre-embryo*. A little while later, the pre-embryo may divide again into four cells. After eighteen hours in the incubator, an embryologist will check the eggs to determine whether they are fertilized. Forty-eight hours after retrieval, these two- and four-celled pre-embryos are transferred into your uterus through the vagina. The transfer is similar to an IUI procedure.

Typically, not all eggs fertilize. Also, some eggs get fertilized by more than one sperm. These *polyspermic eggs*, as they are called, cannot be transferred. But if you've had a large harvest of eggs—say twelve to sixteen—more than likely many have fertilized and divided. The doctor usually will transfer about four to six and freeze the remaining pre-embryos.

Couples who are amazed that doctors can fertilize eggs in the laboratory ask why scientists cannot continue to grow the baby in this carefully monitored environment. The answer is that there is a limit to how much viable embryologic development can take place outside your body. Doctors give your baby a two- to four-celled jump start in the lab and then you take over and grow your baby just as any other pregnant woman would—in your womb.

The two-day period between egg harvest and embryo transfer is filled with suspense. Many questions wander through your mind, not the least of which is: "Can my husband's sperm fertilize my eggs?" IVF is the only way to get a clear answer. To learn how many embryos will be available for transfer, you need merely to hang in there for two days. As you grapple with your anxiety, try to remember that what is happening in that incubator during this critical two-day period can be the catalyst to help you get pregnant when you thought you couldn't.

Embryo Transfer

Embryo transfer requires no anesthesia, although some patients prefer to have a mild sedative. The transfer procedure is very similar to what happens during an intrauterine insemination.

You will be asked to lie on a table or bed with your feet in stirrups. The doctor will use a catheter loaded with one or more pre-embryos that have been suspended in a drop of culture medium. The doctor inserts the catheter into the cervix and deposits the pre-embryos into the uterine cavity. The procedure takes ten to twenty minutes. Some clinics recommend that you remain on your back for two to four hours following the transfer.

Medically, a pre-embryo transfer is fairly simple. Emotionally, it is rather complex. As these pre-embryos enter your body, you may begin to think you are pregnant. After all, your body now contains fertilized eggs. Many women become convinced that they have finally succeeded— they are now "with embryo." Unfortunately, implantation is the aspect of ART that is least understood. Despite their ability to fertilize and transfer pre-embryos, doctors are frustrated by their inability to exercise comparable control over the implantation process. Everyone involved must wait apprehensively for the next two weeks to see whether a pregnancy has occurred.

Post-Transfer Hormonal Support

Even though doctors cannot ensure that your pre-embryos will implant successfully, they can help increase the odds. They know that an ample supply of progesterone increases the likelihood of a successful pregnancy. When a woman becomes pregnant on her own, the corpus luteum produces progesterone, which helps keep the uterine lining conducive to pregnancy. Sometimes, however, ART procedures can affect the ovary's progesterone production. Because of a diminished internal supply of progesterone, you must get it externally. You can take injections, use vaginal suppositories, or even take pills to get the needed supply of progesterone.

You will use progesterone supplements up until you have your pregnancy test. If the test result is positive, you will continue to take progesterone for twelve weeks or as long as your doctor deems necessary. Statistically, about 14 percent of women who begin a cycle of IVF will take home a baby nine months later. The average cost for IVF is about $7,000.

Cryopreservation

If the first transfer fails, you can avoid another retrieval procedure thanks to *pre-embryo cryopreservation*. This involves freezing pre-embryos under carefully controlled conditions, storing them under liquid nitrogen, and eventually thawing the pre-embryos for use in future cycles, if needed. Extensive research has shown that freezing and thawing pre-embryos does not contribute to birth defects or other fetal problems. On the other hand, you must be prepared for the possibility that some of your frozen pre-embryos may not survive the freezing and thawing process. New developments in cryopreservation techniques are enabling about 80 percent of frozen pre-embryos to survive the freeze-thaw process, however.[5] A 1992 study of IVF procedures in North American IVF clinics found that 12 percent of frozen embryo transfers resulted in pregnancies, and 9 percent resulted in deliveries.[6]

One area of controversy is whether it's better to transfer thawed pre-embryos during a natural, drug-free cycle or during one in which drugs are used. Ask your doctor which is best for you. In either case, you are likely to take progesterone supplements after receiving the thawed pre-embryos just as you would if the pre-embryo was fresh.

Frozen pre-embryo transfers can create some unusual questions. Consider this case, reported in the November 1991 issue of *Fertility and Sterility*.[7] In March 1985, a doctor in Australia collected eggs from a woman, fertilized them, and obtained six pre-embryos. Three were transferred immediately, and the remaining three were frozen. One of the freshly transferred pre-embryos developed into a baby girl who was born in December 1985. In January 1987, the same woman received one of her frozen pre-embryos, which developed into another baby girl, born in October 1987. Finally, in November 1989, the woman had the last two frozen pre-embryos thawed and transferred to her womb. In September 1990, the woman gave birth to a baby boy.

So what are these babies? Are they triplets or three single children? From the point of view of a biologist, they are triplets since they were conceived simultaneously. But from the parents' point of view, these children are singletons, born years apart. For the infertile couple, they are a blessing regardless of when or how they were conceived.

Pregnancy Testing

The most taxing phase of ART procedures is waiting for the results of a pregnancy test. Fourteen days after embryo transfer, your doctor will take a blood sample and analyze your hCG level. If hCG is detected in your blood, you are pregnant. In the next chapter, we offer an activity to help you stay hopeful but realistic during this difficult waiting period.

THE GIFT ALTERNATIVE

Some doctors believe that the fallopian tube is a better, more natural site for fertilization to occur because there may be certain fluids in the tube that help stimulate fertilization. To help infertile couples achieve this goal, medical science has come up with GIFT—Gamete IntraFallopian Transfer. During a GIFT procedure, gametes (sperm and egg cells) are injected into one or both fallopian tubes. If all goes well, fertilization takes place in the tube and the embryo enters the uterus and implants, just as it would in natural, unassisted reproduction.

As in IVF, GIFT begins with drug-induced superovulation and its accompanying monitoring process. When the egg follicles reach the optimal size, ovulation is triggered by an hCG injection. Approximately thirty-six hours after the hCG shot, the eggs are retrieved either by the transvaginal procedure or through laparoscopy. Before the gametes are placed in the fallopian tube, the sperm sample is washed and the eggs are examined by an embryologist, who selects only the best ones. The eggs and sperm are then introduced into the top end of the fallopian tube through a special double-barreled catheter during a laparoscopy.

In choosing which procedure to try, remember that GIFT requires surgery and general anesthesia, while IVF is a *minor surgical* procedure.[8] Unlike IVF, where the transfer is done two days after egg retrieval, GIFT takes place within hours after the eggs are harvested, thus sparing the couple an additional trip to the hospital. A disadvantage to GIFT is that you cannot know how many—if any—eggs become fertilized after being transferred to the fallopian tube.

You are a candidate for GIFT if you have at least one healthy fallopian tube—even if your infertility is unexplained or you have mild endometriosis or a cervical or immunological problem. Per-cycle success rate for GIFT is about 22 percent. Cost of the procedure is about $9,000.

THE ZIFT ALTERNATIVE

ZIFT—Zygote IntraFallopian Transfer—involves the transfer of a zygote, the medical term for a fertilized egg before it begins to divide. ZIFT is sometimes called PROST, or PROnuclear Stage Transfer. The pronuclear stage occurs approximately fourteen hours after the sperm fertilizes the egg.

For ZIFT, your eggs are retrieved transvaginally and fertilized in a laboratory dish. The next day, you return for a laparoscopy, during which the zygotes are placed into your fallopian tubes. ZIFT is essentially a combination of IVF and GIFT. Like IVF, eggs are fertilized by sperm in a laboratory dish and you must undergo procedures on two separate days. Like GIFT, ZIFT involves surgery, and the embryonic material is placed directly into your tubes, not into your uterus.

A variation of ZIFT is called Tubal Embryo Transfer, or TET. During TET, a two- or four-celled pre-embryo is transferred to the fallopian tubes by means of a laparoscopy. Both ZIFT and TET require the use of anesthesia and the same recovery period as a GIFT procedure, about one to four days.

ZIFT and TET are recommended in cases where the husband has below average sperm and in cases where there is an immunological factor preventing pregnancy. ZIFT and TET enable doctors to confirm that fertilization has occurred while providing the natural environment of the fallopian tubes to nurture the pre-embryo.

Figure 7.1 summarizes the differences between IVF, GIFT, and ZIFT.

SUCCESS STATISTICS OF ART PROCEDURES

Every January, the journal *Fertility and Sterility* publishes the results of the United States IVF-ET (embryo transfer) registry. According to the January 1992 report, summarizing data from 1990, there were 175 clinics performing IVF procedures. These clinics performed a total of 16,405 egg retrievals, from which 2,345 babies were born, for an overall delivery rate of 14 percent.[9]

That same year, 135 clinics performed at least one GIFT, according to the journal. These clinics performed a total of 3,750 retrievals, which resulted in the birth of 842 babies, for a delivery rate of 22 percent.

Finally, 90 clinics stated that they performed ZIFT. From the 1,370 ZIFT retrievals that were done, 215 babies were born—a 16 percent delivery rate.

The report provides additional information about the success of IVF and GIFT (but not ZIFT) as a function of the patient's age. For both IVF and GIFT, success rates drop dramatically when the woman is over forty. So in contrast with the overall 14 percent delivery rate for IVF, women over forty have a delivery rate of only 7 percent. And in contrast to the 22 percent overall delivery rate for GIFT, only 9 percent of the procedures done on women over forty resulted in a live birth. For women under forty, the success rate ranges from 21 percent to 30 percent.

What's the Difference?

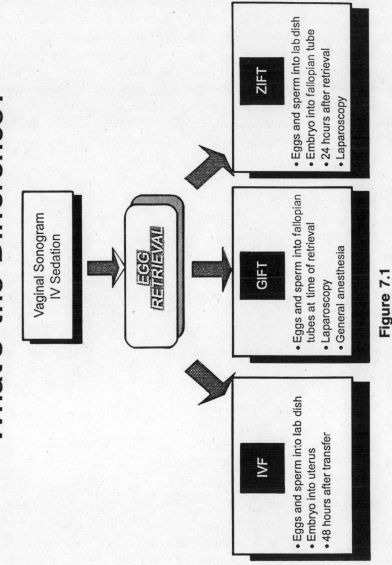

Figure 7.1
Comparison of IVF, GIFT, and ZIFT

IVF
- Eggs and sperm into lab dish
- Embryo into uterus
- 48 hours after transfer

GIFT
- Eggs and sperm into fallopian tubes at time of retrieval
- Laparoscopy
- General anesthesia

ZIFT
- Eggs and sperm into lab dish
- Embryo into fallopian tube
- 24 hours after retrieval
- Laparoscopy

Vaginal Sonogram
IV Sedation

EGG RETRIEVAL

Many patients seeking ART overestimate their odds of success. Part of our job at IVF New Jersey in Somerset is to help these couples become more realistic. (One couple we counseled thought they had an 80 percent chance of getting pregnant on their first ART attempt.) By understanding that the odds are always against you for any given cycle, you can avoid becoming overly distressed if the procedure fails.

It's important not to blind yourself with unrealistic hope. But we also urge you not to despair over the statistics. In the next chapter, we will give you some activities to help you balance hope and despair and to realistically assess your odds of success with repeated ART attempts.

WHICH ART PROCEDURE IS FOR YOU?

Your doctor is the best judge of which procedure is most appropriate in your case. To help you become a Partner in Your Treatment, however, Drs. Michael Darder and Susan Treiser of IVF New Jersey offer the following recommendations:

You can benefit from IVF if:

- Your FSH on Day 3 is under 20;
- You have blocked or damaged fallopian tubes;
- You have severe endometriosis;
- Your husband has a low sperm count and poor motility; and
- You've tried GIFT without success.

You can benefit from GIFT if:

- Your FSH on Day 3 is under 20;
- You have *at least one* normal fallopian tube;
- You have mild or moderate endometriosis;
- Your husband has a mild sperm problem; and
- You have a cervical or immunological problem, or you have unexplained infertility.

You can benefit from ZIFT if:

- Your FSH on Day 3 is under 20;
- You have *at least one* normal fallopian tube;
- You have mild or moderate endometriosis;
- Your husband has a severe male factor problem;
- You have a cervical or immunological problem, or you have unexplained infertility; and
- You've had a failed GIFT cycle.

Cost is another factor in decision-making. Generally, GIFT and ZIFT are more expensive than IVF because both involve surgery and the use of anesthesia. All three procedures have indirect costs of about $3,000 for hormonal monitoring, ultrasound scans, and pregnancy testing.[10] In addition to the $3,000, expect to pay about $3,500 for the IVF cycle, $4,200 for a GIFT cycle, and $6,500 for a ZIFT cycle. These additional charges cover operating room costs for egg retrieval, the doctor's fee for retrieving the eggs, the embryology lab fees, the operating room fee for transferring the embryos, and the physician's fee for performing the transfer.

When general anesthesia is used, expect to pay an additional $800. Finally, expect to pay about $1,000 to freeze your embryos, $300 to thaw embryos for one transfer cycle, and about $500 per year to store your frozen embryos. While many couples can clear the emotional hurdles to ART, they are stymied by the price tag on these high-tech treatments. In the next chapter, we will share some tips to increase your chances of getting insurance coverage for these procedures.

SELECTING AN IVF PROGRAM

In Chapter 6, we talked you through the process of choosing an infertility specialist. Two important aspects of this process were constructing and using a guide to interview the doctor and using decision-making skills from the Getting Pregnant Workout to help you make your choice. We recommend you reread this material before selecting an IVF program.

In many instances, however, there is no choice to be made because there is only one IVF clinic within driving distance. But in large, metropolitan areas there are likely to be several clinics and hospitals offering ART. When researching them, ask:

- What are the qualifications and experience of the doctors in this practice?
- Are they treating patients who have your kind of problem?
- What are the success statistics of this clinic? (Caution: Don't rule out a clinic simply on the basis of low rates of success. Patient selection can influence success rates. Some clinics turn away older patients or patients with problems that are difficult to treat. For this reason, they may boast high success rates. Other clinics treat challenging cases and therefore have comparably lower success rates.)
- Are support services available? For example, does the program include psychological counseling or support groups to help you get through difficult times?
- What treatment options does the program offer? Do they perform IVF, GIFT, and ZIFT? Do they offer donor egg and sperm for patients who need them? Do they freeze embryos?
- How do the costs compare with other clinics?
- Is the procedure performed in a hospital operating room or in the operating suite of a free-standing facility devoted exclusively to IVF?
- How convenient will it be to work with this program given your time constraints? Do they have early-morning and weekend hours? How far do you have to travel to get to the clinic?

ART ISN'T EASY

Some people are reluctant to try ART because they view it as unnatural or as meddling with nature. Others are reluctant to give up on ART despite repeated failures. For them, abandoning treatment means giving up their dream. Regardless of where you are on this spectrum, expect to encounter a certain degree of emotional turmoil as you venture into the world of high-tech infertility treatment. The next chapter can help you cope.

CHAPTER EIGHT

HELPING YOURSELF THROUGH ART— FINANCIALLY AND EMOTIONALLY

WHEN KRISTEN'S doctor suggested she take Clomid after failing to conceive after twelve months of trying, Kristen was shocked. "How could I manipulate my menstrual cycle like this?" she thought. As time went on with no pregnancy, Kristen slowly accepted the logic of her doctor's advice and began taking Clomid. When Clomid didn't work, Kristen's doctor recommended she advance to Pergonal. But again, Kristen was reluctant.

"I can't believe I'm doing some of the things I'm doing now," Kristen told us during a counseling session. "I said I'd never take Pergonal, and then I did. Six months later, the doctor told me I needed to have inseminations. I said, 'No way, I'll never do it' . . . and I did it."

Kristen also had recoiled at the thought of advanced reproductive treatments (ART). But eventually she did that, too.

What allowed Kristen to change her attitude and reconsider something she previously considered repugnant? According to social psychologist Kurt Lewin, the key was Kristen's ability to remove roadblocks that prevented her from trying something new.[1]

Generally speaking, people feel most comfortable maintaining the status quo. It's easier to stay in a job that is not boosting your career than it is to quit and look for something more fulfilling. Likewise, it is far easier to repeat Pergonal/IUI cycles month after month than it is to abandon the familiar routine and take the emotional and financial risks involved with ART.

If you have been engaging in low-tech treatments for six months to a year and still haven't had a baby, you have reached a set of crossroads— and a daunting one at that. Your choices: Continue your current treatment; move to more advanced treatment; or give up trying to become pregnant altogether. If everything else has failed and you still want to give birth, ART may be your only viable alternative.

MOVING FROM LOW-TECH TO HIGH-TECH TREATMENT

As much as you want to be pregnant, the idea of taking massive doses of fertility drugs and then having your eggs plucked out of your ovaries might paralyze you with fear.

In addition to fear, there are two other major roadblocks encountered by most people considering ART: insufficient finances and lack of family support. In this chapter, we will show you how to break through those roadblocks. We also will teach you how to remain optimistic but realistic while engaging in these exciting new treatments.

Identifying Roadblocks

Let's look at two diagrams that we helped Kristen prepare. The act of making the diagrams helped Kristen conquer her fears and move from Clomid to Pergonal, and then to add inseminations to her treatment regimen.

Kristen was stuck in the Clomid treatment status quo. She was telling herself: "Pills are one thing, but injections are something else. I am drawing the line at Clomid." Kristen needed to Change Her Thinking. She used Getting Pregnant Self-Talk (GPST) to help move her line in

MOVING THE LINE

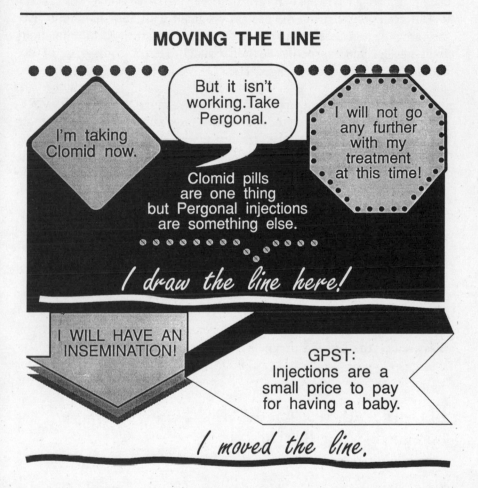

Figure 8.1

the sand. She told herself: "Injections are a small price to pay for having a baby. I will take Pergonal."

Unfortunately, Kristen did not get pregnant with Pergonal alone. Her doctor said she needed to combine Pergonal and artificial inseminations with her husband's sperm. Kristen balked. Here's a diagram of her thoughts and how she Changed Her Thinking to once again move the line.

Kristen used the same approach to help her move the line to try ART. You can use Kristen's method to help you change your mind-set—to help you try the more advanced treatment your doctor may be suggesting. We've provided a blank form for you to fill out that can help you move on.

Having changed her attitude, Kristen now needed to remove the roadblocks to ART and get psyched up for the rigors of high-tech treatment. Like Kristen you need to:

- Educate Yourself about medical insurance for infertility;
- Manage Your Social Life by garnering the support of your family; and
- Motivate yourself to hang in despite setbacks: Don't Give Up.

To accomplish these goals, we ask you to draw upon the skills you mastered in the Getting Pregnant Workout.

BLOOD AND MONEY: PAYING FOR INFERTILITY TREATMENT

By the time you've begun thinking about ART, you've probably gotten used to having blood taken out of your arm for various tests. While parting with a vial of your blood has become second nature, parting with your money gets more and more difficult as infertility treatment goes on. Even if you are insured, many policies have limited benefits for infertility treatment. For most people, then, the high cost of ART becomes the major roadblock to getting pregnant when they thought they couldn't.

Scores of patients we have interviewed ranked money as the No. 1 or No. 2 factor (behind psychological or physical trauma) that prevented them from pursuing ART. Every aspect of high-tech treatment costs

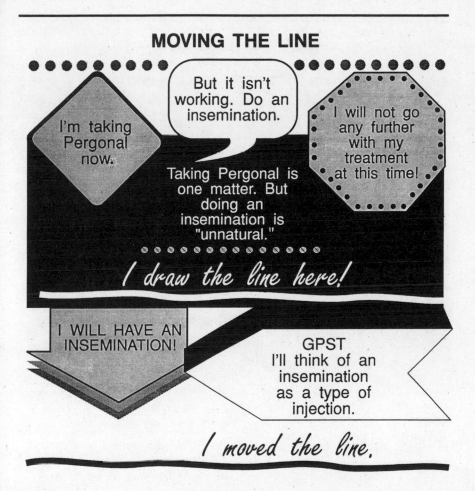

Figure 8.2

MOVING THE LINE

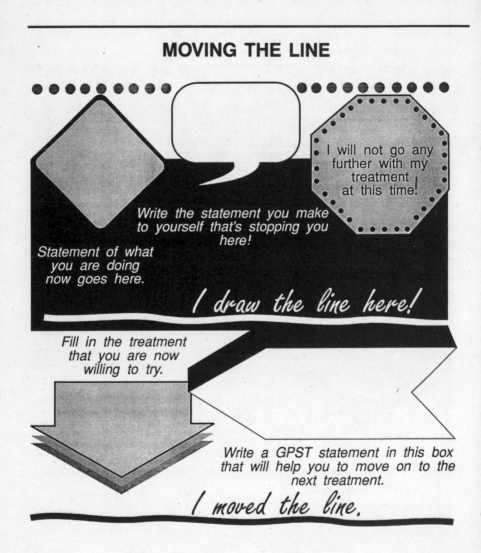

Figure 8.3

money: drugs, hormonal studies, ultrasounds, interpretation of results, professional fees, the operating room, freezing and thawing embryos, and sperm-washing, to name a few.

You can't completely begrudge infertility doctors and technicians for charging so much. Thanks to their knowledge and training, many infertile couples are getting pregnant. Certainly, you want your doctor to be the best that money can buy. But you also wish his fees weren't so steep. When presented with the bill, it is easy to succumb to the unfairness of it all: People lucky enough to get pregnant the "regular" way can spend their money on baby furniture and college funds. You, on the other hand, are spending your hard-earned money on Pergonal and surgeries. And unlike fertile couples, you aren't even guaranteed success.

We can offer no simple explanations for the inequities of life. We can encourage you, however, to face the issue of money in a pragmatic manner, separating your grief over your infertility from a rational approach to money management.

For many couples, ART is simply too expensive to try more than once, if at all. Other couples who can afford ART fail to investigate the various ways of keeping costs as low as possible. They may be embarrassed to work with their doctor and insurance company to enhance their reimbursements. Instead of fighting for what rights or services are theirs, they withdraw, give up, and mourn their predicament. They are engaging in what psychologist Martin Seligman, author of *Learned Optimism*, calls *learned helplessness*.[2] Learned helplessness is the tendency to expect that bad things will happen to you and that nothing you can do will prevent them from happening. A person who has failed to influence others on numerous occasions may conclude that nothing he or she can do will ever make a difference.

In contrast, we urge you to be assertive and leave no avenue unexplored that might help you loosen ART's financial pinch. While the following section emphasizes ART insurance coverage, it also pertains to coverage for low-tech infertility treatments.

Some Facts About Insurance and Infertility Coverage

Insurers and infertile couples always seem to be battling over costs. Until infertile couples took on the roles of advocates, few, if any, insurers automatically paid for infertility treatment. In the last several years, however, infertile couples have been successfully lobbying state legislatures to pass laws requiring insurers to cover their medical bills.

As of March 1992, twenty-one states had introduced legislation that requires insurance coverage for the diagnosis and treatment of infertility. Of these, ten had enacted infertility insurance legislation: Arkansas, California, Connecticut, Hawaii, Illinois, Maryland, Massachusetts, New York, Rhode Island, and Texas.

The first state to revise its insurance laws in this manner was Maryland, which mandated low-tech treatment and IVF coverage in 1985.[3] Under the Maryland law, married couples were entitled to some reimbursement if they have been:

- Infertile for five years;
- Have infertility due to endometriosis, DES exposure, or blocked or missing fallopian tubes;
- Have tried less costly treatments unsuccessfully;
- Used their own gametes; and
- Tried IVF at clinics approved by the American Fertility Society.

Shortly after Maryland's law was passed, Texas passed an almost identical law. Massachusetts passed a law that requires all infertility diagnosis and treatment, including IVF, be considered for insurance reimbursement. Connecticut, Rhode Island, and Illinois subsequently passed laws similar to the one passed by Massachusetts.

In 1987, Arkansas enacted a law that included embryo freezing but set a maximum benefit for IVF coverage at $15,000. Legislation passed in Hawaii in 1987 provided for a one-time-only IVF reimbursement. California and New York require coverage for diagnosis and treatment of infertility but exclude IVF. Interestingly, however, New York legislation requires coverage for GIFT procedures.

In a recent RESOLVE of Central Jersey newsletter, attorney Raymond Godwin summarized differences in the various state laws dealing with infertility insurance. According to Godwin: "Other differences include, for example, the length of time a couple has experienced infertility (Arkansas: two years; Maryland: five years) before coverage is allowed; the exemption of employers with a certain number of employees (California: fewer than twenty; Illinois: fewer than twenty-five); and whether only the husband's sperm can be used with IVF and GIFT."[4]

If you live in any of these ten states, you probably have a better chance of having some of the costs reimbursed than if you live elsewhere. But if you do not meet all the conditions set forth under the law (i.e., length of time, medical condition, or use of your own gametes), then the law may work against you. On the other hand, insurance may in fact cover your diagnosis and treatment, even if you live in one of the other forty states.

At the time of this writing, the majority of insurance carriers cover between 50 percent and 80 percent of conventional infertility treatments.[5] In terms of in vitro fertilization, 41 percent of commercial health insurance carriers provide coverage. One in four do so as a standard practice, and the remainder do so on a case-by-case basis.[6]

For lesser, low-tech procedures, most Blue Cross and Blue Shield plans cover much of the diagnostic testing. As long as the insurance company can justify a treatment as leading up to the diagnosis of an illness or condition, the company will reimburse you for surgeries, blood tests, diagnostic tests (like the HSG or endometrial biopsy), and ultrasound scans.

Insurance companies do not consider infertility to be the illness itself; their argument is that most procedures bypass rather than cure the problem and are experimental in nature.

But don't lose hope or make assumptions. There are various ways to find out definitively what, if any infertility tests and treatments your policy covers. One couple we know assumed that their insurance would not reimburse them for $700 of out-of-pocket expenses for Lupron during an IVF cycle. The insurer had initially turned down their claim, but they resubmitted it, pointing out that the FDA had recently approved the Lupron for the treatment of endometriosis, a recognized contributor to infertility. The argument was convincing enough that the insurer reimbursed their $700.

Finding Out What Your Insurance Company Covers

If you and your husband are covered by different health plans, be sure to investigate both. One policy may be preferable for low-tech treatment, the other for high-tech. One policy may even consider reimbursing you on the unpaid balance of your claims. So Company A may pay 80 percent of a procedure and Company B may pay 80 percent of the 20 percent you paid out-of-pocket, giving you effective insurance coverage of 96 percent.

Finding out which infertility treatments your policy covers can be tricky. On one hand, you want accurate information. On the other hand, you risk alerting your insurer to the fact that you are about to undergo infertility treatment. If you are covered by a group plan, you cannot be disenrolled for medical reasons. But if you have individual coverage, there is always the possibility that the insurer will try to cancel your policy if it anticipates costly claims on the horizon. But there are ways to make inquiries about coverage *without* jeopardizing your policy.

The first step is to read your claims booklet carefully. This booklet may contain statements like, "The treatment of infertility is not provided through the general policy, but may be part of a rider clause negotiated by a specific group." Your personnel manager should be able to give you a copy of the rider. Even though infertility treatment (particularly in vitro procedures or even inseminations) may not be covered, try to find out if diagnostic blood tests and ultrasound procedures are, and if so, how many are covered. From the booklet, you may be able to deduce which diagnoses are more likely than others to be reimbursable.

You also will want to know what percentage of treatment costs are typically covered by the policy. Sometimes, instead of paying a percentage of a medical bill, some companies offer a flat fee. They may, for example, pay up to $45 for any blood analysis, even if your analysis costs $100. Try to find out what the general fee schedule is, particularly if you have ever seen the following explanation (or one like it) from the insurer when it only partially reimbursed you: "This charge has been declared over and above the customary fees charged by medical professionals in your area." Finally, try to find out about deductibles and at what ceiling your coverage changes. Many companies begin to offer a higher percentage of coverage when your co-payment ceiling is reached. For example, our carrier pays 80 percent of specific charges until the total bill reaches $2,000, at which point they cover 100 percent of certain charges.

Also try to find out which drugs may be covered. Pergonal, Metrodin, and Lupron are all costly. Some insurers cover them, others do not. Some policies have an annual dollar limit for prescriptions. If you are lucky, your policy includes a liberal prescription plan that covers almost all prescription medications (except birth control pills), with a small co-payment by you. If your claims booklet fails to answer all your questions about covered medications, your pharmacist—who deals with numerous insurance carriers every day—may be able to answer some of your questions.

If you are still baffled after reading the claims booklet (some of them are notoriously vague and confusing), schedule an interview with the benefits representative or personnel manager at your and your husband's workplaces. Begin at the workplace that provides your primary coverage, and then move to the workplace that provides your secondary coverage. Even if you've chosen to keep your fertility problem a secret from your boss and co-workers, we encourage you to level with your benefits representative, urging him or her to maintain your confidentiality. By giving the representative specifics about your condition, you are apt to walk out of the meeting knowing exactly how much—if any—money you will personally have to fork over for your treatment. Also, knowing exactly how many of those treatments are covered can help you Make a Plan.

Another good source of information is a co-worker or friend who has the same policy as you and has undergone infertility diagnosis and treatment. This individual should be able to give you the lowdown on the insurer's payment record and can alert you to any land mines. Even if this person is only an acquaintance, remember that there is an allegiance, of sorts, among infertile people. Having suffered and survived the experience, most of us are eager to help and comfort others in any way we can.

If all else fails, you may have no choice but to call your insurance company, which probably provides a toll-free number for its policyholders. If the insurance representative tells you something is covered either by the general policy or under a rider to that policy, write down the representative's name, exactly what he or she told you, and the date and time of your call. If possible, have the representative confirm your conversation in writing. This letter can become invaluable should you need to appeal a claim denial in the future. Some insurers require a letter from your doctor estimating the cost of an ART treatment prior to considering any claims related to that treatment. The request for such a letter doesn't necessarily mean your claim will be turned down. It's a tool insurance carriers use to budget for their future outlays.

Reducing the Stress of Financial Strain

Going in the hole to finance infertility treatment is stressful and can provoke marital strife. For example, if you and your partner have agreed to set aside money for important life goals, your suggestion that you allocate that money for ART can spur an argument about priorities. Even if your heart is set on ART, your husband might argue that the money you spend on treatment will render you unable to afford an adoption should the procedure fail.

To minimize or even prevent these conflicts, we urge you to employ the skills described in the Getting Pregnant Workout. You and your spouse must listen and level with each other about how to handle this financial crisis. We further recommend using the decision-making exercises described in this book to decide whether to pursue ART or to spend that money on adoption.

It is at this point that you may decide that enough is enough. The money crisis may be the straw that breaks the camel's back. You may have been able to bounce back from failed cycles, cope with injections and medication, and deal with the disruption in your social life. But spending your last penny or borrowing money you don't even have may just be more than you can handle. If you are unable to continue treatment because the costs are beyond your means, you are not giving up—merely being realistic. But if, somehow, you are able to hang in financially, you need to consider ways to finance your ART treatment.

How Deep Are Your Pockets?

Before you begin an IVF cycle, make sure you have enough money to pay for it should the insurance company fall through or fail to fully cover all your medical bills. You may want to sell some stock, dip into your savings account, borrow money from a bank or relative, skip a vacation (or two), or otherwise modify your lifestyle to shore up the necessary funds.

In examining your current financial wherewithal, first look at your savings accounts, CDs, and money market funds, and decide if you can liquidate any of these assets. Are you expecting any lump sums this year, such as an inheritance or lawsuit settlement? One couple told us they waited until they got their tax refund every year and used that money for several Pergonal/IUI cycles.

Next, explore loan programs at your workplace or through the bank where you do business. Also ask your IVF clinic if it can give you access to a low-interest loan to pay for your treatment. Family or friends may be able to lend you money at very low interest. Some lucky couples have well-to-do family members who are happy to make a monetary contribution toward their pregnancy quest. As a very last resort, you can charge ART to your Visa or MasterCard. While this option gives you quick money, don't forget that consumer credit interest rates are extremely high, almost 20 percent in some cases.

Before you borrow money, even at low interest, try to think ahead of how you will pay back the loan. And brace yourself for the possibility that you may wind up making loan payments for a procedure that failed to get you pregnant.

An alternative to dipping into your savings or borrowing money is to take an extra job or become involved in a project that generates money, such as selling Tupperware or your baked goods to a local gourmet shop. If you choose this route, discipline yourself to put your entire extra paycheck into a "getting pregnant account" each week. Also, begin and finish your additional job *prior* to undergoing high-tech treatment. Maintaining an additional job at the same time you are involved in ART can raise your level of stress to the point where it may diminish your chances of becoming pregnant.

Reducing the Cost of ART

A different approach to making ART more affordable is getting your doctor or IVF clinic to reduce fees. Recently, some of the larger clinics have developed so-called scholarship programs and sliding-scale fees based on a couple's need and ability (or inability) to pay. Such programs are designed to assist infertile people who desperately want treatment but who have exhausted their insurance coverage and personal resources. Clinics tend to favor couples who have already completed several cycles there and who are believed to have good potential for success if they try one or two more times.

If your insurance will pick up part of the cost, and you anticipate that you'll have trouble making up the difference, you might be able to persuade your doctor or clinic to accept as payment in full whatever your insurance company is willing to reimburse. Always talk to the doctor *before* you begin a cycle about any arrangement of this sort.

Finally, some women who have produced many eggs in a previous IVF cycle may be able to work out an agreement to finance their next cycle by donating any extra eggs in exchange for free medication or a lowering of fees.

Preparing to Submit Your Bills to Insurance

Many infertility doctors and programs are willing to work with insurance companies and couples to help obtain the maximum coverage to which their patients are entitled. Toward this end, many doctor's offices and clinics employ a benefits counselor to help patients navigate the insurance maze. Be sure to discuss your ideas and concerns with this individual *before* your bills are prepared.

Here are some tips:

- Don't use "infertility" as a diagnosis. Use instead the *cause* of your infertility, such as endometriosis, endocrine dysfunction, ovarian failure, tubal occlusion, fibroids, polycystic ovaries, or low sperm count. The reason is that insurers are more apt to cover treatment for precise diagnoses than they are for infertility in general.
- Break down a particular procedure into its smallest components. Instead of insemination, for example, which may or may not be covered by your policy, the bill should reflect a series of less costly items such as cervical dilation, mucus check, sperm washing, office visit, and other procedures or charges. Always use as many treatment codes (called CPT codes) as possible.
- Specify dates. If you are having a series of ultrasound scans, blood tests, or office visits, make sure each bill states the date and the individual costs for each, instead of lumping all the scans and tests into a single day's billing.
- Don't overlook the potential to be reimbursed for office visits. If you are seeing your doctor frequently, ask the billing manager to vary the CPT code number of the office visits. Office visits are listed with numbers such as 90020 (initial visit), 90060 (office visit), 90080 (comprehensive visit), and other numbers between 90020 and 90080. Insurance companies are more likely to cover CPT codes that are in the middle range (not initial consultation or comprehensive office visit)—code numbers such as 90030, 90050, or 90060.
- If you are undergoing various procedures over a two- or three-week period, submit insurance claims on different forms in separate envelopes.
- If you are having a first GIFT and you have never had a diagnostic laparoscopy, ask the doctor to perform both procedures at the same time, but bill the surgery as a diagnostic laparoscopy.

Try not to view insurance companies as the bad guys. It's more beneficial if you play their word game, using their parlance in all your verbal and written contact. Remember, your claim is handled by a person who is administering a rigorously designed policy. By following insurance industry rhetoric, you won't call undue attention to your claim. Also remember: Never lie. Outright cheating is insurance fraud. Your goal is to enable your claims to be considered easily and quickly.

Keeping Track of Insurance Payments

If you submit claims in the manner we recommend, within a few weeks your reimbursement checks will begin to trickle in. (Almost all doctors demand payment at the time of treatment and let you play the waiting game.) In some cases, you may have to resubmit claims to major medical or your secondary insurer. It is at this point where the shoe box organization system—the one in which you stick everything into a box—grows into a hurricane of paperwork. The number of claims at different stages of processing can become overwhelming and extremely stressful, especially if you lose or misplace a bill or correspondence.

Lori, a participant in one of our support groups, shared with us her relatively simple system of keeping track of insurance claims. She set up three file folders.

- Folder 1 contains bills that have not been submitted to insurance yet. It is labeled: "Bills to Be Submitted."
- Folder 2 contains bills that have been submitted, but no word has been received concerning their payment. It is labeled: "Bills Pending."
- Folder 3 is for bills that have been reimbursed. It is labeled: "Bills Reimbursed."

As soon as Lori gets a receipt from her IVF clinic, she fills out an insurance form and immediately photocopies both the form and the receipt. The photocopies are for her records, to be used should any question arise. If she can't mail in the claim that day, she places the originals and the photocopies in folder 1.

After she mails in the claim, the copy of the receipt goes into folder 2. When the reimbursement check arrives, or the doctor receives payment from the insurer, Lori staples the check stub or record of payment to the copies of the receipt and insurance form and transfers all documents to folder 3. Lori told us that Getting Organized in this manner helped her keep track of a very complicated process and gave her a welcome sense of control.

Contesting a Claim

If you are undergoing long-term infertility treatment, chances are you eventually will exceed your coverage limit. When this happens, you can contest or appeal the denial of your claim. There are two basic ways of accomplishing this: by telephone or by letter.

Appealing by Phone: Before you make your call, have handy all the relevant information: your policy number, copies of the bills, and notification of denial. Ask the insurance representative to explain why your claim was denied. If the representative is unsure, ask to speak to his or her superior. If the superior cannot make a determination, ask what information you and your doctor must submit to ensure that the claim is covered.

Appealing by Letter: Your letter should state clearly that you want your claim reevaluated because your doctor maintains that the treatment was medically necessary. If you received reimbursement for the same treatment previously, mention that unless the contract stipulates a cash ceiling or a number limit on treatments, insurance cannot stop paying for that procedure if the medical necessity continues. Even if there is a number limit, say three IVFs, explain that the prior procedures were diagnostic in nature and that the information gleaned from those procedures suggested modifications in the current treatment. In addition to your letter, most insurers also require a letter written by your doctor explaining why he or she believes continued treatment is necessary.

Some words of caution: Don't be greedy. If your insurance company paid for a large portion of a treatment, don't push for complete coverage if your co-payment was just a few hundred dollars. One woman who had just undergone a successful IVF got reimbursed in full by her insurer even though the procedure was not fully covered by her policy. The $5,000 reimbursement was a result of some error on the part of the insurer. When the woman received a subsequent $300 bill for the embryo transfer, the clinic's benefits counselor advised her not to submit the bill for reimbursement. This particular bill, with the words "embryo transfer" on it, the counselor explained, might trigger an investigation of the prior claim because embryo transfer is clearly an element of IVF. The woman made a claim on the bill anyway. After a lengthy investigation by the insurance company, the woman was required to repay to the insurer all fees to which she was not initially entitled—a total of $2,500. Even though the woman is thrilled about her pregnancy, she worries about her ability to come up with the money for a second IVF should she want another child.

PSYCHING YOURSELF UP BEFORE, DURING, AND AFTER TREATMENT

Many psychologists tell their infertile clients to be pessimistic. "Don't get your hopes up because if the procedure fails, you will be too disappointed," they warn. Perhaps these psychologists fear that they will somehow be blamed if the procedure fails to result in a pregnancy.

We encourage our clients to be hopeful. We find it hard to imagine how anyone would endure the ordeal of infertility treatments if they believed from the outset that all the pain and sacrifice was to be in vain.

While we tout optimism, we also ask our clients to adopt the realistic view that the procedure might, indeed, fail. We believe that having a good balance of hope and realism has helped our clients better cope with the despair brought on by a failed ART attempt or insemination. Staying hopeful is time-consuming and takes work, but the work of hoping can have a positive impact on your emotional and physical health.

A key ingredient to our philosophy is one of the strategies that permeates this book: Don't Give Up. Infertility specialists agree that both low- and high-tech treatments take time to work, and while your chances of pregnancy are fairly low for each individual cycle, the chances increase dramatically when these attempts are repeated. The vast majority of our clients firmly believe that optimism and hope enabled them to withstand the rigors of treatment.

This is not to say you should continue battling infertility until you are emotionally and financially bankrupt. But neither should you engage in treatment if you aren't able to temper your pessimism with hope. Hope is a powerful motivator. But hope needs to be realistic—not blind.

Models of Hope

People vary in how much weight they give to hope and its counterpart, despair.[7] We present three cases below, each of which balances the prospect of success and possibilities of failure in different ways. Consider these three characters, each of whom is about to have a second ART procedure. Try to decide which of these models best describes you.

Rosie Sunshine: Rosie sees everything through rose-colored glasses. Her hopeful outlook filters out all information that pertains to potential failure. When Rosie undergoes an ART procedure that has a 25 percent pregnancy rate, she tells herself: "I know it will work." She never considers the 75 percent chance that it will fail. She never prepares herself for despair in the event of failure. While she is pleasant company, Rosie is deluding herself. Surely she cannot continue ignoring negative information indefinitely. If her ART procedure fails, her strategy of unabridged optimism could collapse, crushing her will to give it another try. *Rosie hopes for success and denies the possibility of failure.*

Gladys Gloomsbury: Gladys's outlook is steeped in pessimism. Facing the same ART procedure that Rosie tried (with its 25 percent chance of success), Gladys focuses solely on the 75 percent chance of failure. She says: "I'm sure this procedure won't work for me. Other procedures have failed in the past, why should this one work?" In her mind, she changes the failure rate from 75 percent to 100 percent. Psychologically, Gladys has given up. She avoids any information that might remind her that there is a one in four chance of success. Her point of view bodes ill for the future. *Gladys excludes hope from her life and focuses on impending failure.*

Olga Optimistic: Olga pays attention to both success and failure rates. When Olga participates in the ART procedure discussed above, she tells herself: "I'm real hopeful that this procedure will work. Sure, there's a 75 percent possibility that it won't work this time. But there's also a 25 percent chance that it *will* work. And if it fails, I can always try again." She permits herself to entertain negative information, but invests energy in the positive elements. Hers is a mature hope. *Olga hopes for success but accepts the possibility of failure.*

Obviously, the healthiest strategy is Olga's. Like Olga, you need to have hope, but not at the expense of distorting reality. Olga is savvy without being so negative that she can't get out of bed or so positive that she has already furnished the nursery. If you are feeling more like Gladys or Rosie, here are some ways you can begin to see your world through Olga's eyes.

Using the Odds to Help, *Not* Hinder You

As you begin to incorporate hope into your life, you must first learn your personal odds for success. Consider the following scenario. You are about to undergo a GIFT procedure. Your doctor estimates that your odds of becoming pregnant through GIFT are 25 percent for each attempt. Now, 25 percent is not a high probability. In fact, it means that you have a 75 percent chance of failure.

But your doctor also tells you that you must be patient and give GIFT a chance. "If it doesn't work the first time," he tells you, "try it again. I know that your insurance will pay for at least four attempts. I think you should consider that you will try GIFT four times before giving up." He also points out that, although the odds are only 25 percent *on any given try,* in four tries the odds increase to about 68 percent. So if you play the odds, after four attempts, you will have almost a 70 percent chance of success and only a 30 percent chance of failure. Clearly there is a chance of failure, but the odds of ultimate success are certainly worth shooting for.

Next you must change the way you look at the odds to have them to work *for* you, not *against* you. We have developed a simple exercise called Counting Backward to help couples accomplish this goal. Counting Backward helps you Change Your Thinking. Beginning with your first GIFT procedure, say to yourself, "By the end of the year, I have a good chance of being pregnant." Then, if your first GIFT does not lead to a pregnancy, say, "One down, only three more to go until my odds of being pregnant are very high." With each failed procedure, focus on how *your pregnancy is now more likely to happen* rather than focusing on how many times you have failed. The odds, as well as how you look at them, are an important piece of information that can help keep you reality-based, yet hopeful, through repeated attempts at getting pregnant through ART. This tactic works equally well with inseminations and other low-tech treatments.

Hoping Through a Procedure:
Working at Being Realistically Optimistic

The work of hoping is an ongoing process. One important facet of the work of hoping is sequencing the focus of attention from the possibility of failure to the likelihood of success—throughout the progression of treatment. Through sequencing, you can balance hope and realism and avoid being overwhelmed by the enormity of what you are doing. Because so many infertile couples feel they are on an emotional roller coaster, we use that metaphor to divide that roller-coaster ride into four phases:

- Before the procedure: standing on line to board the roller coaster.
- During the procedure: riding the roller coaster.
- Waiting for results: getting off the ride and waiting to either feel invigorated and elated or sick to your stomach.
- Reassessing before the next treatment: psyching yourself up to get back on line for another roller-coaster ride.

Here's how sequencing might go for the GIFT procedure, with its 25 percent chance of success:

- *Before the procedure,* think about the potential for success (25 percent) *and* failure (75 percent). By doing so, you can start on level ground. Say, "Realistically, the odds are more in favor of failure than of success. I'm prepared for that. But I do know that I have a chance for success. Maybe this will be my month."
- *During the procedure* work at being as hopeful as possible. Since you've already allowed yourself to entertain the possibility of failure, you have protected yourself emotionally. Now is the time to let yourself rise to the peak of hopefulness. During the procedure, be as hopeful as possible. Concentrate *only* on the possibility of success. Repeat to yourself: "I know this will work."
- *While waiting for the results,* you must be hopeful but also begin to prepare yourself again for the possibility of failure. You feel yourself slowly descending from the summit of hope you attained during the procedure. The potential for failure begins to loom large

again. Work at focusing predominantly on the positive side, but also entertain a few negative thoughts. Try to say, "I've got a good chance. I know it might fail, but I hope this will be my month."

- *If the procedure fails,* let your negative thoughts flow freely, even if they pull you to the depths of despair. This is your legitimate time to grieve. Give yourself permission to feel sad. At the same time, try to muster some positive thoughts. After a while, those positive thoughts will help you accept the failure and become strong enough to try again. Tell yourself: "I'm so disappointed that it didn't work last month. I need time to deal with this. I'm not giving up, but I'm not ready to make any plans."

Couples who can equip themselves to handle the roller-coaster emotions of infertility treatment are the least likely to suffer the devastation that ill-equipped couples can experience when a procedure fails. By learning to balance hope and reality, you are developing a psychological arsenal to protect yourself from serious emotional wounds.

AN ACTIVITY TO HELP YOU SEQUENCE HOPE AND DESPAIR

This activity will help you do the work of hoping. It requires a significant investment of psychological energy. But the payoff is grand. It can release you from constant worry and brighten your morale.

Stage 1: Prior to the Procedure

1. Collect information that leads you to believe that the procedure may fail. Record this data in a column labeled "Failure Ideas."
2. Collect information that leads you to believe the procedure will succeed. Record this data in a column labeled "Success Ideas."
3. Look over the list, and make sure you've included *more information about failure than about success.*
4. Now write a Getting Pregnant Self-Talk (GPST) statement that is hopeful but realistically reflects a balance between failure and success.

Here is a sample of how to do this. Look it over and use it as a model to fill in your own statements.

Stage of Procedure	Failure Ideas	Success Ideas	GPST Statement
Prior to procedure	Louise had five GIFTs and she still isn't pregnant.	Bonnie kept saying she could never get pregnant, and she just gave birth.	"I know it's a long shot, but maybe this is the month I'll get pregnant."
	I know the chances of failure this first time are quite high.		
	Even if it works, there's still a chance of miscarriage		

Stage 2: During the Procedure

Prepare the statements that you will use for this stage just as you did for Stage 1. The only difference is that you reverse the balance between failure and success ideas. The following table illustrates how you do it.

Stage of Procedure	Failure Ideas	Success Ideas	GPST Statement
During the procedure	(No failure ideas. This is the point where you allow yourself to believe completely in success.)	My doctor has a high success rate with this procedure.	"I just know this is my month."
		My response to Pergonal has never been better.	"I believe I'm going to get pregnant."
		Everything about this cycle is perfect.	"I deserve to have this work finally."

Stage 3: Waiting for the Results

You now must become more realistic. Try developing an equal number of success and failure ideas.

Stage of Procedure	Failure Ideas	Success Ideas	GPST Statement
Prior to getting results	This wasn't my husband's best sperm sample. Maybe that's why it won't work.	My estradiol level was good this time.	"I need to keep hoping that it will work."
	Maybe my endometrium wasn't perfect. I have had difficulty before.	My nipples feel really tender.	"By doing this procedure, I'm upping my odds."
	Sometimes the first test is positive and then you get a negative result the second time.	I had some spotting. Maybe that means the embryo was trying to hook up.	"If it doesn't work this time, it can always work next time."

Stage 4: If the Procedure Fails

At this point, you can give yourself permission to feel disappointed and very sad. Write down statements indicating how badly you feel. You might say, "It will never work," or, "I must be kidding myself. Why do I go on with these treatments?" *No statement at this stage is too negative.* Allow yourself to grieve. But at the same time, keep in mind that after you've given yourself sufficient time to mourn, you can psych yourself back up and board that roller coaster again. Remind yourself that the next ride can end differently.

Incorporating Hope into Your Treatment

We've helped you reconsider your misgivings about ART. We provided information to help you optimize your insurance coverage. We showed you ways to strike a healthy balance between being hopeful and realistic.

The final push must be yours. As you embark on ART, it's your job to find the best way to meet the demands of treatment and to stay optimistic even in the face of failure. Photocopy the following chart. Fill in your chart at the various phases of your treatment. Throughout all the stages of your treatment, never forget that your goal—to conceive and bear a child—deserves every bit of effort you are putting into it.

Enough Is Enough

Even though you have managed your social life, coped with Pergonal injections and repeated doctor's visits, and bounced back from a half dozen or more failed IUIs, you may simply be unable to afford ART either financially or emotionally, under any circumstances. There is no shame in deciding that you've reached the end of the line. If you arrive at this conclusion, you must accept the fact that you may never give birth. It will take a great deal of time and emotional energy to get past this crisis. You and your partner should give yourselves time to heal. Work as a Team to support each other.

Stage of Procedure	Failure Ideas

Charlotte Rosin, past president of RESOLVE of Central Jersey, discusses this so-called resolution phase with great sensitivity in the afterword of this book. We are confident that couples who end treatment at this point will find comfort in her words.

GETTING THE SUPPORT YOU NEED

If you decide to pursue ART, it is vital that you elicit support from others, especially your parents, siblings, and in-laws. Sometimes families can be wonderfully supportive. Two days after one of our clients received an embryo transfer, her mother-in-law asked her to hold the telephone to her belly so she could offer the embryos verbal encouragement to implant. On the other hand, another client told us that her own mother refused to lend her money for ART even though she had set up trust funds for the client's two nieces.

To help sensitize your family to what you are going through, we have prepared a guide that you can fill in, photocopy, and give your family members. Titled "About *(fill in your name here)'s* Infertility," the guide is designed to help open the topic for discussion. Write your name in the appropriate blank spaces to make the guide more personal. You may also rewrite the following pages to express yourself in your own way.

uccess Ideas	GPST Statement

To:_____

*Because you care about_____ and her
happiness.*

_____ knows that you love her and want her to be happy, to be her "old self" again. But lately she seems isolated, depressed, and obsessed with the idea of having a baby.

You probably have difficulty understanding why getting pregnant has colored virtually every aspect of her daily life. _____ hopes that by reading this booklet, written by counselors with both personal and professional experience with infertility, you will better understand the pain she is feeling. The booklet also will tell you how you can help her.

Some Facts About Infertility

It may surprise you to know that *one out of six women who wants to have a baby cannot conceive.* There are many possible reasons for this dismal statistic: blocked fallopian tubes, ovarian failure, hormonal imbalances, husband's low sperm count, to name just a few. Moreover, after a woman turns thirty-five, it becomes difficult to have a baby primarily because many of the eggs she has left are defective.

All these barriers to pregnancy are physical or physiological, not psychological. Tubes don't become blocked because a woman is "trying too hard" to get pregnant. Antibodies that kill sperm will not disappear if a woman simply relaxes. And a man cannot make his sperm swim faster by developing a more optimistic outlook.

Well-Meaning Advice

When someone we care about has a problem, it is natural to try to help. If there's nothing specific that we can do, we try to give helpful advice. Often we draw on our personal experiences or on anecdotes involving other people we know. Perhaps you recall a friend who had trouble getting pregnant until she and her husband went to a tropical island. So you suggest that _____ and her husband take a vacation, too.

_____ appreciates your advice, but she cannot use it because of the physical nature of her problem. Not only can't she use your advice, the sound of it *upsets her greatly*. Indeed, she's probably inundated with this sort of advice at every turn. Imagine how frustrating it must be for her to hear about other couples who "magically" become pregnant during a vacation simply by making love. To_____, who is undergoing infertility treatment, making love and conceiving a child are unrelated now. You can't imagine how hard she's been trying to have this baby and how crushed she feels every month she learns that she's failed again. *Your well-meaning advice is an attempt to transform an extremely complicated predicament into a simplistic little problem.* By simplifying her problem in this manner, you've diminished the validity of her emotions, making her feel *psychologically undervalued.* Naturally, she will feel angry and upset with you under these circumstances.

The truth is: There's practically nothing concrete you can do to help _____. The best help you can provide is to be understanding and supportive. It's easier to be supportive if you can appreciate how being unable to have a baby can be such a devastating blow.

Why Not Having a Baby Is So Upsetting

Women are reared with the expectation that they will have a baby someday. They've thought about themselves in a motherhood role ever since they played with dolls. A woman may not even consider herself part of the adult world unless she is a parent. When _____ thinks she cannot have a baby, she feels like "defective merchandise." Not having a baby is literally *a matter of life and death.* In the Bible, Rachel was barren. She said to Jacob "Give me children or I die..." (Genesis 30:1.) Commenting on this, some sages said, "One who is childless is considered dead." So powerful are the feelings connected with barrenness that the person feels dead or wants to die.

Worse, _____ *is not even certain* that she will never have a baby. One of the cruelest things one can do to a person is give them hope and then not come through. Modern medicine has created this double-edged sword. It offers hope where there previously was none— but at the price of slim odds.

What Modern Medicine Has to Offer the Infertile Woman

In the past decade, reproductive medicine has made major break-throughs that enable women who in the past were unable to have children to now conceive. The use of drugs such as Pergonal can increase the number and size of eggs that a woman produces, thereby increasing her chances of fertilization. In vitro fertilization (IVF) techniques extract a woman's eggs and mix them with sperm in a "test tube" and allow them to fertilize in a laboratory. The embryo can then be transferred back to the woman's uterus. There are many other options as well.

Despite the hope these technologies offer, they are a hard row to hoe. Some high-tech procedures are offered only at a few places, which may force _____ to travel great distances. Even if the treatment is available locally, the patient must endure repeated doctor's visits, take daily injections, shuffle work and social schedules to accommodate various procedures, and lay out considerable sums of money—money that may or may not be reimbursed by insurance. All of this is preceded by a battery of diagnostic tests that can be both embarrassing and painful.

Infertility is a highly personal medical condition, one that _____ may feel uncomfortable discussing with her employer. So she is faced with coming up with excuses whenever her treatment interferes with her job. Meanwhile, she is devoting considerable time and energy to managing a mountain of claims forms and other paperwork required by insurers.

After every medical attempt at making her pregnant, _____ must play a waiting game that is peppered with spurts of optimism and pessimism. It is an emotional roller coaster. She doesn't know if her swollen breasts are a sign of pregnancy or a side effect of the fertility drugs. If she sees a spot of blood on her underwear, she doesn't know if an embryo is trying to implant or her period is about to begin. If she is not pregnant after an IVF procedure, she may feel as though her baby died. How can a person grieve for a life that existed only in her mind?

While trying to cope with this emotional turmoil, she gets invited to a baby shower or christening, learns that a friend or colleague is pregnant, or she reads about a one-day-old infant found abandoned in a Dumpster. Can you try to imagine her envy, her rage over the inequities in life? Given that infertility permeates practically every facet of her existence, is it any wonder why she is obsessed with her quest?

Every month, _____ wonders whether this will finally be her month. If it isn't, she wonders if she can muster the energy to try again. Will she be able to afford another procedure? How much longer will her husband continue to be supportive? Will she be forced to give up her dream?

So when you speak with _____, try to empathize with the

burdens on her mind and on her heart. She knows you care about her, and she may need to talk with you about her ordeal. But she knows that there is nothing you can say or do to make her pregnant. And she fears that you will offer a suggestion that will trigger even more despair.

What Can You Do for _____?

You can give her support and not criticize her for any steps she may be taking—such as not attending a nephew's bris—to protect herself from emotional trauma. You can say something like this:

I care about you. After reading this booklet, I have a better idea about how hard this must be for you. I wish I could help. I'm here to listen to you and cry with you, if you feel like crying. I'm here to cheer you on when you feel as though there is no hope. You can talk to me. I care.

The most important thing to remember is that _____ is distraught and very worried. Listen to what she has to say, but do not judge. Do not belittle her feelings. Don't try to pretend that everything will be okay. Don't sell her on fatalism with statements like, "What will be will be." If that were truly the case, what's the point of using medical technology to try to accomplish what nature cannot?

Your willingness to listen can be of great help. Infertile women feel cut off from other people. Your ability to listen and support her will help her handle the stress she's experiencing. Her infertility is one of the most difficult situations she will ever have to deal with.

Problem Situations

Just as an ordinary room can be an obstacle course to a blind person, so can the everyday world be full of hazards for an infertile woman—hazards that do not exist for women with children.

She goes to her sister-in-law's house for Thanksgiving. Her cousin is breast-feeding. The men are watching the football game while the women talk about the problems with their kids. She feels left out, to say the least.

Thanksgiving is an example of the many holidays that are particularly difficult for her. They mark the passage of time. She remembers what came to mind last Thanksgiving—that the next year, she would have a new son or daughter to show off to her family.

Each holiday presents its own unique burden to the infertile woman. Valentine's Day reminds her of her romance, love, marriage—and the family she may never be able to create. Mother's Day and Father's Day? Their difficulties are obvious.

Mundane activities like a walk down the street or going to the shopping mall are packed with land mines. Seeing women pushing baby carriages and strollers strikes a raw nerve. While watching TV, _____ is bombarded by commercials for diapers, baby food, and early pregnancy tests.

At a party, someone asks how long she's been married and whether she has any kids. She feels like running out of the room, but she can't. If she talks about being infertile, she's likely to get well-intentioned advice—just the thing she *doesn't* need: "Just relax. Don't worry. It will happen soon." Or, "You're lucky. I've had it with my kids. I wish I had your freedom." These are the kinds of comments that make her want to crawl under the nearest sofa and die.

Escape into work and career can be impossible. Watching her dream shatter on a monthly basis, she can have difficulty investing energy in advancing her career. All around, her co-workers are getting pregnant. Going to a baby shower is painful—but so is distancing herself from social occasions celebrated by her colleagues.

The Bottom Line

Because she is infertile, life is extremely stressful for _____. She's doing her best to cope. Please be understanding. Sometimes she will be depressed. Sometimes she will be angry. Sometimes she will be physically and emotionally exhausted. She's not going to be "the same old _____" she used to be. She won't want to do many of the things she used to do.

She has no idea when, or if, her problem will be solved. She's engaged in an emotionally and financially taxing venture with a low probability of success. The longer she perseveres, however, the greater her chances of pregnancy become.

Maybe someday she will be successful. Maybe someday she will give up and turn to adoption, or come to terms with living a child-free life. At present, though, she has no idea what will happen. It's all she can do to keep going from one day to the next. She does not know why this is her lot. Nobody does. All she knows is the horrible anguish that she lives with every day.

Please care about her. Please be sensitive to her situation. Give her your support—she needs it and wants it.

CHAPTER NINE

THIRD PARTY PREGNANCY: MEDICAL AND PRACTICAL CONSIDERATIONS

FOR MANY would-be parents, the desire to have children is intertwined with the wish to pass their genes on to the next generation. Part of the joy of parenthood is having a son or daughter with your eyes, nose, hair color, and even a semblance of your personality.

Unfortunately, some couples are incapable of conceiving a child who carries both the husband's and wife's genes. Fortunately, modern medicine can give them the next best thing: a baby with either the wife's or husband's hereditary makeup. The rest of the baby's genes come from a *third party donor.* The fetus may be carried by the wife or by a surrogate. The sperm donor may or may not be known to the infertile couple. It's even possible for the wife or a surrogate to carry a pregnancy spawned in a test tube with both donor sperm *and* a donor egg.

As part of our Educate Yourself Pointer, this chapter covers the various forms third party donations can take, the legal and financial considerations involved, how to find a clinic or agency that specializes in third party donations, and other nuances and risks involved in achieving pregnancy by use of a third party.

THERAPEUTIC DONOR INSEMINATION (TDI)[1]

What Is TDI?

TDI—the use of donor sperm when the husband's sperm is inadequate—has been used as a treatment for male infertility for more than a hundred years.[2] An estimated thirty thousand babies are born annually in the United States as a result of TDI.[3] Of all the third party procedures described in this chapter. TDI has the highest success rate and is the simplest to accomplish, medically speaking.

One reason for TDI's popularity is its versatility. Donor sperm can be used in cervical inseminations, intrauterine inseminations, during natural menstrual cycles, or during cycles stimulated by fertility drugs. Donor sperm can even be used with in vitro fertilization. In fact, if your doctor determines that all or part of your infertility is male-factor-related, you can substitute your husband's sperm with that of a fertile donor in any of the low- or high-tech procedures described in earlier chapters of this book.

Who Qualifies?

TDI is the only option for the wives of males who are completely without sperm (azoospermic). TDI is also a treatment option for males whose semen is oligospermic (few sperm present), but you may want to use donor sperm only if you have tried unsuccessfully to get pregnant with your husband's sperm using various kinds of inseminations or advanced reproductive techniques. The one circumstance in which couples may go directly to TDI is when the husband has a genetic defect he does not want to risk passing to his offspring.

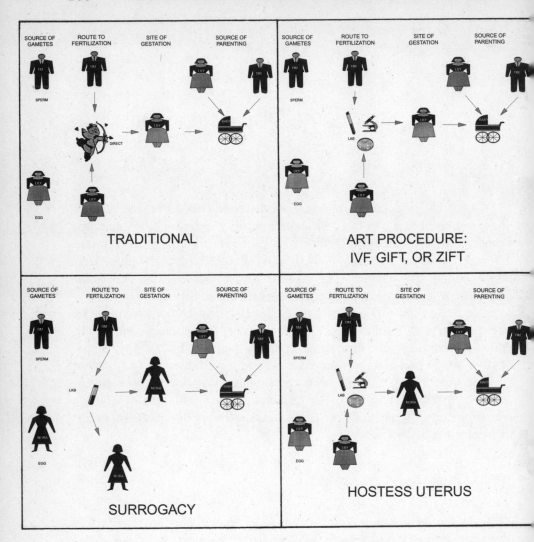

Figure 9.1

PATHS TO PARENTHOOD

This figure depicts the various paths to parenthood. Each path involves four variables:

- The source of the gametes
- The route to fertilization
- The site of gestation
- The source of parenting

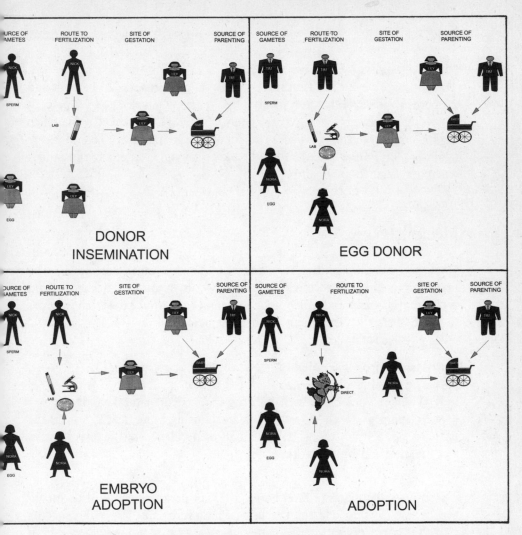

DONOR INSEMINATION

EGG DONOR

EMBRYO ADOPTION

ADOPTION

The figures allow you to compare each of the options and show you the differences among the different paths to parenthood. For example, compare egg donation and adoption. In egg donation, Tim and Nora provide the gametes. Nora is *not* Tim's wife. The gametes are fertilized in the lab and the resulting embryo is placed in Lily's uterus. Lily gestates and gives birth to the baby. Lily and Tim (the husband and wife) are the parents of the baby. In comparison, in adoption, Nick and Nora provide the gametes. Fertilization takes place naturally in Nora's body. Nora gestates and gives birth to the baby. She then gives the baby to Lily and Tim (husband and wife), who become the baby's parents. PLEASE NOTE: These figures depict "traditional" family units. However, other arrangements are also possible, such as the adoption of a baby by partners who are not married, by partners of the same sex, or by a single parent.

Success Rate

Most women who conceive with TDI do so within the first six cycles. The success rate for the first three cycles ranges between 20 percent and 25 percent per cycle. After six months of trying, more than 70 percent of women who try to get pregnant using TDI succeed. Statistics demonstrate continuing success even after six months.[4] The message again is Don't Give Up. You need to keep trying as long as your spirits and your finances will allow.

Medical Issues

Once you have opted for TDI, there are several other decisions to be made. In making the following choices, we urge you to Work as a Team with your husband and voice your preferences to your physician in order to be a Partner in Treatment. You must decide:

- The type of insemination (intracervical or intrauterine);
- The number of inseminations per cycle;
- Whether your cycle will be drug-induced or natural; and
- Whether you will monitor your cycle using home test kits or at the doctor's office using a combination of ultrasound scans of your ovaries and blood work.

You also may be asked to choose whether donor sperm will be mixed together with your husband's sperm. Mixing tends to lower the success rate, but some doctors believe that there is a psychological benefit of thinking that your husband's sperm, helped by the donor's, was the ultimate sperm that impregnated you. Other doctors ignore potential psychological benefits and refuse to mix the sperm, saying that the husband's sperm may cause an antibody reaction in the donor sperm. If your doctor feels this way, you and your husband can certainly have intercourse on the night after the insemination. Then you can choose to believe that the donor sperm cleared the pathway and your husband's sperm fertilized the egg.[5]

One decision you need not make is whether to use fresh or frozen donor sperm. Since the AIDS epidemic, the American Fertility Society has developed insemination guidelines that all but eliminate the use of fresh sperm.[6] All reputable sperm banks test donors for HIV, keep HIV-negative donors' samples frozen for six months, then retest the donor before allowing the sperm to be used. Six months between collection and retesting allows any HIV virus in the donor to produce enough antibodies to be picked up by an AIDS test. The only time that fresh sperm is used is when the donor is known (such as your husband's brother) to the recipient, and the donor is known to be free of the HIV virus.

Practical Decisions

SELECTING A SPERM BANK

Most large metropolitan areas have at least one sperm bank. But even if there is no sperm bank nearby, be assured that sperm banks routinely ship their frozen sperm in freezerlike thermos containers right to your doctor's doorstep. A list of selected sperm banks, addresses, and telephone numbers appears at the end of this book.

As you shop around for a sperm bank, ask whether it tests all donors not only for HIV, but also for syphilis, gonorrhea, hepatitis, and chlamydia. The bank also should tell you whether the donor has ever fathered a child in the past. Many sperm banks are members of the American Association of Tissue Banks, an organization that provides quality screening. You can also ask the bank to do genetic studies called *karyotyping* to learn whether a donor you are considering has some hidden genetic disease or defect. If the bank refuses, you may wish to take your business elsewhere.

Cost, while fairly standard, is another consideration, but not one that should deter you from proceeding. A typical cost is $350 for two vials of sperm. Your doctor may also charge a $100 storage fee to keep your sample until you are ready for insemination. No sperm bank guarantees that the sample you choose will get you pregnant, nor is your health insurance likely to cover the cost of the sample itself. High cost does not guarantee that the sample will work nor does low cost mean that you are getting a less potent sample.

Often your doctor may only work with one or two banks. If you are unhappy with the screening process of those banks, ask your doctor to find you another bank or to use sperm from the one you have selected.

As we have advised, *be assertive*. You may wish to bring up other issues of screening, such as the minimum sperm motility they find acceptable or the overall success rate of the bank or a particular donor's success rate. Remember, just because a man provides sperm to a sperm bank, it doesn't necessarily mean his sperm is capable of fertilizing an egg.

According to the American Fertility Society guidelines on donor insemination, the sperm bank should stop selling the sperm of one man after his sperm have resulted in ten pregnancies.[7] If only ten babies from any given donor are born, there is a low probability that these offspring will meet and marry. You may want to buy enough sperm for a series of inseminations or to ensure that you can use the same donor again if you want another child.

SELECTING A SPERM DONOR

The manner in which information is provided varies little from sperm bank to sperm bank (See Figure 9.2 for one example). Sperm banks assign a number to each donor and provide the prospective recipients with a list of donors' characteristics. The kind of information provided typically includes a donor's height, weight, ethnic origin, body build, skin color, eye color, hair color, blood type, career or college major, education, and hobbies.[8] A few sperm banks will provide additional information, including personality type, results of psychological or cognitive testing, career of parents, or reasons for donating sperm.[9] It helps to learn as much as possible about the donor, but if you are confident that the bank is highly selective to begin with, then you know that all the donors accepted by the sperm bank have numerous desirable traits.

Legal Considerations

The official view is that your husband is the legal father of the TDI-conceived child. Currently, twenty-nine states have laws on donor insemination that make the consenting husband the legal father of a TDI baby.[10] It is nevertheless important to protect yourself and your future child with a legal document that can be used should a custody or child support battle loom in your future. The most common agreements, signed by the couple, the doctor, and another witness, if you so choose, state that:

DONOR LIST

Complete Donor Medical History Available Upon Request

Specimen Releases Quarantined 180 Days
Donors Tested Monthly for HIV & STD

Donor	Race	Ethnic Origin Mother	Ethnic Origin Father	Religion	Skin Tone	Hair	Txt	Eyes	Hgt	lbs	ABO	Rh	Bone Size	CMV	Ed	Occupation	Hobby
1010	CAU	PUERT RIC	DOMINICAN	CATHOLIC	M	BRN	C	HAZ	6.2	195	O	P	L	N	15	STUDENT:LAW	SPORTS-READING
1030	CAU	SPANISH	FRENCH	CATHOLIC	M	BLK	W	BRN	6.0	165	O	P	M	N	14	STUDENT:ENGINEER	TRACK/FIELD-SWIM
1100	BLK	AFRICAN	AFRICAN	BAPTIST	M	BRN	W	BRN	5.8	148	A	P	M	N	16	MILITARY OFFICER	FOOTBALL-BOXING
111	CAU	GERMAN	ITALIAN	CATHOLIC	F	BRN	S	BRN	5.9	160	A	P	M	N	16	FOREMAN	SKIING-POOL
12	CAU	FRENCH	GERMAN	PRESBYTERIAN	M	BRN	S	BRN	5.10	170	A	P	M	N	16	INTERIOR DESIGN	SWIMMING-TENNIS
175	CAU	ITALIAN	ITALIAN	CATHOLIC	M	BRN	S	BRN	5.11	185	O	P	M	N	16	DENTAL SALES	SKIING-READING
188	CAU	IRISH	HUNGARIAN	CATHOLIC	M	BRN	S	BRN	5.10	175	A	P	M	N	14	JEWELER	FITNESS-READING
200	CAU	SICILIAN	SICILIAN	CATHOLIC	M	BLK	S	HAZ	5.8	170	O	P	S	N	16	COMPUTER SALES	BROADCASTING
220	CAU	IRISH	GERMAN	CATHOLIC	M	BRN	S	GRN	5.7	150	O	P	S	N	16	COMPUTER SALES	SPORTS
266	CAU	CZECHOSLO	ITALIAN	CATHOLIC	M	BRN	S	GRN	6.0	230	O	P	L	N	14	DISPATCHER	ASTRONOMY-WOODWK
30	CAU	ITALIAN	IRISH	CATHOLIC	F	BRN	W	BRN	5.11	180	O	N	M	N	16	MECH. ENGINEER	GOLF-COINS-BOAT
317	CAU	ROMANIAN	RUSSIAN	CHRISTIAN	M	BLK	W	HAZ	5.10	160	B	N	M	N	16	SELF-EMPLOYED	MUSIC-SPORTS
340	CAU	POLISH	GERMAN	JEWISH	F	BRN	S	BRN	5.10	170	O	P	S	N	16	INSURANCE BROKER	SPORTS-MUSIC
366	CAU	ENGLISH	SCOTTISH	NON-SECT	F	BRN	W	BRN	5.9	140	AB	P	S	N	16	FINANCIAL SERVICE	RUNNING-FISHING
377	CAU	ITALIAN	ITALIAN	CATHOLIC	M	BRN	S	BRN	6.0	215	O	P	M	N	16	PROPERTY MANAGER	SPORTS
395	CAU	NORWEGIAN	SICILIAN	CATHOLIC	M	BRN	W	BRN	5.10	175	O	P	M	N	16	STUDENT:FINANCE	SPORTS
404	CAU	GERMAN	SCOTTISH	PROTESTANT	F	BLD	W	BLU	5.10	170	A	N	M	N	18	BIOCHEMIST	MUSIC-SPORTS
414	CAU	IRISH	DANISH	CATHOLIC	F	RED	S	BRN	5.9	175	A	P	M	N	15	STUDENT:ECONOMICS	SAILING-SPORTS
42	CAU	GERMAN	GERMAN	LUTHERAN	F	BLD	W	BLU	6.2	220	A	P	S	M	15	COMPUTER ANALYST	AUDIO/VIDEO
430	CAU	IRISH	GERMAN	CATHOLIC	M	BLD	C	BLU	6.0	158	O	P	M	N	15	GEN. CONTRACTOR	BOATING-GUITAR
440	CAU	ITALIAN	ITALIAN	CATHOLIC	M	BRN	S	BRN	5.7	171	B	P	M	N	13	REGISTERED NURSE	READING-RUNNING
450	CAU	ITALIAN	NORWEGIAN	CATHOLIC	M	BRN	S	BRN	6.0	165	B	P	S	N	16	STUDENT:BUSINESS	BICYCLING-SKIING
485	CAU	CZECHOSLO	GERMAN	PRESBYTERIAN	F	BLK	S	BLU	6.0	175	B	N	L	N	16	AUTO MECHANIC	SPORTS-CARS
62	CAU	GERMAN	IRISH	PRESBYTERIAN	M	BRN	S	BLU	6.0	200	A	N	M	N	16	SELF-EMPLOYED	ALL SPORTS
633	CAU	POLISH	ITALIAN	JEWISH	M	BLK	C	BRN	6.3	180	A	P	M	N	19	STUDENT:MEDICAL	READ-MUSIC-POETRY
645	CAU	ITALIAN	IRISH	CATHOLIC	M	BRN	S	BRN	5.6	165	B	P	S	N	14	JEWELER	SKIING-SWIM-TRAVEL
655	AMA	JAPANESE	IRISH	CATHOLIC	M	BLK	S	HAZ	5.11	179	O	P	M	N	16	MECH. ENGINEER	BODY BUILDING-ART
675	CAU	SWEDISH	POLISH	CATHOLIC	M	BRN	W	GRN	5.11	195	B	P	S	N	19	STUDENT:ENVIR.ENG	SPORTS
690	CAU	ITALIAN	ITALIAN	CATHOLIC	M	BRN	S	BLU	6.5	210	O	P	L	N	16	RECREATION DIRECT	SPORTS-FISHING
735	CAU	IRISH	DANISH	CATHOLIC	M	BLD	S	BLU	5.11	170	O	P	M	N	16	BIOLOGIST	BIKE-SOCCER-SWIM
755	CAU	POLISH	IRISH	CATHOLIC	F	BLD	S	BLU	5.10	175	A	P	S	N	14	STUDENT:BUSINESS	SPORTS-MUSIC
800	CAU	ITALIAN	IRISH	PROTESTANT	M	BRN	W	BRN	5.9	170	O	P	M	N	17	STUDENT:MEDICAL	TENNIS-PHOTOGRAPHY
855	CAU	PORTUGUES	PORTUGUES	CATHOLIC	M	BLK	S	BRN	6.2	210	AB	P	L	N	14	TRUCK DRIVER	TROP FISH
870	CAU	CANADIAN	IRISH	EPISCOPALIAN	M	BRN	S	BLU	6.0	171	O	F	M	N	16	POSTAL SERVICE	GOLF-TENNIS

Abbreviations

Race: CAU-Caucasian BLK-Black ORN-Oriental
ASN-Asian AMA-Amerasian

Skin Tone: F-Fair M-Medium D-Dark

Hair Color: BLD-Blond BRN-Brown BLK-Black RED-Red

Hair Texture (Txt): S-Straight C-Curley K-Kinky W-Wavey

Eye Color: BLU—Blue BRN-Brown HAZ-Hazel GRN-Green

Weight (lbs.): Weight in pounds

Height (Hgt)-Feet-Inches
Blood Type (ABO): A B AB O
RH: P-Positive N-Negative
Bone Size: S-Small M-Medium L-Large
CMV (IgM): P-Positive N-Negative
Ed: Education # of Years

AATB accredited sperm bank.
New York State licensed sperm bank.

Figure 9.2

- Any children produced by TDI will be the couple's own legitimate children and heirs;
- The couple waive forever the right to disclaim such children as theirs; and
- The agreement will be confidential among couple and doctor.

Of course, any agreement is only as good as the parties involved. No legal document can ensure emotional attachment to your baby. Only a positive, loving attitude, commitment, and couple unity can do that.

Your doctor will probably provide you with an agreement form. Here's a sample agreement. Always remember, however, that you are in the procedure together. If you Work as a Team, you will significantly reduce the stress related to selecting a donor, undergoing the procedure, and waiting for the results.

OVUM DONATION

What Is Ovum Donation

As women age, so do their eggs. An egg of a twenty-five-year-old is more likely to be fertilized than an egg of a forty-year-old. Even though countless women in their forties have used their own eggs to give birth to healthy infants, the eggs in some women—no one knows how many—are no longer viable, or perhaps never were to begin with.

For some of these women, obtaining an egg, or ovum, from a donor is the answer. The procedure entails harvesting eggs from a donor and giving them to the recipient to be fertilized either inside or outside her body. It is vital that the ovum donor and recipient synchronize their menstrual cycles. The donor eggs are fertilized with the husband's sperm through any of the advanced reproductive techniques (GIFT, IVF, ZIFT) discussed in Chapter 7. Depending on the procedure used, the embryo is either placed into the wife's uterus or implants there after being fertilized in one of her own fallopian tubes.

To optimize the chance of success, doctors generally want the donor to produce a large number of eggs in a given cycle before they perform a harvest surgery. Some donors produce sixteen or more. To generate this many eggs, the donor takes the fertility drug, Pergonal, followed by

THERAPEUTIC DONOR INSEMINATION: RECIPIENT CONSENT FORM

We, _____, hereinafter designated wife, and _____, hereinafter designated husband, authorize Dr. _____, and his/her designated assistants to perform one or more artificial inseminations on wife with the sperm obtained from an anonymous donor designated by code # _____ from the _____ sperm bank, for the purposes of making wife pregnant.

The anonymous donor we select must have the following characteristics: _____. We have been informed that donor # _____ has the aforementioned characteristics. We hold the _____ sperm bank responsible for the accuracy of their description of these donor characteristics. We have been informed that the _____ sperm bank has investigated the background of donor # _____ and to the best of its knowledge has determined that neither he nor his immediate family have a history of any physical or mental defects. We have been further informed that the _____ sperm bank has tested donor # _____ for acquired immune deficiency syndrome (AIDS) prior to obtaining his semen sample. We have also been informed that this semen sample has been frozen for at least six months and that at least six months after the first AIDS test, donor # _____ was tested for AIDS a second time. We have been informed that the results of both of these AIDS tests on donor # _____ were negative. We are aware that any pregnancy carries the risk of birth defects and that approximately 4 percent of the children born to healthy parents have physical or mental defects. On the basis of the accuracy of the information concerning the characteristics of the donor as specified above, and on the basis of the testimony of sperm bank _____ that donor # _____ shows no family history of physical or mental defects and on the basis that donor # _____ had two negative tests for HIV, we agree not to hold Dr. _____ or his/her designated assistants or sperm bank _____ responsible for any defects in a child born as a result of this insemination. We also understand that within the normal population, approximately 20 percent of all pregnancies result in miscarriages and that this may occur after therapeutic donor insemination as well. Similarly, obstetrical complications may occur in any pregnancy. This agreement is not a contract to cure infertility nor a guarantee of conception. Therefore, in accordance with the conditions stated above, we do hereby absolve, release, indemnify, protect, and hold harmless from any and all liability Dr. _____ and his/her assistants from any or all liability for the mental or physical nature or character of any child or children conceived or born as a result of this therapeutic donor insemination procedure.

We understand that, if a woman is artificially inseminated with the consent of her husband, the husband is treated in law as if he were the natural father of a child thereby conceived.

It is further agreed that from conception, I _____, as husband accept the act of insemination as my own and agree:

a. That such child or children conceived or born shall be my legitimate children and heirs of my body, and
b. That I hereby waive forever any rights that I might have to disclaim or omit the child or children as my legitimate heir or heirs, and
c. That such child or children conceived or born shall be considered to be in all respects, including descent and distribution of my property, a child or children of my body.

Husband_____   Wife_____

Date_____, 19____   Witness_____

_____o'clock ___. M.

I consent to the above doctor-patient relationship _____
                                                                    (Doctor)

an injection of hCG, the same protocol used with women undergoing IVF.

The first successful ovum donor procedure occurred in 1983. In the early years, women undergoing in vitro fertilization donated eggs in excess of those they needed for their own fertilization. However, with the development of cryopreservation techniques, these potential donors now opt to freeze their excess embryos for use in future cycles. A second early source of eggs was women undergoing tubal ligation; these women often traded the eggs made in a stimulated cycle for the cost of their ligation surgery. This source too has diminished. Other early egg donors were sisters or cousins of infertile women.

The supply of available donors has not kept up with demand. So in the past few years several IVF facilities began to incorporate an ovum donor program component to recruit young, fertile women willing to give their eggs to infertile couples. Because it is illegal in most states to sell organs or eggs, these donors participate out of kindness, receiving a relatively small fee for their time and inconvenience. (Typical fees for the ovum donor range from $1,500 to $2,000.)

At first glance, ovum donation seems like the female version of sperm donation. Yet because of the drugs, the monitoring, and the invasiveness of the retrieval, as well as the newness of the procedure, ovum donation is truly a pioneer venture. Deciding that ovum donation is for you, locating a program, selecting a donor, synchronizing your cycle—these and other decisions and hurdles all await you. Cost is also high—fees for the drugs, the medical monitoring of both you and the donor, egg retrieval of the donor, embryologist and laboratory fees, and embryo transfer into your uterus can run as high as $12,000. But if you qualify medically and psychologically and you can pay for the procedure, this third party pregnancy option can help you get pregnant when you thought you couldn't.

Who Qualifies?

Ovum donation can help you get pregnant if:

- You have been diagnosed with premature ovarian failure, i.e., your ovaries are not functioning even though you are in your twenties, thirties, or early forties; or
- You have undeveloped ovaries, no ovaries at all, or your ovaries

have been affected by radiation or other medical treatments for illnesses unrelated to infertility; or

- You have a genetically defective trait that you don't wish to pass on to your offspring, such as hemophilia; or
- You are in your late thirties or early forties and have had at least three or four failed in vitro attempts and you or your doctor suspect that many of your eggs are not viable; or
- You are menopausal, but in excellent health.

To receive a donated egg, you must have a healthy uterus, be able to respond to drugs that stimulate the natural estrogen/progesterone cycle, and appear medically able to carry a baby to term. Egg recipients have been as young as twenty-three or as old as fifty-seven.

Success Rate

Reported success rates vary dramatically, as do the statistics for all in vitro attempts. If you have no other fertility problem except a lack of viable eggs, you have about a 30 percent chance each cycle of becoming pregnant with a donated ovum.[11] Of course, if you have additional difficulties, such as problems with progesterone absorption or with the quality of your donor's eggs, your success rate may drop. Also, when in the cycle the procedure is done can affect your rate of success.[12] As in all IVF procedures, your odds of success increase with each attempt. Ovum donation, one of the newer additions to the third party pregnancy menu, seems likely to be a major success in the 1990's.

Medical Considerations

CYCLE SYNCHRONIZATION

The key factor here is to ensure that both the donor and the recipient be at mid-cycle at about the same time. The protocol to achieve synchronization is fairly standard. The table below gives an example of one standard protocol, if the recipient still has ovarian function. If the recipient has no ovarian function, synchronization can occur more easily.

Day of Recipient Cycle	Day of Donor Cycle	Recipient Protocol	Donor Protocol
Day she gets her period			
Next day		Begin Lupron, continuing until donor gets hCG injection	
	Day 21	Continue Lupron	Begin Lupron
	next 6 days	Continue Lupron	Continue Lupron
	next day	Continue Lupron; begin estrogen	Continue Lupron
	Day 1 of period (within next 6 days)	Continue Lupron and estrogen	Continue Lupron
	Day 3 of new cycle	Continue Lupron; gradually increase estrogen dosage	Continue Lupron; begin Pergonal
	Day 12 of new cycle	Continue Lupron and estrogen	Stop Pergonal and Lupron; take hCG injection
	Day 13 of new cycle	Stop Lupron; continue estrogen; begin progesterone	
	Day 14 of new cycle	If doing GIFT, have GIFT procedure; continue estrogen and progesterone	Eggs retrieved; end of involvement
2 days later		If doing IVF, embryo transfer; continue estrogen and progesterone	
Next 2 weeks		Continue estrogen and progesterone	
Day 14 after GIFT or Day 12 after IVF		Pregnancy test; if positive, continue estrogen and progesterone for next 12 weeks	

In essence, Lupron shuts down both the donor's and the recipient's natural FSH/LH function so that their cycles can be artificially stimulated. Everybody's cycle is slightly different. These factors remain fairly constant:

- Both donor and recipient continue taking Lupron throughout the entire protocol, until the donor gets her hCG injection.
- The donor should not begin taking Pergonal until the recipient is taking estrogen for at least four days.
- The length of the artificial follicular phase (taking estrogen) of the recipient is not important; what is important is when the recipient adds progesterone.
- No transfer can take place unless the endometrium is adequately prepared with estrogen and progesterone.
- Estrogen can be taken in the form of patches (Estraderm) or by mouth (Estrace), as long as the estrogen is natural, not synthetic. Usually the program prescribes one or the other.[13]
- Progesterone can be taken by injection, in vaginal suppository form, or by mouth; any form is acceptable as long as the progesterone is natural, not synthetic.

Almost always prior to going through the actual cycle, the recipient must participate in a test cycle to ensure that her estrogen and progesterone levels can be manipulated with drugs. Although a successful test cycle does not guarantee a successful procedure, it rules out certain recipient candidates. At various points during this experimental cycle, you will have your blood tested and your endometrium scanned with ultrasound. You will complete this cycle with an endometrial biopsy.

Practical Considerations

SELECTING A PROGRAM

By 1995, we believe, many in vitro fertilization programs will have an ovum donation component up and running. If your IVF center does not have an ovum donor component, ask when it will, or ask the staff to help you locate such a program. When you select a program, use the same selection criteria you used when selecting an IVF program, with these additional elements. The program should:

- Demonstrate that it can synchronize cycles;
- Have a pool of anonymous donors who meet the minimum requirements for gamete donation as developed by the American Fertility Society;

- Provide counseling during and psychological testing prior to the procedure; and
- Be able to document success rates that are satisfactory to you.

SELECTING AN ANONYMOUS OVUM DONOR

Because egg donors are less plentiful than sperm donors, don't expect to get a list of potential ovum donors from an IVF center. Instead, you will be asked to list characteristics that are important to you, and the program will attempt to find someone who meets some of your essential requirements. Most programs will present one donor to you at a time. Often they will try to find someone who has some physical traits and even personality traits of you or your husband. You will be told about the potential donor's medical, educational, and family history, and you can either accept or reject her. If you reject her, be prepared to wait until the program finds a more suitable donor. A good ovum donor coordinator should be able to match you with a suitable donor in just one or two tries. And remember, any person who is willing to undergo so much to help a couple she doesn't even know already has demonstrated a helping spirit, courage, and perseverance—all desirable traits.

FINDING AN OVUM DONOR

If the IVF program near you has no pool of anonymous donors, you may have to find your own donor. In the past, the largest group of identified donors were sisters, cousins, or close friends of the infertile woman. Since not every potential ovum recipient has a relative or friend who is willing or able to provide eggs, many infertile women have begun networking through friends at churches, synagogues, or universities. Some even take out classified ads to find egg donors. (Interestingly, many couples in their forties who wish to find an identified donor of the right age—twenty-one to thirty-five, for most programs—tell us that they have no relatives or friends in the right age group.)

We advise all our clients seeking an ovum donor to spread the word in their circle of friends and acquaintances. If no volunteers surface, try placing ads in college newspapers or daily or weekly newspapers in your community.

When you find a candidate, set up a face-to-face meeting with her. This enables you and your husband to size up her looks, intelligence, interests, education, family background, and medical history—information you will use to make your selection. You may want to provide a written description of the donation procedure using relevant sections of this book. Also have handy some Pergonal vials and needles; once most potential donors have seen the needles, they are less fearful of the injections. During the interview, be truthful and realistic in terms of the time commitment involved.

Potential ovum donors ask questions in three basic categories: the procedure itself, other women's motivation to become a donor, and you—your fertility and theories of child-rearing. Be prepared to answer questions concerning the number and site of Pergonal injections, potential side effects, how blood monitoring and ultrasound feel, the number and timing of trips to the IVF center, the retrieval operation, and anesthesia.

Although your ovum donation program will carefully screen your donor, you can save time and money by screening out donors on your own. Based on 1990 guidelines issued by the American Fertility Society for sperm donors (there are no guidelines for ovum donors), we urge you to find out whether your potential egg donor engages in behaviors that put her at risk for AIDS; whether she has had a sexually transmitted disease within the last six months; and whether she has a family history of asthma, juvenile diabetes, epilepsy, hypertension, psychosis, or a severe vision or hearing disorder. To get an indication of how fertile her eggs might be, ask her about past pregnancies, abortions, menstrual history, and exercise habits. If she has irregular periods and engages in massive amounts of exercise, you have grounds for ruling her out. If, however, you feel sold on this particular person, your doctor can perform tests to medically determine whether she is good donor potential.

Developing a Legal Agreement with a Known Donor

When you give birth as a result of a donated ovum, you are the child's legal mother. The law does not consider the source of the egg in determining motherhood. This concept must be clear in the donor's mind. She must understand that she is providing a biochemical contribution to you and your husband, not giving you a baby. She must agree to give up all claims, present and future, to her eggs and to any embryos that are made with these eggs.

Because ovum donation is relatively new, few legal precedents exist to help you develop a contract. As of this writing, no ovum donor has

AGREEMENT BETWEEN:

Recipients: MARIA AND CARLOS RUIZ
                  and
Donor: KAREN SILVERA

Karen Silvera, hereinafter referred to as the *donor,* agrees to participate, freely and without duress, with the couple, Maria and Carlos Ruiz, hereinafter referred to as the *recipients,* in an ovum donor procedure, hereinafter referred to as the *procedure.* The procedure will take place at Gotham Hospital in New York City. The procedure is tentatively scheduled to take place during September/October 1993.

The donor agrees to participate in activities required to accomplish the procedure. These activities include, but are not limited to:

1. using drugs prescribed by the Gotham medical staff. These drugs may include, but are not limited to:

   a. Lupron
   b. Metrodin
   c. Pergonal
   d. antibiotics

2. having these drugs administered by means of injections;

3. having her blood levels and ovarian follicles monitored through blood tests and ultrasound on the days designated by the Gotham medical staff;

4. having her eggs aspirated and retrieved at Gotham Hospital on the day determined by the Gotham medical staff;

5. donating these eggs to the recipients for use exclusively by them in an in vitro fertilization (IVF) procedure;

6. agreeing to allow any embryos not transferred during the time of the procedure to be frozen and transferred in a subsequent transfer attempt.

The recipients agree to pay the entire cost of the donor's medical expenses in conjunction with the procedure. These costs include, but are not limited to:

1. diagnostic tests;
2. blood level monitoring;
3. ultrasound monitoring;
4. psychological counseling prior to the procedure;
5. all fertility and other prescribed medications;
6. operating room and anesthesia costs;
7. egg aspiration and retrieval costs;
8. cost of freezing any nontransferred embryos;
9. cost of any medical or hospital expenses arising in connection with any complications resulting from any aspect of the procedure.[15]

The donor will *not* be responsible for any of the financial costs of the procedure.

The recipients agree to provide to the donor, at no cost to the donor, the appropriate medications and injection materials (including needles). Recipients also agree to be responsible for injecting the donor, should she so desire, and to provide her with the necessary information about the date and time of each injection.

The recipients agree to pay to the donor the sum of $2,000 after the egg retrieval for her participation in the procedure. However, should the Gotham medical staff cancel the procedure through no fault of the donor, the recipients agree to pay the donor $1,000 for her participation.

The donor agrees to adhere to the timetable for the procedure established by the Gotham medical staff. This timetable includes but is not limited to:

1. injection dates and times;
2. dates and times of blood and ultrasound monitoring;
3. date and time of egg retrieval.

The donor understands that her pregnancy potential is greatly increased during the month of fertility drug administration and agrees to use condoms/diaphragm both prior to and after egg retrieval, until she menstruates at the end of the stimulated cycle.

The donor agrees to take no other drugs or medications, including aspirin and vitamins, except those approved by the Gotham medical staff during the stimulation cycle.

The donor understands that she is making a biochemical contribution to the potential embryo of the recipients. Consequently, the donor agrees to make no current or future claim to any baby of the recipients resulting from the embryo transfer(s) from this procedure. Also, the donor understands that she is not responsible in any way, financially or emotionally, currently or in the future, for the support or well-being of any child resulting from the embryo transfer(s) from this procedure.

Finally, the donor understands that the recipients recognize and acknowledge her altruistic contribution in participating with them in this procedure.

_____ (Date)   _____ (Witness)

                                                  _____ Karen Silvera, Donor

                                        _____ Maria Ruiz, Recipient (wife)

                                        _____ Carlos Ruiz, Recipient (husband)

made a claim on an infant born from this procedure.[14] You should protect yourself nonetheless. Here is a contract (using pseudonyms) we think you might use. Before you use it or modify it, we advise you to consult an attorney.

SURROGACY

A surrogate mother is a woman who is artificially inseminated with the sperm of a man whose wife is infertile or otherwise unable to carry a pregnancy. In this procedure, both the ovum and the uterus are provided by the surrogate. After the child is born, the surrogate gives the child to the husband and wife, who had legally adopted the infant before it was born.

Another, less common type of surrogacy involves an IVF procedure, during which an egg is aspirated from the wife and fertilized by the sperm of the husband in a petri dish. The resulting embryo is placed into the uterus of the *surrogate gestational mother* (hostess uterus), who carries the baby for nine months and gives birth.

Even though surrogacy has produced more babies than ovum donation or even embryo-freezing techniques, there have been few articles written on the medical procedure and the psychological ramifications of surrogate motherhood.[16] Only when a surrogacy contract fails and a heated custody battle ensues has the media paid close attention to the topic.

Who Qualifies?

According to the American Fertility Society 1990 publication on *Ethical Considerations of the New Reproductive Technologies,* the primary criterion for surrogacy is the inability of the woman to provide either the genetic or gestational component for childbearing. So if you have had a hysterectomy combined with the removal of your ovaries, you are a candidate for this procedure.

If you are unable to carry the baby, you might also wish to consider surrogacy. If you have, for example, severe hypertension, a uterine malformation, or the absence of a uterus, you can participate in either of the two surrogacy options. If you and your husband wish to provide the genetic material, you can create an embryo to be transferred into the uterus of the surrogate.

A third category of candidate is a woman whose ovaries are not present because of removal for medical reasons unrelated to infertility or are not functioning for a variety of reasons, such as premature ovarian failure. Also in this category is the woman who does not wish to risk passing on a genetic defect. If you have ovarian problems or defective genetic traits, you may wish to consider surrogacy. But before you do, do not rule out the ovum donor procedure just discussed. That newer procedure can enable you to experience pregnancy and childbirth as well as control the uterine environment for the growing fetus, neither of which are possible with surrogacy.

A word of caution: The American Fertility Society encourages couples to get a complete medical workup before they consider surrogacy. It is their belief that couples who have fertility problems that could be helped by drugs, surgery, IVF, or other alternatives may be employing a surrogate because they do not realize that they have other options. They also point out their reservations concerning career women using a surrogate to avoid the inconvenience of pregnancy. It is our belief that any woman who does not wish her life to be disrupted by pregnancy will certainly not wish her life disrupted by a child and will most likely be an unfit mother.

Success Rate

As in all other third party pregnancy procedures, the popularity of surrogacy is growing. No statistics are available concerning the percentage of couples attempting surrogacy who eventually take home a baby. Keep in mind that medically it can take several insemination or implantation attempts before the surrogate gets pregnant, and if she doesn't, the couple can find another surrogate. The American Organization of Surrogate Parenting Practitioners reports 1,200 live births via surrogate mothers in the United States, the majority of them since 1980. Of these 1,200 births, seven surrogates have kept their babies and twenty couples report that they are experiencing custody difficulties. Thus 98 percent of surrogacy births are uncontested.[17]

Not counted in the aforementioned statistics are the number of surrogate pregnancies arranged informally among friends or relatives or by the growing number of entrepreneurs entering the field. In any case, the rate of success can usually be increased if all parties have psychological support, legal advice, and a sound legal agreement. Be aware, however, that several states have begun the process of banning paid surrogacy. For example in June 1992, the New York State Assembly passed a law banning surrogate parenting for pay. Also in 1992, a Michigan court upheld a ban on paid surrogacy.[18]

Ethics of the Procedure

Polls show that the general public takes a dimmer view of surrogate mothering than it does of the other third party procedures discussed in this chapter.[19] Be aware of potential negative reactions from friends and family members as you decide whether surrogacy is for you.

Infertility itself can put a tremendous strain on a marriage. But unlike the other third party procedures, surrogacy demands that an outsider become part of your life for at least nine months. Working as a Team, therefore, is critical to keeping your marriage on solid ground. Often the relationship with your surrogate doesn't end at the time of birth. Particularly when the surrogate is a friend, she may become part of your extended family. People opposed to surrogacy fear its potential to destroy or undermine a marital bond. On the other hand, pro-surrogacy organizations report that couples who have used a surrogate rarely divorce (only 1 percent of them have, compared with a 49 percent divorce rate in the general population).

You also must think about your potential child, both medically and psychologically. On the medical side, you must be able to trust your surrogate to avoid drugs and alcohol while the fetus is developing. So far, the American Fertility Society has reported no unhealthy children born to surrogates as a result of substance abuse.

The psychological risks to the future child are complex and largely unknown. It's unclear at what age a child can grasp the notion of surrogacy. Even before you can share the specifics, be sure to emphasize the fact that he or she was a wanted child. Whether fully or half biologically yours, the child certainly will have questions about the surrogate's identity and may even wish to meet her someday. It is wise to figure out how you will handle your future child's inquiries *before* he or she is born.

Medical risks to a surrogate are no different than overall pregnancy risk. Psychological risks are more difficult to assess. Even though most surrogates receive a fee, sometimes as high as $10,000, you should make sure that the surrogate was neither coerced nor solely motivated by money. Surrogacy offers women a chance to be altruistic and to experience pregnancy, which most surrogates report are the main incentives.

Working with an Agency

Unless you already know a woman willing to carry your child, you'll probably want to work with a surrogate agency. While most agencies do all the legal work and medical arrangements, they charge the recipients an enormous fee, which is not covered by insurance. Agency fees can run from $2,500 to $20,000, excluding prenatal care and childbirth, which is paid for by the adoptive couple.

In selecting an agency, look for one that *carefully* screens surrogates and is willing to tell you its screening procedure. If its rejection rate of surrogate applicants seems too small, go elsewhere, no matter how charming its director is. We stress this point because many agencies are notorious for scrimping in this area, a situation that can lead to emotionally and financially devastating custody fights. So, Educate Yourself by interviewing several agencies, and Make a Plan by talking to others who have participated in a surrogacy arrangement and by developing personal guidelines for surrogacy selection. A good agency will provide several references and offer guidance in making your selection.

Once you choose your surrogate, the agency should:

- Facilitate and coordinate meetings;
- Arrange and coordinate a schedule of medical and psychological evaluations;
- Recommend legal counsel for both parties involved and provide a model contract;
- Coordinate medical procedures;
- Act as intermediary between the couple and the surrogate;
- Provide ongoing psychological support for both parties and their families;
- Monitor the pregnancy; and
- Counsel couples on the impact of surrogacy on their social interactions.

To Know or Not to Know Your Surrogate

Most couples select their surrogate, so the issue of anonymous versus identified surrogacy is usually not a factor. What does become a factor, however, is whether you should meet, talk, and have a relationship with your surrogate, or whether you should have as little contact as possible. Some couples end up establishing a relationship that is somewhere in between.

The more involved you are with the surrogate prior to the birth, the more likely you are to have a continuing relationship with her after the baby is born. Be aware that some surrogates have difficulty breaking the bond with the baby, especially if she contributed half of its genetic material.

What Your Surrogate Will Be Like

According to the American Fertility Society, the average age of paid surrogates is twenty-five. More than one half are married, one fifth are divorced, and about one fourth are single. More than 50 percent are Protestant and 42 percent are Catholic. More than one half are high school graduates and more than one quarter went to college. Other studies indicate that 96 percent had at least one previous pregnancy and 80 percent had at least one previous live birth.[20]

Surrogates' motivations vary. Some who have had abortions or had given up a baby for adoption view surrogacy as a way to absolve themselves of guilt or relive the pregnancy experience in a more positive way. Others are adoptees or know someone who is adopted and want to make a childless couple happy. Or they know other infertile couples and simply wish to help. Almost all surrogates report that they have had easy pregnancies and enjoy being pregnant. Many surrogates report that they need the money received to enable them to stay home while pregnant and care for their own young children.

Whether you meet your surrogate or select her through photos, it's important that you like her looks and feel comfortable about her other attributes. Most importantly, you must feel that she can be trusted and is willing to carry your child for the right reasons.

Developing the Contract

Because the success of surrogacy depends more on legal issues than on medical ones, be sure you have a solid contract. Your surrogate must sign the contract before she becomes pregnant, not after. The reason for this is that the surrogate is to be paid in exchange for her help in creating a child, not in exchange for your taking possession of an already existing child. The contract signing must be witnessed by a third party, and you and your surrogate must have different attorneys.

EMBRYO ADOPTION

The newest third party pregnancy option is embryo adoption, a procedure in which an embryo, produced by another couple, is transferred into the womb of another woman whose uterus has been prepared through drug and hormonal therapy. The primary source of these embryos are those that have been frozen and stored when they were not needed by couples undergoing IVF. Because these couples have had several pregnancies from a particular batch of embryos and no longer wish to pay to keep them "on ice," they donate their frozen embryos to another infertile couple. As in adoption, the baby is genetically unrelated to the couple. Unlike adoption, the adoptive mother gets to experience pregnancy and childbirth.

Who Qualifies?

Although anyone can adopt an embryo, it is most likely to occur when:

■ You are unable to produce your own eggs and cannot find an egg donor; or
■ You have had many failed attempts at in vitro fertilization using your own or donated eggs, and there is no clear-cut reason for these failures.

Success Rate

Because so few such procedures have been recorded, there is no data about the success rate. It is possible that the success rate could equal the success rate of other frozen embryo transfers.

Practical and Ethical Issues

FINDING AN EMBRYO TO ADOPT

Many IVF clinics are developing embryo adoption programs out of necessity. IVF America, for example, affectionately calls their proposed program "The Full Tank Program." This approach is bound to become more popular in years to come.

Another way to find embryos is to contact couples directly. Through RESOLVE Inc. or other infertility support groups, you may meet couples who are willing to have their embryos adopted. Before donating frozen embryos, however, the couple must be certain that they have had as many successful pregnancies as they want through the program. Feel free to inquire about their intentions.

"WHERE DID I COME FROM, MOMMY?"

On the surface, embryo adoption seems less emotionally complicated than adoption of an infant, since the biological mother has no contact whatsoever with the fetus or the newborn. But there are unique aspects to embryo adoption that can pose difficulties, particularly in the area of telling your future child about his or her origins. There is no research on the psychological impact of embryo adoption on these children, since carrying a fetus completely unrelated to you or your spouse is still an extraordinarily rare phenomenon.

Fortunately, books on rearing adopted children are plentiful. When the time seems right, explain things in a way he or she can understand, perhaps noting that, like you, the child is a pioneer of sorts. Eventually, your child may ask about his or her biological parents, siblings, and, of course, the embryo adoption procedure itself. Although answering such questions will be hard, try to explain about the procedure as simply as possible and only tell your child as much as he or she can understand. And, of course, always stress how much you and your husband wanted to have him or her for your child!

CHAPTER TEN

THIRD PARTY PREGNANCY: THREE COUPLES' STORIES

By THE TIME you begin considering a third party pregnancy, you have probably endured months, if not years, of frustration trying to have a baby. The temptation to throw in the infertility towel and adopt a child—or give up trying to become parents entirely—may be stronger than ever. Many couples who easily moved from Clomid to Pergonal and then from IUI to IVF draw the line at using a third party procedure. Not surprisingly. When faced with the possibility of having a baby that is conceived or gestated in a nontraditional, highly controversial way, adoption is certainly a safer, more acceptable alternative. And adoption is the answer for many couples who want to expand their families.

Yet some infertile couples still don't want to relinquish their *pregnancy* quest. In this chapter, we present three stories from actual couples who took the third party pregnancy route. We show how they coped by using elements from our Nine Pointers and our Getting Pregnant Workout. We urge you to read this chapter, as well as Chapter 9, *before* you decide to attempt any of these procedures, even if someone in the medical community has been quick to propose one of them to you. The baby made through a third party procedure will be part of your life forever, so give yourself time to prepare.

While none of the couples' stories will fit your situation precisely, they reveal many common emotions inherent in third party pregnancies. We tell these stories in the hope that they will serve as role models of how to keep emotionally healthy while engaging in these pioneering reproductive methods. As with the other anecdotes used in this book, we have changed the names to protect our clients' privacy.

MICHAEL AND SUSAN

Michael and Susan are in their forties. Michael has two daughters, ages twenty-one and fourteen, from his previous marriage. This is Susan's first marriage. When they took their vows in 1989, Susan and Michael intended to have a baby as quickly as possible. After six months of failing to conceive, they sought medical attention.

Their formal diagnosis is unexplained infertility, but Susan's doctor surmised that her eggs are probably of poor quality because of her age. During the last two years, Susan has undergone seven IUIs, two GIFTs, two IVF procedures, and two frozen embryo transfers. No pregnancies resulted.

After these failures, Susan read an article in a woman's magazine about ovum donation, a new procedure in which younger, healthier donor eggs are used with a husband's sperm to make embryos that are placed into the woman's uterus. Despite their continued failures to make a baby, Susan and Michael are eager to give ovum donation a try. They are prime examples of a couple who Don't Give Up.

Before proceeding, however, Susan and Michael spent several months actively contemplating ovum donation. Of critical importance for Susan and Michael, and probably for many couples considering any of the third party options discussed in this chapter and the last, was comparing the third party procedure to adoption. In telling this particular story, we point out how adoption and ovum donation compared for Susan and Michael. We believe, however, that every couple feels differently about this issue. For many couples, adoption is clearly the right choice. For Susan and Michael, *not* to pursue adoption at this time was the better option. We present their decision-making charts as models for your own.

Because Susan and Michael had used the decision-making activity many times before during other critical junctures in their treatment, they found it to be helpful for this decision as well. They sat down together and began to compare ovum donation to adoption. First, they made a list of all the factors that were important to them in their quest for parenthood, in terms of both adoption and the ovum donation procedure. Then they assigned a grade from 1 (worst) to 10 (best) to indicate how each option (adoption or third party) affected that factor.

Factor	Choosing Adoption	Choosing Ovum Donation
1. Potential for the couple to make a genetic contribution.	1	10
2. Potential to control the environment of the growing fetus.	3	9
3. Opportunity to personally experience a pregnancy.	3	10
4. Probability of success.	9	6
5. Availability of role models.	10	2
6. Social acceptability of the procedure.	10	2
7. Cost.	2	2

The very process of making the list stimulated discussion and helped the couple begin to explore their feelings and think clearly about the two options. Looking at their chart, they drew their first conclusion—that the only factor on which the two options were similar was their high cost, upward of $10,000. Next, Susan and Michael assigned a weight from 1 (least) to 10 (most) to the importance of each factor. This weighting reflected how the couple viewed both the good points and the bad points of each item on their list. For Susan and Michael, the four most important factors were: potential to make a genetic contribution to the pregnancy, potential to control the uterine environment during pregnancy, personally experiencing the pregnancy, and probability of success. When they disagreed on how much weight to give a particular item, they talked it over and compromised.

Then they calculated a score for both adoption and ovum donation. To determine each factor score, they multiplied the weight by the rating for each option, then added up the totals.

Factor	Weight for this factor	Grade for adoption	Factor score for adoption	Grade for ovum donation	Factor score for ovum donation
1. Potential for the couple to make a genetic contribution.	10	1	10	10	100
2. Potential to control the uterine environment of the growing fetus.	9	3	27	9	81
3. Opportunity to personally experience a pregnancy.	9	3	27	10	90
4. Probability of success.	9	9	81	6	54
5. Availability of role models.	3	10	30	2	6
6. Social acceptability of the procedure.	2	10	20	2	4
7. Cost.	5	2	10	2	10
TOTAL SCORE			205		345

For Susan and Michael, the total scores indicated that they should proceed with the ovum donor procedure. In addition to helping them make an exceedingly difficult choice with confidence, the process reduced their stress tremendously because they knew they were employing their thoughts and feelings to steer them down a path that was right for them.

Initially, Susan and Michael seemed to find the next step fairly easy. Unlike most couples who decide to use an anonymous donor, Susan and Michael felt confident that they wanted to know their donor. They wanted to know all about their donor and even involve their donor in their lives if the donor felt comfortable with that arrangement. Since Susan had no sisters or cousins of the right age (twenty-one to thirty-five), she began to inquire among her friends. Following the Manage Your Social Life Pointer, Susan and Michael talked to all their female friends in their early thirties, and Karen, one of Susan's closest friends, who had in fact driven Susan home from one previous embryo transfer, agreed to participate.

What happened next was startling and unexpected and threw Susan into a real tizzy. Susan, who believed she could cope with anything, began to have feelings that she found overwhelmingly unsettling. Susan described how she began to see her relationship with her longtime friend Karen changing. Susan started to feel as if she had to "court Karen" and make herself "appealing and desirable" so Karen would feel confident in allowing her eggs to go into Susan's womb. In the several sessions that Susan described what she was feeling, we helped Susan to understand that she did not have to entice Karen to provide the eggs. Karen, like any ovum donor, was a willing and altruistic person. We also helped Susan value her own contribution to the pregnancy: carrying the baby for nine months.

To further cope with the trepidation of having a third party take on such an intimate role in her life, we coached Susan to use mental imagery techniques that focused on the notion that she and Karen were joining forces with Michael to create a team to form a new life. The idea that three people were merging was initially distasteful to Susan. But through some carefully structured guided imagery activities, Susan was able to come to terms with a revised mental picture of her baby-to-be—one that helped her feel connected to the procedure.

"I would relax and conjure up an image of my father playing the piano and me playing the violin," Susan recalls. "I'd take this picture and transfer it to my situation at hand, with Michael at the piano and Karen on the violin. A few minutes after they'd begin to play, Karen would hand me the violin, allowing me to play the middle and ending of the concerto. I felt that if I practiced this relaxing imagery every day, the baby would get the best of both me and my ovum donor. The image makes me feel good and helps me feel like I'm in control, orchestrating the whole thing."

CONNIE AND FRANK

Connie and Frank are in their late twenties. At age twenty-one, before she met Frank, Connie had developed Hodgkin's disease. The prescribed treatment at the time was radiation therapy, which the doctors explained carried a potential risk of infertility as a side effect. Although she wanted to bear children someday, Connie felt she had no choice but to undergo the intensive radiation treatments. At the end of her course of treatment, the doctors felt that Connie had been cured of this once-fatal disease. Unfortunately, the trade-off was the destruction of her reproductive capabilities.

As soon as she fell in love with Frank, Connie leveled with him about her inability to have children. "I'm marrying you for you, not your eggs or your uterus," Frank responded. Not surprisingly, Frank and Connie have a wonderful marriage and they would like to have a large family. Since both her ovaries and her uterus were exposed to radiation therapy, Connie seems to be unable to produce eggs or carry a baby. Before taking steps toward adoption, however, Connie and Frank decided to explore surrogacy as an option.

Connie and Frank tried to be open-minded about surrogacy, but also allowed themselves to Get in Touch with Their Feelings. Despite the relatively long history of surrogate parenting, it still carries a social stigma for many people. Connie thought it best to deal with her macabre feelings by "jumping right into the procedure and beginning the search for a surrogate." By seeing what the people were like—the agencies and the surrogates—Connie felt that she "would feel everything, both the good and the bad."

After developing a list of agencies throughout the country and then interviewing two agencies within a hundred miles of their home in New Jersey, Connie reported back to Frank that her "gut instinct" was to look for an agency outside the metropolitan area. Together they decided to seek out a surrogate from the Midwest. Connie felt that women from the Midwest were "more down-to-earth" than the Easterners and "would become a surrogate for better reasons." Also, Connie wanted the surrogate to look different from her so that "Frank wouldn't have to feel he was doing it [having sex] with my substitute," she said. "I wanted a blonde, not a little Italian girl like me for our surrogate." Clearly, the couple had begun to Make a Plan.

Based primarily on its comparatively low fee, location, and compassion, the couple selected a surrogacy agency in the Midwest, which then helped them select a suitable surrogate. Connie and Frank paid the agency $2,500 up front, started a fund of approximately $5,000 to cover medical expenses for the surrogate, and put a $10,000 fee into an account for the surrogate, who would receive that money once the couple had custody of the baby. Both Frank and the surrogate had all the appropriate medical tests and all three the psychological screenings. When the surrogate's cycle was ready, Connie and Frank would fly from New Jersey to the Midwest, and Frank would produce a semen sample in a doctor's office where the surrogate would be inseminated.

To keep control over negative feelings during all the tests, ovulation and airplane schedules, and pregnancy/no pregnancy results, Connie tried to remain in touch with how she was feeling—which was often excited and sometimes "a little scared." Connie also reported that she tried hard to stick to her plan—which included overseeing the legal work and accompanying Frank to the insemination. All along the way, Connie was straightforward with her family and friends about why she was pursuing surrogacy. Paramount to the couple, she would explain, was that "the baby would be genetically connected to Frank." Being honest and forthright precluded the gossip and embarrassing questions that might have plagued Connie and Frank otherwise.

MARILYN AND STAN

Marilyn and Stan are in their thirties. They have been trying to get pregnant for more than four years. Doctors have diagnosed their problem as a low sperm count and even lower motility of Stan's sperm. Clomid and other drugs failed to improve his sperm quality or quantity. Doctors believed that Stan was not a candidate for a varicocelectomy.

After many cycles of various combinations of drugs and IUIs, Stan and Marilyn's doctor suggested they try inseminating Marilyn with sperm from a sperm bank. Stan initially liked the idea; Marilyn was not so sure. To reach a decision, we helped Marilyn and Stan Work as a Team.

Even though therapeutic donor insemination (TDI) seemed the obvious choice for Marilyn and Stan, neither were able to verbalize what they were feeling. When Marilyn first came to see us, all she could do was cry. Finally, we helped Marilyn understand why she was crying. Knowing why would ultimately help her make a decision. "I just wanted to be like everyone else," Marilyn lamented. "I want to make love and have a baby—Stan's and my baby. I've always been part of the crowd. I never was a nonconformist. Why do I have to consider donor sperm? It's weird and creepy; we're not weird and creepy. We're regular. I want a regular baby."

The perceived strangeness of making a baby with donor sperm plagued Marilyn for many months. She wanted very much for her life to proceed according to a plan that had been stuck in her head since childhood. The fact that this major life goal would not happen in the way it does for most people made Marilyn miserable and depressed. Conforming to the norm was so important that she lost sight of her ultimate goal: having a baby and becoming a parent.

Before she could embrace TDI as an option, Marilyn needed to mourn—for Stan's "crooked smile and his long legs and his skinny hips" her child will not inherit. Although she told us that she had married Stan for his good looks, Marilyn allowed herself to get in touch with what really mattered about Stan—that he was calm and dependable and that he always made her feel special. As she reached resolution concerning TDI, Marilyn decided that even if their baby didn't look like Stan, Stan could be calm and dependable as a parent and make their baby feel special. And since many personality traits are learned, it is entirely possible that her future child will resemble Stan in many ways.

Marilyn balked at our suggestion that she use GPST because she felt it was embarrassing to talk out loud when no one was in the room. So we had her write down a statement describing her grief for Stan's lost biological contribution. We explained that writing can be just as cleansing as talking and that she could keep her statements to share with Stan if she ever felt the need.

Marilyn's statement was simple, but lovely. "I love Stan. I feel that Stan is so much better than me in many ways. He's so smart and so good-looking. I want our baby to look like him. I'm very sad that won't happen. But also, I want my baby to be like Stan: calm and steady, not high-strung and moody like me. With Stan as the father, everything will be all right."

Soon afterward, the couple felt ready. They phoned their doctor, who sent them lists from the two sperm banks he used on a regular basis. Marilyn and Stan chose four donors, all blue-eyed blondes, whose hobbies and education seemed similar to Stan's. A few weeks later, just as Marilyn was due to ovulate, her doctor placed the donor sperm from their No. 1 choice into her cervix and inserted a cervical cap to ensure nothing would spill out: a classic intracervical insemination with donor sperm. Everything went smoothly—until that night when Stan had second thoughts about parenting a child who was not biologically his own.

Stan and Marilyn came to see us the next day. We insisted that they openly discuss all their fears and turnoffs concerning TDI. Marilyn disclosed that she felt as if she had been raped or had been seduced by another man. Stan felt as though he were condoning rape and irrationally feared that Marilyn would run off with the donor even though neither of them even knew his name. Even though Stan was expressing very negative feelings, at least he was expressing himself to Marilyn, something he had not been able to do throughout the whole ordeal.

Luckily, perhaps, Marilyn did not become pregnant that cycle, which gave the couple more time to explore their feelings. They took a month off, decided to remove that particular donor from their selection list, and renewed their marriage vows during a weekend getaway. In a sense, they were purging themselves of their negative feelings in order to begin their efforts with a positive attitude.

As they prepared for the second TDI, they used their GPST skills to develop a script that put them in touch with what they called "their real-life life." They developed a "Toast to Donor 607," and recited it over glasses of nonalcoholic champagne the night before the procedure. Here is what they said:

"We've never met. We know so little about you. But that's more than you know about us. Yet we feel you are with us tonight and will be there to help us tomorrow. Wherever you may be, know that we are grateful to you for helping make our dream come true. Cheers!"

By acknowledging the donor's spirit of giving and verbally expressing their appreciation, Marilyn and Stan no longer saw him as a threat. You too may wish to use a ritual of this sort the night before a third party medical procedure. We've shared this toast with many couples after Marilyn and Stan and they found it a compelling way to thank the donor in spirit as a couple.

GRIEVING FOR A LOST BIOLOGICAL CONNECTION

Before you can openly accept and nurture a third party pregnancy, it's important to grieve for the genetic line you will be unable to pass to the next generation. If you are the one whose line will not be passed down, you must say goodbye, in a sense, to that baby—the one who would have had your dimples or your eyes. By working through your grief, only then can you recognize the many nongenetic characteristics you can give your child.

You probably have asked yourself, "Why me? Why can't I have the same opportunity that other parents have to pass down their traits?'' There are no answers to these questions. Sometimes life is not fair; we urge you to make peace with this injustice. Also realize that deprivation sometimes fosters a greater appreciation for the other opportunities you have. Perhaps because you cannot pass down some of your traits, you will work harder than other parents to set examples for your baby that will teach him or her to be a warm, loving person.

For Susan, grieving the biological loss was relatively easy. Even before she chose ovum donation, she realized that she could pass on her very best characteristics to a child—her appreciation for art and music, her sense of humor—even without being genetically bonded to that child. Susan had the advantage of raising one of her stepdaughters, Jessy, Michael's younger daughter from his first marriage. Although Susan was not Jessy's biological parent, everyone who met them thought that Susan, not Michael, was Jessy's biological parent. Jessy dressed like Susan, told jokes like Susan, and seemed even to look like Susan.

Despite the fact that Susan's and Jessy's features were different, Susan saw herself in Jessy through facial expressions and gestures. When she learned she couldn't have her own biological child, Susan initially was sad. ''I liked myself so much,'' she says, ''I loved my dimples. I thought I was very bright. I wanted my baby to have my dimples and to be smart. I cried for a while, and then I thought about Jessy and what I had done for her. I knew that no matter who contributed the egg, this baby would be terrific. Michael and I would parent this baby in the same way we did Jessy.''

The critical step here is that Susan allowed herself to Get in Touch with Her Feelings—to be sad and to confront what was being lost. Only then was Susan able to get past these feelings and conclude that a major part of parenting is daily interaction with the child as he or she grows up.

Before her ovum donor procedure, Susan engaged in a ritual to let go of grief. A form of GPST, this statement helped Susan bid farewell to her biological contribution and to the genetic connection her beloved late father would have had to the child. Alone, Susan read her statement in her backyard at twilight, her favorite time of day. She performed her ritual as a symbolic gesture on the night before she was to begin her ovum donor cycle.

On page 242 is the activity designed by Susan to help Change Her

Thinking and gain a new, healthy perspective on having children using an ovum donor. You can also use the activity if you are doing a surrogate procedure. With slight modifications, your husband can use it before undergoing TDI.

GIFTS FOR MY BABY

This activity is designed to help you come to terms with the realities of a third party pregnancy. Although each procedure prohibits one of you from making a genetic contribution to your baby, each of you can give your baby some very precious gifts by the examples you set and the ways in which you raise your baby.

You probably have asked yourself, "Why me? Why can't I have the same opportunity to pass down my traits that other parents have?" It is impossible to find answers to these questions. Sometimes life is not fair; all you can really do is make peace with this injustice. On a more positive note, sometimes being deprived can make a person appreciate all the more the opportunities she has been given. Perhaps because you cannot pass down some of your traits, you can work harder than most people to set examples for your baby that will teach him or her to become a wonderful person. This activity helps you to gain perspective on what you can and cannot give to your baby and to feel resolved about this reality.

PREPARING THE LIST OF WHAT YOU CANNOT PASS DOWN GENETICALLY

The first part of the activity helps you to determine what you cannot give your baby and then to put these traits away. In the next part, you determine what gifts you can give by the way you raise your baby and concentrate on these qualities.

List the names of each relative who had a feature that you hoped to pass down to your baby. These features can be physical traits, mental abilities, or characteristics of temperament. Next to this person's name, list the feature you wanted to pass down. We will give an example.

WHAT I CANNOT PASS DOWN GENETICALLY

Name of Relative

Feature This Person Had That I Hoped to Pass Down to My Baby

Aunt Joan — Her wavy brown hair (a physical characteristic)
Dad — His mathematical mind (a mental ability)
Mom — Her boundless energy (a temperament characteristic)

_____ _____

_____ _____

_____ _____

_____ _____

_____ _____

Now do the same for *your own* features that you hoped to pass down to your baby.

Me — My manual dexterity
Me — My creativity

_____ _____

_____ _____

Now fill out the form on page 244 entitled "What I Cannot Give My Baby." If you are having trouble, use Susan's GPST statement as a model.

WHAT I CANNOT GIVE MY BABY

I believe that I have wonderful traits and abilities that I could have passed on genetically to my baby. Many of these traits and abilities came from _____, (an) important person(s) in my life. In preparation for what I am about to do, I am giving myself time to think about all that is good and wonderful and special about _____. I like to think that I am like _____ and can carry _____ with me in my heart. Not just through _____'s genes, but also through what _____ taught me, which helped me to become who I am.

I also believe that I have much that I could have passed on genetically to my baby. I am a _____ person. I have great _____ and a good _____. I hoped that my baby would be all of this—and more—but I will not be able to give my baby my genes. I feel sad that I cannot genetically contribute to my baby. But I will provide this baby the best uterine environment and transfer what I can in utero. And by the way that I raise him or her, I will ensure that this baby can have the best of me. Together with my husband _____, we will raise a baby with a love of life.

Signed_____

Date _____

PUTTING MY GENES AWAY: THE CEREMONY

Now take the signed and dated document, "What I Cannot Give My Baby," to a quiet place where you can be alone. Read the document out loud. When you have finished reading this form out loud, take a few minutes to look at it. Form a picture of this document. Take a special envelope, place the document inside it, and seal it. Then gently and lovingly put it away in a special place.

PREPARING THE LIST OF WHAT YOU CAN GIVE YOUR BABY BY EXAMPLE

Now list those things that you *can* give to your baby by the way you raise her or him and by the example you set for your baby. We will provide some examples.

What I Can Give My Baby:

My honorable character

My love of art

Now, on the following form, "Setting Examples: My Gifts to My Baby," fill in the information you just listed in the appropriate place. Then sign and date the form.

SETTING EXAMPLES: MY GIFTS TO MY BABY

I believe that I have many gifts that I can give to my baby. By setting an example, I can teach him or her to be_____, to love _____, to value _____, and to know how to _____. I can raise my baby with love and build up our baby's sense of self and love of humanity.

Signed_____
Date _____

THE AFFIRMATION CEREMONY

Find a special place in which you can read aloud the "Setting Examples" document you just prepared. Take a long look at the document and form a picture of it in your mind. Then place it in an envelope in a special place that you reserve for important and valued documents.

DEALING WITH THE LINGERING FEELINGS OF LOSS

Even after completing these exercises, there will be moments of grief. You will remember those items you listed on your "What I Cannot Pass Down Genetically" form. Don't fight these feelings. Allow yourself to go with them. Then relax yourself with your deep breathing and picture the "Setting Examples" document and the second ritual. Let the positive statements override the negative thoughts by concentrating on or even rereading the list of gifts you can give your baby.

GRIEVING FOR YOUR SPOUSE'S LOST BIOLOGICAL CONNECTION

Sometimes it's easier to say goodbye to your own lost contribution than to the potentially lost contribution of your mate. It seems that women in particular need time to mourn the loss of their husband's genes. If you are contemplating TDI, you have probably already begun to think about what you find so attractive about your husband. All those physical and temperament characteristics, which have a genetic component, cannot be passed down—genetically at least—to your baby.

At this time, it's important to separate the genetic characteristics from the everyday life skills that your spouse possesses. These skills are the ones that your spouse will rely upon to help shape the growing child and will be the skills your baby will likely learn to imitate.

STRANGE EMOTIONS

As you contemplate a third party pregnancy, unexpected or frightening thoughts may enter your mind. These thoughts are common among the people we counsel. TDI and surrogacy, in particular, carry sexual connotations in the minds of many people unfamiliar with these procedures. Like Marilyn and Stan, for example, you might equate TDI with rape. Hiring a surrogate may conjure up images of your husband having an extramarital affair instead of a doctor simply injecting your husband's sperm into a surrogate's uterus. Perhaps your husband is struggling with the widely held, yet erroneous, belief that a low sperm count diminishes a person's virility or sexual attractiveness. Likewise, you may fear that hiring a surrogate implies to outsiders that you are unwilling to have sex with your husband.

Our advice: Don't try to squelch these unusual or bizarre thoughts. Instead, talk them out with someone—a counselor, a psychotherapist, your husband or a close friend or relative—you trust. Once you articulate your feelings, you can use the information in this book to negate any erroneous beliefs. By thinking of a sperm donation as though it were a life-sustaining blood donation, for instance, you can no longer equate it with rape. You are now viewing TDI in its proper medical perspective.

Strange emotions are part and parcel of third party procedures. Just as physical pain signals you to take protective actions to prevent damage to your body, so do disturbing emotions serve as signals to warn you to work through troubling beliefs. In fact, if you have *not* experienced these strange emotions, you probably have not come to terms with your third party decision. You must be aware that these emotions may revisit you even after the pregnancy is in progress. If you continue to be bothered by recurring bizarre or unsettling emotions, seek advice and support outside your family and circle of friends. In addition to psychologists and other mental health professionals, clergy members and attorneys specializing in reproductive law also may be of help.

RELIGIOUS ISSUES: FINDING THE RIGHT ANSWERS

Susan and Michael practice Conservative Judaism, and they are committed to following traditional Jewish law concerning permissible third party pregnancy practices. So before they made their decision, Michael consulted his rabbi to find out whether ovum donation was permissible under Jewish law. Would a union of his sperm with the egg of a woman to whom he is not married be considered adultery? If so, would their baby be considered a bastard? Would the baby be Jewish if the ovum donor was not?

As it turned out, there were no cut-and-dried answers since Michael's inquiries involved such new scientific developments. The rabbi promised to study the issue.

Several months later, just before the Sabbath, the rabbi phoned Michael with good news. He said he had consulted rabbinic authorities and had determined that the procedure was permissible, and the child would be Jewish since a Jewish woman (Susan) would give birth to it and be the baby's legal mother. The rabbi also determined that ovum donation is not adultery. The donated gamete is treated as though it were a donated organ. The rabbi closed with some wise advice. "Don't concern yourself with the religion of the donor. Instead, try to find a woman who can make a positive contribution to the gene pool you are giving your baby.'' Michael and Susan spent a joyous Sabbath knowing that an important hurdle had been cleared.

Because they agreed not to tell anyone, Marilyn and Stan did not seek the advice of a rabbi before opting for TDI. Even though a rabbi, like a lawyer, is committed to maintaining confidentiality, they felt uncomfortable letting him know of their plan. Rather than asking their rabbi, they read a book, *And Hannah Wept,* by Rabbi Michael Gold,[1] recommended by someone they met through RESOLVE Inc. The book deals with the Jewish perspective on third party pregnancy as well as adoption and child-free living. Reading this book, they learned that a baby born through TDI is considered legitimate. But Rabbi Gold cautions that it is a good idea to use an anonymous donor since he will be unable to claim paternity. Stan and Marilyn were surprised to learn that Gold saw merit in using a Gentile rather than a Jewish donor. Since Jews are encouraged to marry other Jews, the risk of an unwittingly incestuous marriage for the baby is reduced when the donor is Gentile. After reading the book, Stan and Marilyn chose an anonymous Gentile to be their sperm donor.

Frank and Connie, who opted for surrogacy, are practicing Catholics. They talked to Father Francis, their parish priest, who pointed out that in 1987 the Congregation for the Doctrine of the Faith issued a document entitled *Instruction on the Respect for Human Life in Its Origins and on the Dignity of Procreation.*[2] That document set out the Vatican position on assisted reproductive technology. The doctrine expressed sympathy for couples who are unable to have children. But it rejected many aspects of assisted reproductive technology, including third party procedures. According to this document, a child must be conceived through an act of love, which is expressed as sexual intercourse only. This position ruled out artificial insemination *even with the husband's sperm*. The document also suggests that the use of third party gametes can damage family relationships. Surrogacy, therefore, flies in the face of the Vatican.

Frank and Connie felt crushed. Father Francis could see how upset they were. As they walked out of the church, Father Francis shook Frank's hand and whispered, ''Do what's in your heart, and confess it later.'' They followed that advice, but not until after they had suffered much anguish as they wrestled to bring their actions in line with their beliefs.

Problems of religious bioethics are serious and difficult to resolve. Religious leaders as well as laypersons are struggling to find solutions to these problems. Each individual finds peace in his or her own way. Sometimes it is helpful to talk with several clergypersons to get varying words of advice.

LEGAL ISSUES: THE TIE THAT MAY NOT BIND

The legal status of third party procedures has been examined closely by the Ethics Committee of the American Fertility Society. This committee included a professor of law and the project director in medical law of the American Bar Foundation.[3]

Earlier we mentioned how several of the third party procedures connote sexual misconduct. This view was promulgated by laws and legal findings such as a 1954 Illinois decision declaring that a woman who underwent TDI with her husband's consent had committed adultery.[4] A 1963 New York State ruling held that a child born from a TDI procedure to which both husband and wife consented was considered illegitimate.[5]

Much has changed recently, however. As of 1984, twenty-eight states have enacted statutes stating that a child born from a TDI procedure is the legal offspring of the sperm recipient and her consenting husband.[6] In states without such a statute, problems can arise. There is a presumption that without evidence to the contrary, a sperm recipient's husband is presumed to be the legal father. This is fine, providing the husband is capable of producing *some* sperm, regardless of how few or how poor their quality. But if the husband can be proven to be azoospermic (making *no* sperm), a judge may find that he cannot be the father.

For TDI, the husband must sign an agreement consenting to the procedure. There are few, if any, cases of the anonymous donor claiming the child, because he is never told who his sperm is given to or if conception took place. If you use an identified donor, you need a good contract, but as with any contract, the document is only as good as the people who sign it.

For ovum donation, the legal issues are less complicated. The law recognizes that the mother who gives birth to the baby is legally its mother. Nonetheless, for an identified donor, it is advisable to have a legal document. When we prepared for our own ovum donor procedure, we had no model of a legal document to consult. We spoke to several lawyers, and with their advice constructed the agreement, which is similar to the model offered in the previous chapter.

Surrogacy poses a potential legal nightmare, like the famed Baby M case in which Mary Beth Whitehead attempted to claim the baby she bore under contract with a New Jersey couple in the mid-1980s.[7] The same law that protects the recipients of donated sperm or ova puts the recipients at risk if they participate in a surrogacy arrangement. Since the birth mother is considered the legal mother, the woman hiring the surrogate may have a weaker claim on the baby than the surrogate has. Likewise, if the hired surrogate is married, the husband donating the sperm risks having the surrogate's husband declared the legal father. The ideal surrogate candidate is one whose husband has had a vasectomy.

A second legal problem connected with surrogacy concerns payment to the surrogate because such a payment can be construed as child-selling. A Michigan Supreme Court ruled that it is,[8] but a Kentucky Supreme Court ruled it is not.[9] The judge in Kentucky said that the surrogate was not being paid to get rid of an unwanted child, but rather to "assist a person or couple who desperately want a child but are unable to conceive one in the customary manner to achieve a biologically related offspring."

Despite the questionable status of each party's rights in a surrogacy procedure, only about 2 percent of the arrangements fall through. Nonetheless, nobody wants to be the one whose arrangement failed to materialize. If you are considering surrogacy, protect yourself by carefully investigating the agency with whom you will work, as well as spending as much time as possible selecting and getting to know your surrogate. You might also reassure yourself by speaking with an attorney who specializes in reproductive technology and adoption.[10] By Educating Yourself about the potential pitfalls of surrogacy, you may be able to avoid them.

TO TELL OR NOT TO TELL

For third party pregnancy procedures, disclosure, or telling people what you are doing, is at the core of our Managing Your Social Life Pointer. Deciding *not* to tell is usually the more difficult choice. Not disclosing can narrow your options substantially, particularly in terms of finding an identified ovum donor. If you decide not to tell, then you have to take care to select an anonymous donor of the appropriate blood type and ethnic type, and with the right physical characteristics so no one will guess the baby is not fully yours biologically. If you and your husband both have blue eyes, for example, take care to select a donor who also has blue eyes.[11] If you are not concerned about secrecy, then factors like eye color are not important.

Deciding not to tell also affects how much support you can get from family and friends. Certainly, while undergoing TDI, you could say you were being inseminated with your husband's sperm. Likewise, while undergoing ovum donation, you could say you were using your own eggs in an IVF procedure. But tales of deception are hard to keep straight, particularly when you tell half truths. We believe that it is better either to tell no one or to tell everyone. Of those two options, it's easier to tell everyone. Yet many couples decide that they are more comfortable telling no one.

Marilyn and Stan decided to tell no one about their therapeutic donor insemination. "My sister's my best friend. She keeps giving me articles about donor sperm because she knows about how bad Stan's sperm count is," Marilyn says. "And she knows how much we want a baby. I want to tell her we've been having inseminations for four months now. Every month when I get my period, I want to cry to her, but I can't. It's only me and Stan, and of course the doctor, who know. I'm feeling lonely at a time when I should be feeling hopeful." We advised Marilyn and Stan to Work as a Team and develop and stick to the same story when questioned about developments in their pregnancy quest.

Marilyn also was worried about what she'd say if her baby doesn't look like any family member. To ease her fears, we asked Marilyn and Stan to write down some of the comments they expected to hear. Then we urged them to write down and rehearse their responses. This Managing Your Social Life activity seemed to relieve both of them. We have incorporated some of their statements into the following exercise entitled Ready Retorts.

READY RETORTS

People who decide not to disclose their third party pregnancy worry about being caught off guard. Friends, colleagues, and relatives may often ask embarrassing questions or make comments that put you on the spot. Keep in mind that your questioner is probably not trying to be mean. Many people just say the first thing that comes into their head. But you, on the other hand, need to be ready and armed with comments. Just as you used GPST to dispute your negative self-statements, you need to prepare yourself with responses to these questions and comments. We will give you some sample questions and comments and ways to respond to them. Notice that our retorts are not out-and-out lies. You can tell half the story and satisfy your questioner.

1. Together with your husband, read the sample comments and retorts.

COMMENT	RETORT
Well, what a surprise. You said you couldn't get pregnant. What happened?	We showed them, didn't we? We spent all that money on these hotshot experts who said we'd have trouble. But we got pregnant!
Your baby doesn't look like either one of you.	Actually, he looks more like my side of the family. He's the spitting image of my uncle Mel when he was a baby.
You and your wife are such bad athletes. How come your son is the star of the Little League team?	We're lucky I guess. Must be those pediatric vitamins they give nowadays.

2. Think about the questions and comments you may encounter. Here are some situations in which you are likely to have to deal with these comments. Look them over.

Situations:

a. A comment made about differences between the baby's appearance and the parent's appearance.

b. A comment about how you are late to work all the time when you are going for treatment.

c. A question your child might ask you about why he or she has different abilities than you or your husband have.

3. Now, together with your husband, make up a list of comments you think you might have to respond to. Then make up your retorts. Use the table below to list the comments and your retorts.

COMMENT

4. The final step is to use mental rehearsal. Imagine you are actually in each of these situations. Then role-play the situations. Have your husband be the commenter; have him make the comment. Practice making the retort. Then switch roles. You be the commenter and let him make the retort. Try doing it with style! Feel confident and happy.

DECIDING TO TELL

Susan and Michael decided to talk openly about their ovum donor procedure. As in all other aspects of their lives, they felt that discussions provided them with information and that leveling with people gave them feedback. In addition to their rabbi, they discussed the implications of their ovum donation with their mothers, their colleagues, and friends.

Predictably, they got plenty of feedback, both negative and positive.

Therefore, well before the baby was to be conceived, they had ample opportunity to deal with every potential inquiry and judgment and prepare a response. Even though they would have preferred to make a baby the "regular" way, they were not ashamed. And when their first ovum donor procedure had to be canceled because the donor failed to respond to fertility drugs, Michael and Susan received tremendous emotional

RETORT

support from everyone who knew about it, even from those who initially viewed ovum donation as weird. Friends and colleagues could see how much Susan and Michael wanted this option to work for them, and some even offered to help them find another donor.

Susan and Michael also decided to tell their child as soon as he, she, or they (ovum donor procedures often result in multiple births) were able to grasp certain aspects of it. They'd never tell too much too soon. But as soon as the baby was able to listen to stories, about age three or even younger, they'd tell one called "The Right Seed," which they wrote before the baby was conceived. Gradually, as the baby got older, they would share more medically accurate details. We liked their story so much we offer it here for anyone who would like to use it with their third party child. With slight modifications, the story can be adapted for children born through TDI.

THE RIGHT SEED
A Story to Tell Your Donor Baby

It is said that babies wait in a place called Baby Heaven for their Mommies and Daddies to come to get them. When we decided we wanted to have a baby, Mommy and Daddy planted their seeds together in the ground and waited for a stalk to grow so they could climb up the stalk to get you in Baby Heaven. Every month Mommy and Daddy planted their seeds. Some months the seeds would grow into a tiny little stalk, not big enough to get us to heaven to get you. Some months no stalk would grow at all. We were very sad. We knew you were up there waiting for us, but we just couldn't get to you. Our seeds didn't seem to grow right.

Then we had an idea. "What if we looked for a friendly person to help us? Maybe that person could give us some of her seeds to help us make a good strong stalk so we could climb up that stalk and finally get you," Mommy said to Daddy. "Great idea," Daddy said, "let's look around." So we looked and looked. Then we found a very friendly lady who said, "I'll help you. I like to help people. I have good seeds." The lady's name was Karen.

The three of us planted our seeds together and what do you think happened? The seeds grew into the best and strongest stalk. These seeds were the right seeds. The stalk grew way up into Baby Heaven. Mommy and Daddy climbed up the stalk. We were very happy. When we got to Baby Heaven, we were a little worried at first. There were so many babies. "How will we know which one is ours?" Daddy said to Mommy. Mommy reassured Daddy: "We'll just know." And then we saw you. You were standing there smiling and waving at us. You knew too that you were our baby and we were your right Mommy and Daddy. So all of us went down the stalk and moved into our house. We were so happy that we had found the right seeds to grow the stalk. So we could get the right baby. You. You are the baby that was meant for us.

# UNEQUAL CONTRIBUTION

The final, and perhaps the most difficult, aspect of a third party pregnancy is the unequal biological contribution that each of the partners makes. For TDI, the wife supplies the egg, but a donor supplies the sperm. The husband, therefore, makes a "lesser" contribution. For ovum donation, the husband supplies the sperm and a donor supplies the egg. The wife supplies a uterus but no gamete. For traditional surrogacy, the man supplies the sperm, and the surrogate provides the egg. The wife is completely left out, supplying neither the egg nor the womb. Conflicts, therefore, are likely to arise over the inequities of third party pregnancy. By Working As a Team, you are less likely to blame the other person for their inability to provide a gamete or a womb, and instead you will always view the third party pregnancy as it really is—a quest you are pursuing together—with equal stakes in the outcome.

Like so many aspects of third party pregnancy, the psychological ramifications of the unequal contribution may be overlooked until after the baby is born. Then they may hit home with great force. It is necessary for the husband and wife to deal with them in advance and feel comfortable with their contribution. To help you, we have developed an activity entitled Fair Shares.

FAIR SHARES

Here is a list of statements you may say to yourself regarding unequal contribution and retorts to these statements. In the spaces provided (after these examples), you and your husband can each construct your own statements and counterarguments. The examples are based on couples pursuing various third party procedures.

STATEMENT	COUNTERARGUMENT
It's not fair that my husband can make a genetic contribution and I cannot. (*Woman with ovum donor*)	I get to carry the baby for nine months inside me. His contribution only takes a few moments.
I feel like I'm contributing nothing to this pregnancy. My wife is giving her eggs and her uterus, and all I have to give is my consent to a sperm donor. (*Man using TDI*)	I'll never understand why it worked out this way. But I will work especially hard to be a major force in this child's life. In that way, she will reflect me.
When I look at my baby I will see my husband in him but nothing of me. (*Woman pursuing surrogacy*)	I will look at this baby as a unique individual—not as an extension of anyone else. He will be himself.

Now construct your own statements and their counter arguments. Use the boxes below.

STATEMENT	COUNTERARGUMENT

After creating individual lists of statements and retorts, read them to each other, using the active listening skills covered in Chapter 2. Try to communicate empathy for your partner's sense of loss. Don't try to talk him or her out of these feelings. Instead, offer your support and encouragement. If you do this with sensitivity and caring, you can get past this hurdle and may even further solidify your marital bond.

HOW OUR THREE COUPLES FARED

Much to her delight, Susan conceived during her second attempt as an ovum recipient. At this writing, Susan and Michael are preparing for the birth of their twins.

Connie and Frank are getting ready to travel to the Midwest for their surrogate's fifth insemination. They plan to be on hand at delivery. As for Marilyn and Stan, they achieved pregnancy with their second TDI procedure. Marilyn and Stan await the birth of their baby, scheduled to be born just a month after Susan and Michael's twins.

ARE YOU A PIONEER?

As you consider a third party procedure, bear in mind that it is *nontraditional*. Are you willing to be a pioneer? Can you picture yourself taking a path less traveled, being the first in your family or community to trek into the unfamiliar territory of third party pregnancy? The path may be risky but the rewards can be great.

CHAPTER ELEVEN

SECONDARY INFERTILITY: THE LONELIEST KIND

CARRIE, a thirty-two-year-old homemaker and mother of one, was on the verge of tears. She never before sought the help of a psychotherapist, but her problem was growing unbearable.

"I'm sort of embarrassed to say he was an accident because of what's happening now, but he was," Carrie said of her five-year-old son, Bobby, who was conceived shortly after she married Chuck in 1985. "We thought we'd get pregnant just as quickly this time. We started trying when Bobby was two. A year later when I wasn't pregnant, I went to my doctor, who told me we should 'just relax.' We did relax, but I knew something was wrong."

Like tens of thousands of parents, Carrie and Chuck suffer from secondary infertility—the inability to conceive a second child to term and live birth after bearing a first child.[1] There are two types of secondary infertility: one where pregnancy came easily the first time but is elusive the second time; the other where primary infertility plagued the first pregnancy and is resurfacing as the couple try to conceive again. In the latter case, the couple is actually having primary infertility the second time around.

As many as 70 percent of all couples who are infertile already have at least one child, according to a 1988 national survey.[2] Women with secondary infertility, however, are only *half as likely* to seek medical treatment as women with primary infertility, the researcher who conducted the survey discovered. Because these couples already have at least one child, they may believe that either nothing can be done to help them or that they shouldn't tamper with nature.

But the urge to enlarge your family can be just as compelling as the urge to have your first child. And the inability to have more children can be just as psychologically and socially devastating as being childless against your will. Despite the enormous problems it can cause for couples, secondary infertility is arguably the least explored aspect of infertility—medically, psychologically, and socially.

The lack of research in this area leads many busy OB-GYNS to view the secondary infertility patient as a pain or impatient. So many of their patients have second or even third pregnancies that they assume this patient will also conceive. They tend to postpone diagnostic testing that might uncover the problem, or they neglect to prescribe therapy that might solve it.

Outside of the doctor's office, your problem is even less visible. Acquaintances, friends, and even some family members might assume you don't want any more children or that you're simply waiting for the right time to get pregnant again. In the throes of raising two or more youngsters themselves, some friends may be unable to empathize with your plight; they might even envy your relative freedom.

People with secondary infertility often tell us that they have trouble fitting in with any group. They don't feel they're part of the infertile world because evidence of their earlier fertility is scampering around the house. Yet they don't feel they're part of the fertile world either because they can't get pregnant again. It's not unusual for people with secondary infertility to avoid women with children, pregnant women, and babies because it makes them feel blue. The only person you may feel comfortable talking with at this point is another woman with secondary infertility, if you can find one.

If you feel this way, you are what social psychologists define as a "marginal woman," someone who "stands on the boundary between two groups." You do not belong to either group, or you are uncertain of your "belongingness."[3] You have lost membership in the primary infertility group by attaining the dream that these women still long for. How can you ask them to understand the anguish that you feel at not having a second child? Yet you feel you do not really belong to the world of the fertile. They can choose the size of their family, whereas you cannot increase the size of yours.

Many of our clients describe superstitious thoughts and behavior patterns that are fairly unique to secondary infertility. For example, couples may try to re-create the conditions of the first conception by revisiting the romantic restaurant they ate in the night they conceived, by listening to the same music, or even traveling to a distant hotel. Many people with secondary infertility also begin to wonder whether their first child was a fluke. They may even feel they are somehow being punished for not raising that child properly.

Others view secondary infertility as an omen: "Stop trying. Be satisfied with the child you have. Don't tempt fate, or you'll give birth to a defective baby," are some of the notions that wander through their minds.

Yet it's perfectly reasonable to want to expand the size of your family. Carrie and Chuck both came from large families and desperately wanted Bobby to grow up in a similar environment. Carrie grew extremely jealous of fertile women. She also grew angry with herself. In a sense, secondary infertility was appropriately named since it made Carrie feel like a second-class citizen.

While these feelings are common and perfectly understandable, it's important to move beyond them so they don't stand in the way of your treatment and ultimate success. Through this chapter, we will try to help you help yourself out of this rut.

A COUPLE'S PROBLEM

Like primary infertility, secondary infertility is a couple's problem, not an individual problem. Yet more likely than not, the woman struggles alone. The most common reason: Men and women have diverging needs with respect to parenthood. Both want to be parents because parenting confers adult status, among other reasons. And both want to be able to pass on their genetic lineage to the next generation. So when a couple is childless, both the husband and wife feel equally invested in conquering the fertility problem. In most cases, the childless husband is fully supportive of his wife's efforts, needs, and concerns.

After their first child is born, however, most men's parenting needs are fulfilled. Women, on the other hand, may have an entirely different and more enduring image of what a family should be with regard to size. Usually, it is an image of two parents and two or more children. The inability to have a second child distorts that image and leaves a gaping hole in her emotional life.

Not so with many men. For them, a second child is desirable but not critical. Women with secondary infertility, therefore, are more likely to lose their husband's support and are at higher risk for marital conflict.

If that weren't enough, women yearning for more children also may lose the support of friends, relatives, physicians, and women with primary infertility. Friends and relatives often say the wrong things because they cannot comprehend that you have a medical problem. In contrast to the primarily infertile woman, who can elicit sympathy because she has repeatedly failed to conceive despite heroic medical efforts, the secondary infertile woman appears to have living evidence that her infertility problem is all in her head. The most common, and for many, the most exasperating advice women hear is: "Relax, and you can do again what you did before."

THE MEDICAL FACTS

After a year of secondary infertility, Carrie changed doctors. This new physician put her on Clomid and "told me to have sex a lot when I was ovulating," she related. "I wasn't sure I was even ovulating, but the doctor told me I just had to look at Bobby to know I was fertile."

It didn't work. Looking at Bobby with no brothers and sisters only made Carrie cry. "My mother told me I was ruining my marriage and upsetting Bobby because I cried so much," Carrie said. "My younger sister, who has three kids, told me how grateful I should be that I only had to buy one pair of shoes and one load of toys instead of three."

After Carrie failed to conceive after several months on Clomid, her doctor performed some tests, which revealed a fibroid in Carrie's uterus. Since a fibroid may prevent an embryo from implanting, the tissue was removed surgically. Now three years had passed since Carrie and Chuck began trying to have their second child.

Diagnosis had been delayed because Carrie's first two doctors assumed the possibility of a medical problem was remote. As Carrie's case proves, that assumption is not always correct. Most specialists we know agree that there is no one problem typical in the secondary infertility population. In fact, the breakdown of problems mirrors that of the primary infertility population.

It's also important to realize that people's bodies are not static. Couples get older. Their health may have deteriorated. Adhesions and fibroids can develop after a first pregnancy, but not necessarily as a result of that pregnancy. Environmental contaminants, leisure activities, and medications all can contribute to a change in fertility status. If your doctor is still pooh-poohing your infertility a year or more since you began trying for a second baby, it's definitely time to find a specialist who cares.

Even if nothing else in her life has changed, a woman's fertility declines as she ages. The 1988 survey cited previously showed that 8.3 percent of women between ages twenty-five and thirty-four and 8.8 percent of women between ages thirty-five and forty-four had secondary infertility.[4] While the difference between 8.3 and 8.8 may seem small, it actually represents nearly 100,000 additional infertile women.

Their problems may include:

- Poor ovulatory function;
- An increased number of eggs with genetic abnormalities that prevent fertilization;
- Decreased implantation rate caused by these genetic abnormalities or by a poor endometrium caused by hormonal problems;
- Increased pregnancy loss (see Chapter 12).

Life experiences that occurred since your last conception also may have diminished your fertility. Both men and women may be exposed to environmental toxins in their jobs, have illnesses that affect their fertility, or may have taken prescription or even illicit drugs that can hurt their ability to produce a baby.

While researching this book, we met Mandy, who had contracted Hodgkin's disease after her first pregnancy. Even though her medical team tried to modify the radiation therapy to protect her fertility, Mandy's ovaries were damaged by the treatment. We also met Jack, who was treated for Crohn's disease with medications that reduced his sperm count.

Other life experiences can affect fertility temporarily. As already described, men and women who engage in too much exercise or who are under too much stress can have difficulty conceiving until they reduce their activity or stress level. For men, taking too many hot baths or spending long periods in a Jacuzzi can temporarily reduce sperm production. Riding a bicycle or a motorcycle for extended periods can similarly diminish sperm count.

Often these changes are subtle or so integrated into a person's lifestyle that they may be missed as a contributing factor to infertility. Unless they've suffered a devastating illness or a trauma, most people expect their bodies to work as well now as they did three, five, or even seven years ago.

For those in their second bout with infertility, being familiar with treatment doesn't make things easier. In fact, sticking to your treatment protocol while rearing a child can be more difficult than ever. Try taking your temperature religiously every morning when your child is screaming for you in the next room. Or try keeping your five-year-old out of the bedroom when your husband is giving you a Pergonal shot. These are tough challenges. And don't expect much sympathy. People who supported you emotionally during your first round of fertility treatment may find it hard to believe you're doing it all again.

COPING WITH YOUR NEGATIVE EMOTIONS

"Why aren't I pregnant?" Definitive answers to this question are rare. The best most of us can do is guess. A primarily infertile person guesses that the reason is medical. But a woman with secondary infertility is more likely to resort to nonmedical guesses to explain why it worked the first time but not now. Often she will invoke a superstitious or other bizarre explanation.

Primitive cultures feel compelled to use symbols and potions in an attempt to cure childlessness. At the beginning of the twentieth century, infertile women spit to deter the evil eye, slept with an egg under their bed, or kept a child's photograph under their pillow.

The same psychology can propel modern-day infertile people to seek out a magic cure; they will believe in anything—fertility earrings and herbs, astrologers, psychics, fortune cookies, magic nighties, making love on the anniversary of their last conception, sleeping on the same bed sheets—purported to make a difference.

If you act on these impulses, relax. You are not going crazy. You are just trying to find a greater truth or appeal to a greater power, whatever that may be. We know one couple who bought three fertility dolls, two pairs of fertility earrings, one bottle of fertility-inducing mineral water, went to several fortune-tellers, and saved fifty fortune cookie fortunes. Quests for a magic cure can help mask the gnawing fear that maybe a second pregnancy will never happen.

Women with secondary infertility can experience other alien feelings, such as being repulsed by an infant or pregnant women. While such aversions seem logical for those battling primary infertility, it seems less logical (to the outside world) that someone who once had a pregnancy and a newborn can no longer tolerate them in others.

To further explore this phenomenon, we asked a woman in our secondary infertility support group to write down her feelings about fertile women with several children. She wrote: "I *am* a member of your club, but I'm not a member. I *am a parent* (like you) but *I can't have another baby* (so I'm not like you). I want to be like you and I can't, so I hate you for having what I don't. But I can't take responsibility for that hatred without ambivalence because I do have what you have, in part at least." In contrast, the primarily infertile woman can hate another's pregnancy unequivocally because she completely lacks what the other person has.

Another set of contradictory emotions that can plague a woman with secondary infertility is resenting her only child because the child impedes her ability to have a second one. She has difficulty justifying treatment when it means finding a baby-sitter and spending time away from her child. She can afford artificial inseminations but feels angry when her parents say she should be saving the money for her existing child's college education instead. She dreams of a family vacation in Disney World but resents her child's asking for it now when her family is not yet complete. Some women wish their son or daughter would disappear long enough for them to finish their infertility treatments. The guilt, as you might already know, can be debilitating.

As we counseled Carrie and Chuck, many emotions—ones neither ever expected to feel—came out. Carrie admitted that she often felt guilty about wanting a child. Few couples experiencing primary infertility feel that their desire to have a child is inappropriate. They may feel guilty about their behavior prior to their diagnosis of infertility, but rarely do they feel that their wish for a child is unjustified. On the other hand, couples with secondary infertility often feel that one should be enough.

Like Carrie and Chuck, you may feel that you are being greedy. Looking at the childless women in your doctor's office, you may feel that they are more deserving than you to become pregnant. In situations like these, try to remind yourself that there is no pregnancy quota or lottery. One woman's pregnancy has nothing to do with another's. You are not in a game show with just one winner. Whether you are trying for your first, second, third, or fourth child, each person's desire is as important as any other's.

When we asked Carrie why she felt guilty for wanting another child, she pointed to the torment her childless neighbor was going through. We helped Carrie change her thinking patterns in order to believe that she is *entitled* to have as many children as she wants. So are you.

It is irrational to believe, like Carrie and Chuck did, that "nature is trying to tell you something" because you are not yet pregnant. While subscribing to this notion may help you accept your predicament, there is no reason to believe that you are trapped in it, considering all the medical means available to help. If technology does not foster your pregnancy, it is you who will decide when or if to stop trying—not some greater power.

USING GPST TO DISPUTE IRRATIONAL BELIEFS

Getting Pregnant Self-Talk is particularly helpful for secondary infertility because so many of the statements you are making to yourself are probably irrational or superstitious.

GPST FOR SECONDARY INFERTILITY:
AN ACTIVITY

Make a list of all the negative statements you are making to yourself about your infertility. These statements could be about the medical procedures, your state of mind, or your relationship with your husband, child, or other family members. In the box on the next page, write these statements in the left-hand column. To give you an idea of what we mean, we have printed some of the negative statements that members of our secondary infertility group have generated.

NEGATIVE STATEMENT	COUNTERARGUMENT
I don't think I can take my temperature one more time.	
I don't think I can handle being infertile much longer.	
I don't think I can keep going for these high-tech procedures forever.	
I don't think I can get pregnant.	
I don't think I can manage much more disappointment.	
I'm afraid I will never carry a baby to term.	
I'm afraid I will never have a second child.	
I'm afraid I will never get pregnant.	
I don't want to get my hopes up just to have them dashed.	
I don't want to not have another baby.	
I don't want to mix with fertile people.	
I think that a miscarriage will happen again.	
I seem to always view my self-worth by the number of children that I have.	
I don't want to ruin my son's childhood over something that may never be.	
I don't want my son to be an only child.	
This can't be happening.	
I'm scared of what the future holds.	

Now use the chart below to fill in your statements. Just fill in the negative statements. Later, we'll talk about disputing these statements with counterarguments.

NEGATIVE STATEMENT	COUNTERARGUMENT

Now it's time to dispute these statements. On the next page, we provide what our group members said to help you create counterarguments to your own negative statements.

NEGATIVE STATEMENT	COUNTERARGUMENT
I don't think I can take my temperature one more time.	By taking my temperature I up the odds of getting pregnant.
I don't think I can handle being infertile much longer.	I'll be as strong as I need to be.
I don't think I can keep going for these high-tech procedures forever.	I think I can psych myself up for three more tries.
I don't think I can get pregnant.	I can get pregnant when I take charge of my treatment.
I don't think I can manage much more disappointment.	Every disappointment is a step closer to success.
I'm afraid I will never carry a baby to term.	I know I will find the answer to this puzzle of miscarriage.
I'm afraid I will never have a second child.	At least I was able to have one child.
I'm afraid I will never get pregnant.	By pursuing treatment, I'll be satisfied that I tried everything humanly possible to get pregnant again. Anyway, research shows that only children often are more secure and have higher IQs. We can make our daughter's life rich and full.
I don't want to get my hopes up just to have them dashed.	Perhaps getting my hopes up will help me get through the next procedure.
I don't want to not have another baby.	I will be happy with my family.
I don't want to mix with fertile people.	The future is bright. I have a loving husband and a wonderful child. Technology is developing at such a rapid rate that the chances are I'll get pregnant eventually.
I think that a miscarriage will happen again.	I am strong enough to deal with another disappointment.
I seem to always view my self-worth by the number of children that I have.	I am a worthwhile person in my own right.
I don't want to ruin my son's childhood over something that may never be.	I'm doing this because I want my son to have a sibling. Maybe he'll understand someday.
I don't want my son to be an only child.	If my son is an only child, he'll be happy and well adjusted anyway.
This can't be happening.	This is not a punishment or a curse but a fact of life.
I'm scared of what the future holds.	This experience, in a bizarre way, has made me a stronger person.

Now, in the right-hand column of your chart, fill in your counterarguments.

COMMUNICATING WITH YOUR SPOUSE: GETTING PREGNANT LISTENING AND LEVELING

As we alluded to earlier in this chapter, staying united in the face of secondary infertility is often more difficult than uniting to combat primary infertility. While husband and wife generally are equally committed to having a first child, one member—usually the husband—is apt to feel less strongly about the importance of the second.

Certainly, if this second child came easily, your husband would happily participate in the pregnancy. But since pregnancy is not happening quickly, your husband probably does not share your pain. Your long-held images of motherhood—two sons fishing together, a brother and sister sharing friends in high school, everyone piling into a station wagon for a family vacation—is shattered. Since these images are so hard to surrender, you are driven to make them a reality.

Your husband's notion of family, meanwhile, has probably been more vague. His desire for children probably isn't as strongly tied to number and age spread. Having one child made him a father, so he may wonder: "Why all the fuss to have another child?"

Chuck's sadness is triggered by Carrie's sadness, not by the secondary infertility. Sure, he fantasizes about taking two sons fishing, and how nice it would be to cuddle a little girl. But he says, "I figure we don't have a six-figure income; we don't have a five-bedroom house; we don't have a Mercedes or even a van, so a second baby is just one more thing that we don't have."

That is not to say men are neutral toward secondary infertility. It's just that the lack of a second child does not contradict long-held fantasies of ideal family size, nor does it suggest a lack of sexuality to the outside world. As long as your husband has proved that he can father at least one child, the world thinks he could still do it, but he has decided not to have any more children. The wife, on the other hand, typically endures comments such as "When is the next baby coming?" Men generally are not asked these kinds of questions.

The discrepancies can be a recipe for marriage problems.

"I love Carrie and I want to be supportive," Chuck says. "I've gone along with all of her requests for treatment. We've been through all kinds of treatments for many years. But at some point, you just have to say enough is enough. I think we've given it a fair chance. It hasn't worked. It's time to quit."

Carrie vehemently disagrees. "I refuse to give up," she says. "I'll do this until I've tried everything. As long as I have strength and we have money, I'll keep trying."

Husband-Wife Negotiation Activity

In order to keep your marriage happy, you and your husband must find a way to negotiate a consensus on whether to begin or to continue infertility treatments. Negotiation is an important skill in building a good working team.[5] It is built on Listening and Leveling and asserting yourself—two Getting Pregnant Workout skills introduced in Chapter 2. Negotiation requires that each of you understand how the other person's desires are reasonable for them, *even if you have a different set of wishes*. You then must strive to be flexible in your demands, by using trade-offs, for example. Remember to be as honest and specific as possible when telling your spouse what you want.

It is a mistaken assumption that your desires are not legitimate because your husband refuses to abide by your requests. And it is human nature to believe that if he doesn't value your wishes, he doesn't value you as a person. To help avoid these traps, begin by communicating your love and respect for each other.

No matter how long you two have been together and how well you think you know each other, neither of you can crawl into the other's head and experience their emotions firsthand. Your job, therefore, is to try to explain the reasons behind your wishes, such as why it makes sense to you to continue treatment rather than give up. Your husband's job is to listen carefully and to ask himself, "Do I really understand why she feels this way?" By asking you questions and sharing his reactions with you, he can come closer to understanding your needs from *your point of view*.

At this stage, he should *not* try to convince you to adopt his point of view. You will know he has completed his tasks successfully when his words indicate he believes your wishes are reasonable. The following example addresses disagreement over continuing treatment, but the exercise can be adapted to any issue about which you and your husband disagree.

PART 1:
STATEMENTS OF WISHES AND REASONS

For the Wife: Write down why you feel it's important to continue treatment and how you would feel if treatment were to be stopped. Since you will be giving this statement to your husband, write it in a way that will lead him to conclude, "Now I understand why my wife wants to keep trying. Her wishes are reasonable. She's not off the wall for wanting to go on."

Wife's Statement:

Why I want to continue treatment.

For the Husband: Write down why you wish to stop treatment and how continuing treatment would make you feel. When your wife reads what you have written, she should be able to conclude: "Now I understand why my husband wants to stop. His wishes are reasonable. He's not off the wall for wanting to stop."

Husband's Statement:

Why I want to stop treatment.

PART 2:
COMMUNICATING MUTUAL UNDERSTANDING

Now comes the difficult part. After reading each other's statement, reiterate to your partner what you understand his or her position to be. Try to convince your husband that you believe his position is a reasonable one, and he should do the same for you. As you move through this part of the exercise, remember that *you don't necessarily have to agree with what the other person wants.* All you have to do is try to see things through their eyes, from their perspective.

To evaluate whether you've achieved full communication, both of you should be able to comfortably sign the statement below. It might help to read the statement aloud.

Statement of Mutual Understanding

We each have legitimate needs and they are in conflict with each other. We are interested in trying to find a solution that recognizes our mutual interests.

_____   _____
Husband's signature   Wife's signature

_____ (Date)

PART 3:
BRAINSTORMING DIFFERENT
SOLUTIONS TO THE PROBLEM

Brainstorming means coming up with creative compromise solutions in a nonjudgmental atmosphere. Come up with as many ideas as you can, but don't hammer them back with a barrage of criticism. Your ideas should focus on four primary concerns: time, money, family, and your child. Here is an example of what we mean:

TIME: How many months or years should be set aside trying to solve the problem?

MONEY: How much out-of-pocket money should be allocated to the effort? If money must be diverted from other expenses to pay for treatment, where should it be taken from?

FAMILY: What family activities are you willing to sacrifice (e.g., traveling out of town for the holidays) to meet the demands of treatment?

CHILD: You each have an image of the kind of parent you want to be to your son or daughter. But your effort may require some sacrifices in your parenting. What are you willing to give up to pursue is effort (such as being unable to chaperon a class trip)?

Keeping these four concerns in mind, continue to brainstorm more solutions to the problem. Write down all ideas. Ideally, you will end up with a list of possibilities.

PART 4:
CREATING AN ACCEPTABLE COMPROMISE

The next step is to hammer out a proposal to solve your problem. The key words here are compromise and trade-off. For instance, you might want to try low- and high-tech treatments for two more years and spend $10,000 of your own money. Your husband might want to try only low-tech treatments for three months and spend $2,000. One acceptable trade-off might be trying for three months, but spending $10,000 on high-tech treatments only. Another compromise might be to try various treatments for a year, but spend no more than $5,000 of your own money.

PART 5:
CREATING THE FINAL AGREEMENT AND SIGNING IT

Once you've negotiated an acceptable compromise, make it official. Write it as though it were a legal document, being as specific as possible. Use the form on the next page. At the end, write: *This agreement was made in good faith. We each commit ourselves to trying to make it work.* After you both sign and date your document, put it in a safe place. If you get into arguments later about the same issue, take out your contract and review it.

FINAL AGREEMENT

This agreement was made in good faith. We each commit ourselves to trying to make it work.

_____   _____

Husband (signature)   Wife (signature)

_____(Date)

DEALING WITH YOUR FAMILY

If families were perfect, your parents, aunts, uncles, and cousins would give you undying support as you grapple with secondary infertility. Unfortunately, it is not always easy to know what to say and not to say to infertile couples, particularly those who already have a child. Carrie and Chuck's relatives think the pregnancy quest is disrupting their family unit and putting unnecessary stress on their marriage and on Bobby, who has begun acting out in school. Bobby, like his grandparents, thinks Carrie and Chuck are somehow unhappy with what they have. Like Carrie and Chuck's relatives yours, too, might wish you would focus on your marriage, or get on with your career and be happy parenting your child, particularly if your child is in kindergarten or grade school.

It may seem impossible, but by Managing Your Social Life, you can turn your family around and win their support. To do this, you must assert yourself.

How your family reacts depends largely on whether you are experiencing primary infertility the second time around or secondary infertility. People in the former category are likely to hear: "Not again. You went through this torture once. Stop. Don't put yourself through it." These relatives may be speaking out of genuine concern for your emotional health, or they might be speaking out of selfishness; perhaps they think they will see your existing child less often while you engage in treatment, or be called upon for baby-sitting services if you do have another child.

Couples battling secondary infertility might hear: "Just relax. You'll get pregnant. You just need to give it time." They can't understand how someone who had a baby can suddenly lose that ability. They can be even less supportive than relatives of couples with primary infertility the second time around.

As you grapple with secondary infertility, we encourage you to make copies of A Family's Guide at the end of this chapter and give them to your relatives. The guide is designed to give your relatives the insight they need to empathize with your plight.

YOUR CHILD'S VIEW OF INFERTILITY

You carry the heavy burden of your secondary infertility in your heart as well as in your head. But your child cannot possibly comprehend the depth of your pain and worry. Your youngster may observe behavioral changes in you that are *consequences* of your inner turmoil. Without a hint as to what's wrong, your child is apt to draw erroneous and potentially damaging conclusions.

A little boy or girl who sees his mother with a sad face or low energy level may worry that Mommy is sick. Your child might think Mommy and Daddy don't love each other anymore if they're arguing over some aspect of the infertility. And a youngster could conclude that babies are despicable creatures because Mommy has begun to recoil in their presence.

If you are spending a lot of your own money on infertility treatments, you may no longer be able to buy your child certain items or take a family vacation. Your child might begin to feel deprived or unloved. Compounding your guilt over this trade-off is the feeling that perhaps you should be saving the money for your child's college education or spending it on him or her instead.

Perhaps the most blatant example is when an insemination or an IVF retrieval conflicts with an activity you planned with your child. Say you promised to attend a school play or birthday party and then leave early or fail to show up. Lacking an understanding that some procedures cannot be delayed, your child may be confused.

Your son or daughter might conclude that Mommy cannot be trusted or depended upon anymore. Children learn ethics and values from what you do as well as from what you say. So by shying away from infants and pregnant women in the presence of your child, the youngster might think something is wrong with them. How should you handle this situation?

As a mother combating infertility, you are left with two difficult options. One, you must monitor your behavior in the presence of your child as much as possible. The goal is to avoid communicating the wrong nonverbal messages, such as babies are bad. Or you must explain your actions to your child. This second option is by no means easy, especially if you are having trouble justifying your actions to yourself. Also, your child might be too young to understand how babies are made in the first place.

Talking with Your Child

Unlike the woman with primary infertility, you have to deal with a child's questions—or lack of them—about your family size, your treatment schedule, and your feelings about both. It is important to be truthful without burdening your child with too much information. Obviously, you can't describe IVF or even IUI to a five-year-old, or even to an eight-year-old, but you can explain that you need to take medicine and visit a special doctor to help you have a baby.

You know your own child better than anyone else does. You are best suited to ferret out the concerns behind your child's questions, and you know how much he or she can grasp. Many children who seem to be asking about the details of IVF really only want to know when their little brother or sister will be born. It's important to answer questions with facts that are appropriate for the child's developmental level and in language that can be understood.

Answering Questions About Treatment

Depending on your child's age and powers of perception, it is possible that he or she already is aware that something is wrong. You get up earlier; you frequent the doctor's office; Mommy and Daddy go into their bedroom at odd hours and lock the door. Such changes in routine might make your child feel angry, and rightfully so. If this happens, it is important that you acknowledge the feelings and explain to the child what's going on.

Hearing pieces of conversations about doctors, blood tests, and shots, meanwhile, can evoke fear in a child. Many children will imagine the worst: that you are dying, that you and your husband are divorcing, or even that you and your husband want a new baby instead of their existing child.

Assure your child that:

- No one is going to die;
- You're taking medicine and visiting the doctor to try to have a baby;

- You love him or her just like before and want another baby *because* you love him or her so much;
- You may sometimes act sad or disappointed because things aren't working out the way you hoped;
- He or she will have to try extra hard to cope with any changes in routine;
- Some people have more trouble than others when they want to have a baby; and
- This information is private so they shouldn't tell their friends or teacher what is happening.

Answering Questions About Your Feelings

Most children are acutely aware of their parents' moods. The rigors of treatment schedules, hormonal shifts caused by medications, and the many losses associated with infertility all can trigger unusual mood swings. When this occurs, assure your child that he or she is *not* the source of your unhappiness. At the same time, *do not* make your child your confidant or give the impression that you need to be taken care of. While it is reasonable to expect your child to be sympathetic, it is inappropriate to let your child bear the responsibility of making you feel better. The only way you should let your child help you is indirectly. You can remind yourself that the joy this child has given you is one of the reasons you want another child in the first place.

When you have trouble hiding your disappointment when you get your period, give your child a basis for your mood change. When your child asks, "Why are you sad, Mommy?" say, "I am sad because I am disappointed that I didn't get what I wanted: a baby growing in my belly." If you are feeling harried, tell your child, "Mommy is going to see a special doctor. I have to go to the doctor very early in the morning, and it's hard for me to get up that early. So, I'm tired and sometimes I'm grumpy. Even though you didn't do anything, sometimes I yell at you. I'm sorry."

Answering Questions About Family Size

Most older children are perfectly satisfied with the size of their family. Being an only child has its advantages: They don't have to share toys or their parents' attention. Still, it's important to explain to them why you want more children while pointing out the positive aspects of being an older sibling.

By contrast, most younger children are upset about not having a sibling. "Bobby's first mention of my infertility came out of the blue," Carrie recalled. "I was feeling very generous one day, and I asked him what he wanted most in the world. I thought he'd say a tricycle or a Nintendo game, but he looked at me with his earnest blue eyes and said, 'I want to be a brother.' It just broke my heart."

Young children, usually between ages four and six, typically ask why they have no brothers or sisters. Such questions can arise in social situations, such as when a friend or neighbor shows up with a baby carriage and other kids in tow. Your immediate response need only be, "We're trying," or "We want a new baby, too." Later in the privacy of your home, you can give your child additional information, if he or she wants to know more.

In cases where your child is clearly perplexed by the changes in your lives but lacks the language to ask you about your fertility problems, it may help to offer information in the form of a fairy tale. We've written one called Maybe Next Year, which is appropriate for three- to six-year-olds. (Some older children like it, too.) After reading it to your child, you can follow up with a discussion.

MAYBE NEXT YEAR:
A SECONDARY INFERTILITY STORY TO TELL YOUR CHILD

The little boy in the blue-striped polo shirt was very sad. His friend with the red hair had a new tricycle. His friend who lived in the green house had a new bicycle. The little boy waited and waited for his mommy to get him a bicycle, too. But no bicycle came. He said, "Mommy, I'm so sad. My friend with the red hair has a tricycle. And my friend who lives in the green house has a bicycle. When will I have a bicycle?" His mommy said, "I'd like to get you a bicycle, but I can't this year. Maybe next year."

The little boy in the blue-striped polo shirt was sad but also mad. He said, "Everybody gets what they want. But not me." His mommy said, "That's not true. Just ask the seal who lives in the zoo who balances the ball on her nose." The boy in the blue-striped polo shirt loved the seal in the zoo who balanced the ball on her nose. He went to visit the seal. "Seal, I'm very sad. I want a bicycle and my mommy can't get me one this year. Did you ever want something that you didn't get?" Seal said, "My little ones love sardines. When we lived in the ocean, I used to catch sardines and give them to my little ones. But here in the zoo I don't have any. My little ones are sad. I told them maybe next year I'd get to the ocean and bring them some sardines."

The little boy in the blue-striped polo shirt felt bad for the little seals. He went home and said, "Mommy, I feel sad. The little seals and I can't get what we want. But everybody else gets what they want." Mommy said, "That's not so. Ask the squirrel who lives in the tree who wiggles his tail." Squirrel lived in the tree in front of the little boy's house. The little boy used to talk to Squirrel. So he went outside and by and by he saw Squirrel. "Squirrel, I'm so sad. I want a bicycle and Mommy can't get it for me this year." Squirrel said, "That's sad. My little ones want acorns. I used to collect acorns from the oak tree across the street. Then last year there was a big storm and the tree was knocked down. Now we have no acorns. I told my little ones that maybe the townspeople will plant a new tree so that in a few years we'll have more acorns."

The little boy in the blue-striped polo shirt was sad. He went home and said, "Mommy, I'm so sad. The little seals don't get sardines and the little squirrels don't get any acorns and I can't get a bicycle. Everybody but us gets the things they want." Mommy said, "That's not true. You never even knew that the little seals wanted something that they didn't get. And you never even knew that the little squirrels wanted something that they didn't get. Everybody wants things that they don't get."

The little boy in the blue-striped polo shirt said, "Mommy, is there anything that you want that you didn't get?" Mommy said, "Yes. I want a baby to be your sister. Daddy and I have been trying to have a baby but we haven't gotten one yet. But maybe we'll get one next year." The little boy in the blue-striped polo shirt said, "Maybe next year Seal and her little ones will get the fish they want. Maybe next year Squirrel and her little ones will get the acorns they want. And maybe next year you and Daddy and I will get the baby sister we all want."

A FAMILY'S GUIDE
TO SECONDARY INFERTILITY

(NOTE: Write your name or the name of your husband or child in the appropriate blank spaces to make the guide more personal, or else rewrite these pages to express yourself in your own way.)

WHAT IS SECONDARY INFERTILITY?

When parents are having great difficulty having a second child, the situation is called "secondary infertility." Some women with secondary infertility also had a great deal of difficulty getting pregnant the first time. If _____ had trouble the first time, it probably won't surprise you that she is having trouble again. But for many other women, the first pregnancy came easily, and trying to have another seems impossible. This guide is aimed at helping you better understand what _____ is going through.

WHY DIFFICULTIES NOW AND NOT LAST TIME?

You're probably asking yourself, "Why are they having so much trouble now when they had no trouble last time?" You don't have an answer—and quite likely, neither do they. There are so many possible reasons.

People change. As they age, their bodies change. Sometimes a woman's hormonal balance changes. Last time, she had the proper hormonal stimulation to make her ovulate. Now something may have changed, and her hormones are out of kilter. The birth of a first child sometimes causes changes. Sometimes changes during a first pregnancy stimulate the production of antibodies that interfere with a subsequent pregnancy. Also, the quality of her eggs may have diminished because she is older.

Not only do changes happen to women, they also happen to men. _____ may have had a good sperm count last time but it has since become poor. Too much exercise, tight underwear, or trauma to the groin area are possible explanations.

In truth, there may be more than one cause of their secondary infertility. The real reason or reasons may never be ascertained. But be assured that they are doing everything they can to find answers.

SHE'S NOT EASY TO GET ALONG WITH, LIKE SHE USED TO BE

Like most people with a loved one suffering from secondary infertility, you probably find _____ extremely difficult to deal with. She is probably depressed much of the time. She probably avoids family gatherings. She may have a strained relationship with her siblings or cousins who have more than one child or who are expecting another child.

WHAT'S GOING ON IN HER HEAD

Perhaps you could be more sympathetic if you knew what _____ is experiencing. She has lots of strange feelings. Probably she is wondering whether her inability to have a second child is an omen. Maybe she thinks she is trying to tempt fate, and she'll be punished by having a child with a birth defect. Maybe she should give up and be satisfied with one child.

She's feeling lots of guilt. By trying so hard to have a baby, she's taking time away from her child, _____. She's spending money on treatment instead of on _____. She devotes her time to treatment instead of spending that time with _____. And when she spends time with _____, she may resent it when it interferes with her treatment schedule. You can imagine how these thoughts must be tormenting her.

She's also hassled by logistical problems. What can she do with _____ when she goes for early-morning treatments or blood tests? What will happen if _____ walks in when her husband is injecting her with a fertility drug?

WHY DO THEY WANT ANOTHER CHILD?

You're probably wondering, "If they're having so much trouble, why don't they just forget about having more children?" The answer is complex.

They love children so much that they want a larger family. Before they got married, they had a vision of the kind of family they would create. That vision included several children. Now they're trying to make that dream come true. The fact that they are having so much difficulty makes them even more intent on achieving their goal.

Also, they want another child as a companion for their son/daughter. Youngsters whose parents suffer secondary infertility often ask for a sibling.

WHY IT'S SO HARD TO GET SUPPORT

_____ is what psychologists call a "marginal woman." She doesn't fit into the infertile world. Those people have no children at all. They can't empathize with her situation. Nor does _____ fit into the fertile world. These people have as many kids as they desire, maybe even more, and have no trouble getting pregnant. Because she's neither fish nor fowl, _____ has few sources of support.

A general lack of empathy for her plight also puts her into uncomfortable or even painful social situations. Well-meaning people ask her, "Why are you waiting so long to have another child?" They figure if she was able to have one, she certainly can have another. Comments like these really hurt.

Sometimes her friends with more than one child tell her, "You're so lucky to have only one kid. You don't have to deal with your children fighting and arguing." Or they say, "I wish I only had one kid. It's so much easier to travel with just one child to worry about." They don't mean to hurt _____. But after hearing remarks like these, she is likely to spend the next few days being depressed.

HOW YOU CAN HELP HER

There are several things you can do to ease her pain. If you live nearby and can baby-sit, offer to watch her child when she goes to the doctor's office. If her treatment is extensive, offer to have her child sleep at your house that night. You can also offer to entertain her child while her husband is giving her an injection.

Don't press her to attend family gatherings that include babies or pregnant women. Understand that being among people who have what she so desperately wants can put her under tremendous stress. Also, you can alert other family members that she is in a difficult phase of her life and to refrain from saying things that might upset or embarrass her.

Be sensitive about the things you say to her. She's doing everything she can to have a baby. Support her. Don't discourage her.

WHAT TO SAY AND NOT TO SAY

Tell her you love and support her. Let her know that you share her anguish and wish her dream will come true. Do say: "I'm praying for you," or, "Next time I see you, I hope you'll be pregnant." Don't say: "What will be will be." And never say: "Maybe you're just not meant to have any more children."

CHAPTER TWELVE

PREGNANCY LOSS AFTER INFERTILITY

FOR MOST women, losing a pregnancy is a tragedy. But losing a pregnancy after months or years of infertility treatments seems the cruelest loss of all. Unfortunately, the same problem that made it difficult for you to become pregnant in the first place may contribute to an increased risk of miscarriage.

Miscarriage, sometimes referred to as spontaneous abortion, is technically defined as the loss of a pregnancy up to twenty weeks after conception. A woman who loses two or more pregnancies in the first twenty weeks has suffered what doctors call recurrent pregnancy loss.[1] After the twentieth week, the loss is called premature labor.

In this chapter, we will address some of the causes of miscarriage, possible preventions, and offer suggestions aimed at minimizing the potentially devastating psychological impact of losing a pregnancy after infertility.

WHAT CAUSED THIS MISCARRIAGE?

The most important thing to remember after suffering a miscarriage after infertility is this: Probably nothing you did—either in the past or in the present—had anything to do with your misfortune. If you find this hard to accept, you are not alone. Many people we talk with believe that the miscarriage, like their infertility, is some kind of punishment for past behaviors. "As a kid I used to misbehave," one woman told us. "My mother used to say to me, 'You'll be sorry. You'll pay for this when you grow up.' My miscarriage is my payment for being a bad girl."

Other people—a much larger group—describe a different source of guilt. They believe the miscarriage is the result of something they did or didn't do, such as sitting too close to a computer screen or taking an airplane trip during their pregnancy. They believe that if they had done things differently, they would still be pregnant.

If you are locked into this kind of mind-set, let yourself off the hook. Recognize and accept the fact that some causes of miscarriage—particularly genetic causes—are beyond your or anyone else's control. And to keep from worrying about future miscarriages, know what medical steps you can take that might prevent a miscarriage in the future.

The Likelihood of Miscarriage

Dr. James Wheeler, a researcher specializing in the causes of recurrent pregnancy loss, describes what he terms "the natural history of spontaneous abortion." He points out that very few of the many sperm and eggs a couple produce are actually used for procreation. Some 10 percent to 15 percent of all *normal* eggs will fail to fertilize. Another 10 to 15 percent of the eggs that do fertilize fail to divide or implant. And of those that do divide and implant, 15 percent to 20 percent (up to one in five) are spontaneously aborted before twenty weeks of pregnancy. "Thus a fertilized egg has, at best, a 60 percent chance of reaching 20 weeks of gestation," Wheeler concludes.[2]

For the infertile population, the miscarriage rate is even higher, although researchers aren't sure exactly why. Here are some of the medical reasons that do have a scientific basis.

Hormonal Causes

Hormonal problems are a possible cause of recurrent miscarriage. A lack of sufficient progesterone is associated with a luteal phase defect. Doctors don't know precisely how a luteal phase defect contributes to miscarriage.[3] They do know, however, that patients with this defect have a high incidence of miscarriage—anywhere from 23 percent to 60 percent. One way to supplement progesterone levels is by giving the woman injections or vaginal suppositories of natural progesterone (the synthetic form must be avoided during pregnancy). If you have had one or more miscarriages, ask your doctor whether progesterone supplementation might be helpful in your case.

Infection

It has recently been discovered that certain types of bacterial infections can cause miscarriage, just as they cause infertility, by hurting the quality of your eggs as well as their ability to be fertilized and implant in the uterus, according to Dr. Niels H. Lauersen, author of *Getting Pregnant: What You Need to Know*. The most common bacteria linked to pregnancy loss are those usually associated with sexually transmitted diseases, including chlamydia, T-mycoplasma, gonorrhea, and syphilis.[4] Dr. Lauersen says that the use of erythromycin, an antibiotic, is "one of the most beneficial treatments in preventing miscarriage."[5]

Having undergone infertility diagnosis, you probably have been tested for bacterial infections already. If you haven't been tested, or if it's been a long time since your initial workup, it cannot hurt to be tested again.

Many doctors do not believe that these infections can cause miscarriage. But being tested and taking antibiotics if indicated, at the very least, will *give you the feeling* that you are improving your future pregnancy outlook.[6]

Anatomic Causes in the Cervix and Uterus

Certain anatomic problems have a high probability for causing miscarriage. A weakness in the cervix, which can be natural or caused by a cone biopsy, is a major cause of miscarriage, particularly after the first trimester. You may have heard that repeated dilation and curettage (D&C) procedures can increase the risk of cervical incompetence. This is certainly not something you want to hear right after you had a D&C for your miscarriage. The good news is that modern D&C techniques use instruments that don't weaken the cervix. The other good news is that before you are about twenty weeks pregnant doctors can put temporary stitches in the cervix to tighten it, thereby preventing this cause of miscarriage.

Another cause of miscarriage is a wall, or septum, in the uterus. Because you've probably had diagnostic testing that included an HSG or a hysteroscopy in order to get pregnant, however, this problem would have been detected and remedied prior to pregnancy. If you are still worried, talk to your doctor.

Women who were exposed to DES (diethylstilbestrol) while in utero also have an increased miscarriage risk. A study that compared DES-exposed women with non-DES-exposed women found that only 54 percent of the DES daughters had live births compared with 82 percent of non-DES-exposed daughters.[7] If you are a DES daughter, insist that your doctor take all steps possible to best manage your pregnancy. Some possible steps include careful monitoring throughout your pregnancy, early ultrasound scans, more than usual bed rest, avoidance of strenuous activities, and frequent cervical examinations.

Immunological Factors

The mechanism by which immunological factors may contribute to miscarriage is not clearly understood. The most reasonable explanation is based on the notion that our immune system protects us from invasion by foreign bodies. When the immune system perceives something as foreign, it mobilizes special cells to attack and destroy it. A reasonable question then is: Why doesn't the woman's immune system perceive an embryo as a foreign body and destroy it?

The proposed answer is that the woman's body produces blocking antibodies, which prevent the immune system's killer cells from destroying the embryo. How these blocking antibodies are mobilized is a mystery.

Perhaps the developing embryo itself sends a chemical message triggering this protection. The special mix of two very different genetic materials, each contributed by one of the spouses, may trigger a "hold-your-fire'' signal. On those occasions when the embryo fails to signal the body to "hold your fire," miscarriage will ensue, according to the theory.

Some experts speculate that an immunological response against an embryo or fetus occurs when there are too many genetic similarities between the husband and wife. Without enough genetic dissimilarity, the stimulus to produce the "hold your fire" signal is perhaps not triggered.

Treatment, albeit a controversial one, involves injecting the wife with her husband's white blood cells. Doctors who prescribe this treatment claim it stimulates the blocking antibodies or at least prevents the attacking antibodies from destroying the fetus.[8] Ask your doctor whether he or she believes the theory and whether immunological treatment might prevent future miscarriages for you.

A different type of immune system deficiency causes a blood-clotting disorder that prohibits the growing fetus from getting enough blood flow to grow and develop. The problem occurs when certain antibodies, most specifically anticardiolipin or cold lupus anticoagulant, cause your body to develop blood clots in the vessels leading to the placenta. The clots prevent the baby from getting the vital nutrients it needs. To overcome this problem, you can take baby aspirin and injections of heparin, an anticoagulant. Again, ask your doctor whether this approach is appropriate for you.

Chromosomal and Genetic Causes

Chromosomal abnormalities are the most common causes of first or isolated miscarriage. Sadly, there is nothing you can do to remedy a chromosomal defect during pregnancy. Dr. Wheeler reports that 40 percent to 60 percent of all first-trimester miscarriages show evidence of chromosomal abnormalities. Many of these abnormalities are *random* (chance) errors that occur during *meiosis* (when gametes lose half their chromosomes before fertilization) or during *mitosis* (when cells divide in half as the embryo grows). Defective genetic material in your eggs or in your partner's sperm can create embryos that are too weak or too deformed to survive. Genetic defects (in contrast to chromosomal abnormalities), however, are very rare.

Sometimes this genetic abnormality may be a statistically uncommon occurrence that will never again happen to you. In other cases, you or your partner may have a chromosomal problem that will cause repeated miscarriages. To find out, you and your husband can have your blood cells tested for chromosomal abnormalities.

Finally, if you are thirty-five or older, your chances of having an embryo with genetic problems, some of which are serious enough to cause a miscarriage, rise substantially. We've included the chart below, not to terrify you, but to apprise you realistically of the odds.

RISK OF SPONTANEOUS ABORTION WITH INCREASED AGE[9]

Maternal Age in Years	Percentage of Spontaneous Abortions
15–19	9.0%
20–24	9.5%
25–29	10.0%
30–34	11.7%
35–39	17.7%
40–44	33.8%
over 45	53.2%

COPING WITH MISCARRIAGE AFTER INFERTILITY: LONG-AWAITED FANTASIES

Infertile couples tend to fantasize about being pregnant beginning with the first Clomid pill or Pergonal shot. As time goes on, however, some couples begin to fight back such fantasies because the treatments have failed so many times. So when pregnancy finally occurs, the fantasy floodgates tend to swing wide open.

Like pregnant women everywhere, you begin to think ahead—to the last months of pregnancy, to the moment you first cradle this long-awaited baby in your arms. You make plans to borrow your sister's maternity clothes and circle your due date on every calendar in the house. You gleefully walk into baby furniture stores and infantwear departments—venues you previously avoided because they were too depressing. You begin to picture yourself playing with your child in the nursery of your dreams. Everything seems to be falling into place.

Then—suddenly or slowly—you're not pregnant anymore. The baby, which may already have been given a name, no longer exists.

If you have miscarried once or several times after infertility, the loss can be overwhelming. Each pregnancy, no matter how brief, gave you permission to believe that this pregnancy would be successful. Each pregnancy, no matter how brief, causes physical, hormonal, and emotional changes, which are very real.

In his book, *Preventing Miscarriage,* Dr. Jonathan Scher states that "the major changes in a woman's hormonal makeup take place *early* in pregnancy, almost just after conception."[10] So when you lose that pregnancy, it can feel as though you gave birth and lost that child. And, in fact, you *have* lost that child.

We lost our first pregnancy in the eighth week—but not until after rejoicing in a positive pregnancy test and the sight of our fetus's heartbeat on a sonogram. April 6 was our due date. We shared our joy with other couples whose pregnancies had occurred around the same time as ours. We allowed ourselves to fantasize with sheer abandon.

In addition to suffering the sadness associated with miscarriage in general, we were further saddened because we realized that not only do we have trouble conceiving, but we also would have trouble maintaining a pregnancy. As we recovered physically and emotionally from the pregnancy loss, we developed many coping activities, which we describe later in this chapter. Many of our clients also found these activities extremely helpful.

Then we got pregnant a second time with a Pergonal/IUI cycle. It was our first attempt after the miscarriage, no less. We charted this second pregnancy, just as we had the first. We calculated a due date: August 27. But this time we were less inclined to talk freely about our pregnancy, although we did confide in a small number of trusted friends, family, and associates.

In the ninth week, we were no longer able to detect a fetal heartbeat. Our recovery from the second miscarriage was slower and more difficult. Unlike the shock we felt with the first miscarriage, this one was characterized by a deadness we both felt inside. We talked to each other about how unfair it all seemed. We thought we were on the brink of winning our war against infertility, but we had only conquered one battle.

Despite all the emotional pain, enduring two miscarriages gave us more knowledge and insight to help ourselves and others through this horrible ordeal. The information contained in the following section summarizes what we have learned through our literature research and from numerous doctors and couples we have talked to.

Getting in Touch with Grief and Loss

If you've experienced a miscarriage after trying so hard to get pregnant, it can be difficult to allow yourself to feel the pain because the loss is so utterly devastating. Another reason the grieving process is especially difficult is that you've worked so hard to stay optimistic for so long. In fact, your pregnancy reinforced the importance of Not Giving Up, because you did get pregnant. You'd learned to move past the devastation of a failed IUI or IVF and steel yourself for the next treatment. You taught yourself to view the period after a failed cycle as one more step toward your goal. Even as you grieved with your period, you reminded yourself that it was also Day 1 of your new cycle: one in which a pregnancy could occur.

With a miscarriage, the end of a cycle is far more profound and overwhelming because it is more closely associated with a real death. The probability of pregnancy had become a possibility and, in so many ways, the baby had seemed a reality-to-be. You had a positive pregnancy test and saw a gestational sac on the ultrasound; you may even have seen a fetal heartbeat. Then the bleeding started. Or maybe there was no bleeding: You got the unforseen news during an ultrasound scan. The news might have come from a radiologist you never met before, and maybe you had no one else around to support you emotionally. To make matters worse, your body may still have felt pregnant, but there was no longer a life growing inside you.

When you are *trying* to get pregnant, the odds, for any given attempt, are *not* in your favor. Even a couple having no fertility problems has only a 20 percent chance of conception for each attempt. The situation is beyond your control. Therefore, although you *hope* you will succeed, you know that the odds are against you, and you don't spend mental energy trying to make it happen.

But once you do get pregnant, the odds of staying pregnant (unless you are over forty-five) *are* in your favor. And for certain conditions, there *are* steps you can take to prevent miscarriage. Therefore, you *hope* you will stay pregnant and you *try to exert control* to make sure that you stay pregnant. Then when a miscarriage occurs, you feel as though your sense of control was just an illusion. This sudden realization that you have no control over your pregnancy can plunge you into a dark depression. In order to get past this experience, you must allow yourself to experience your emotions, to express them to each other, and to ask for what you need from those around you.

Our society has many rituals for mourning death. Wakes, burials, sitting Shiva, and condolence calls are all mechanisms for helping people come to terms with loss. Tombstones, remembrance plaques, and photographs all serve as memorials to the life of the deceased. Unfortunately, society has created no comparable rituals for mourning and remembering fetuses who died. To rectify this problem, registered nurse Pat Schweibert and Dr. Paul Kirk have written a book called *When Hello Means Goodbye*, in which they discuss the mechanisms for dealing with the loss of a fetus.[11] We recommend this book as a supplement to the ideas we discuss in this chapter.

DIFFICULT DATES

Couples who have suffered miscarriage typically describe difficult dates and encounters that seem to halt recovery just as healing begins. The day your baby had been due or the anniversary of the day you conceived can be extraordinarily difficult to get through. Equally difficult is seeing women who got pregnant around the same time you did but are still carrying or have already given birth. Be aware that these circumstances can signal trouble for your emotional well-being. Making a Plan can help you cope with painful thoughts triggered by these dates and encounters. Here is what some of our miscarriage clients listed as difficult dates. At the bottom is space for you to list dates you anticipate to be a problem.

Difficult Dates

Dates our clients found difficult:

- Day your baby was due to be born

- Anniversary of your miscarriage

- Anniversary of a positive pregnancy test

- Milestone for a baby born around the time your baby was supposed to have been born (e.g., christening, bris, baby-naming)

- First day of school

Fill in your difficult dates:

_____

_____

_____

Steps to take:

> *Get in Touch with Your Feelings.* In advance, think about these difficult dates and give yourself time to grieve and mourn the tragedy of your loss.
>
> *Make a Plan.* Tell your husband that these dates will undoubtedly be difficult for you. Use Listening and Leveling skills from Chapter 2 to help him understand why you expect to be upset.
>
> *Work as a Team.* With your husband, plan some activities that you can do together on these dates. You might see a movie, go to a museum, take a walk in the country, go skating, or go out to dinner.

MANAGING YOUR SOCIAL LIFE

It's very difficult for friends to know what to say and what to do after you've suffered a miscarriage. You can help yourself by coaching them about what to say and what not to say. *Don't write people off for their initial insensitive remarks.* Some of your friends may have better instincts than others, but few people are professionally trained to respond to someone in pain.

One of our clients' friends told her, "Sally, we're so sorry about your miscarriage. We can't know the grief you are experiencing. We can only imagine how painful it is. You're in our prayers." Warmed and uplifted by those words, Sally decided that she would tell other friends about the statement and encourage them to take a similar tack should the miscarriage come up in conversation.

Lisa, another client, told us about a particularly disturbing remark made by a colleague who was trying to be helpful. "You're young and healthy," the colleague told her. "You'll have a baby, and then you won't even remember this miscarriage." To alleviate the threat of hearing hurtful comments in the future, we helped Lisa develop a way to teach her friend more helpful responses. Although Lisa initially felt uncomfortable about coaching her friend, she agreed to try. She told her friend, "Yvonne, I know you were trying to be kind, but what you said made me very upset. It's hard for me to imagine that I'll ever forget this miscarriage. So when you say that to me, it makes me very angry."

If people make unsympathetic or otherwise hurtful remarks to you, you cannot change what they actually said. But you can diminish the pain that lingers with the memory of their words. By using mental imagery techniques, you can relive these scenes putting more helpful words into their mouths. The hindsight activity on the following pages helps you do just that.

HINDSIGHT—
WHAT YOU WISH YOU HAD SAID

First list the hurtful statements that were made to you. Then create your response to those statements using 20-20 hindsight. Your response is what you wish you had said. Here are some examples:

Remark:

Did you hear about Carol's pregnancy? She's going to have twins.

Hindsight response:

I'm glad that Carol's pregnancy is going so well, but it's very hard for me to hear about it at this time. Please don't talk to me about people's pregnancies. I'll let you know when I'm ready for that.

Remark:

I'm sorry you lost the pregnancy. But at least you can have fun trying to get pregnant again.

Hindsight response:

Thank you for your concern about my loss. I'm sorry that you didn't realize that I've been undergoing infertility treatment for a long time. In our case, getting pregnant isn't fun, it's work.

Remark:

I heard about your miscarriage. I'm so sorry. But I guess it was just God's will.

Hindsight response:

I appreciate your support and concern. I don't like to think about my pregnancy in those terms. I like to believe that God is on my side. If it helps you to think about tragedies in your life this way, then that's right for you. But it doesn't help me.

Now it's your turn. Recall a situation that happened after your miscarriage that was a particularly painful or difficult one to endure. Allow yourself to go back to that time and place. Try to experience the situation in as much detail as possible. Hear the hurtful statement made by your friend or acquaintance. Take as much time as you need to fully experience the scene. When you have a clear picture in your mind, allow yourself to come back to the here and now. Write down what you found so difficult to hear. Don't be surprised if much of the pain returns as this memory becomes more vivid. Just breathe deeply and let yourself go with it.

Using hindsight, construct a retort. Your retort should let the person know how much what they said hurt your feelings. Take care to construct a statement that you would be comfortable making—one that is assertive and that communicates your feelings.

Now return to the difficult scene in your mind's eye. Recall that scene in as much detail as possible. Hear your friend making the hurtful statement. This time, instead of responding in the way that you did, or not responding at all, make the statement that you just scripted. See your friend's face when you make that statement. Feel better now that you've communicated what you needed to.

Once you've reexperienced the scene on your own terms, return to the here and now. Armed with the language to deal with a similar situation should it arise in the future, you can let go of the pain and move on, putting the hurtful incident behind you.

Should We Try Again? A Husband-Wife Communication Activity

One of the most difficult aspects of your miscarriage can be how differently you and your husband perceive the experience. Many of the women we talk with focus on the emptiness they feel. But more women describe the pain of waiting—waiting for a menstrual period and the chance to try again. Because infertile women who have experienced miscarriage have been actively involved each month in getting pregnant, this waiting time seems like a punishment for failing rather than a time to recover. Getting a period, which is the important first step in trying again, can take up to eight weeks.

To husbands, the loss is altogether different. One male client likened the miscarriage to climbing a rope, almost reaching the top, and then sliding to the bottom again. Another man described how he and his wife had worked so hard to build an elaborate sand castle, then stood back to admire it only to watch the sand castle be carried away by the tide. They feel that all their efforts to overcome great odds against pregnancy were in vain. Perceiving the miscarriage as a failure, many husbands are loath to risk another defeat. As their wives anxiously wait for the opportunity to try again, these husbands want to discontinue infertility treatments.

It is at this impasse that couples come to see us after suffering miscarriage in the wake of extended treatments. Couples who once had no problem Working as a Team now have trouble understanding each other's perceptions and feelings. As you and your husband struggle over whether to give up or try again, we urge you to call upon the communication skills you acquired in the Getting Pregnant Workout. Remember, both of you are:

- Trying to understand your partner's world of experience;
- Conveying information about your own world of experience; and, as a by-product of the first two processes,
- Commenting on the relationship.

Mindy and Stefan, both in their late thirties, came to see us shortly after Mindy's second miscarriage. Mindy was caught up in the interminable wait described above. Stefan was demoralized and frustrated. She wanted to try IVF again; he wanted to quit. Their dilemma was threatening their marriage.

The discussion in our consulting room began with an air of great tension. This couple, who had been through so much infertility treatment together and had comforted and supported each other for years, were now fuming at each other. Each regarded the other as stubborn and irrational. We spent a great deal of time coaching them in Listening and Leveling skills. Despite this coaching, they repeatedly fell back upon former habits of assuming they knew what their partner was thinking and feeling. Their dialogue was merely a recitation of what each wanted, with neither party paying much attention to what their partner was saying:

MINDY: I want to try again.
STEFAN: Enough is enough. We tried so many times. We had two pregnancies and two miscarriages. I'd say that's giving it a reasonable shot.

MINDY: I just want to try one more time. I think it'll work next time.
STEFAN: And then if that doesn't work, you'll want to try again. How
         long will it go on?
MINDY: Why are you being so unreasonable? You used to be so
         supportive.

At this stage in the dialogue, all that was being communicated was
desperation and accusations. We urged Stefan and Mindy to share their
worlds of experience with each other. After much work, they were
finally able to have the following productive dialogue:

STEFAN: Let me tell you what I'm feeling. I'm so frustrated. I feel like
         we've done everything in our power. We've spent tons of
         money. We've devoted four years to this quest. We're getting
         older. We still have time and money to adopt. Two years from
         now, we might be too old and too poor to adopt. Let's get on
         with it.
MINDY: Your points are valid. I know it seems like we've been doing
         this forever. And I appreciate all the support you've given me.
         I love you for what you've done. but I need one more chance.
STEFAN: Why is having one more chance so important to you?
MINDY: Because I feel like a failure, and I need one more time before I
         can allow myself to give up the idea that I can be a biological
         mother. It's hard to explain, I know, but one more try will
         make all the difference in how I see myself.
STEFAN: Well, I can't say I understand your reasons, but I'm willing to
         accept what you say. The thing that's worrying me, though, is
         that if we try and you miscarry again, you'll come back with
         the same statement again: "I need just one more time." Then
         we're right back on the merry-go-round.
MINDY: But there's one difference. We still have one more IVF attempt
         that insurance will cover. Please, let's try that one last time,
         and if it doesn't work, we'll quit.

Now they were making some progress. They understood each other,
but they still were unable to resolve their differences. As a result of their
discussion, however, they were aware of the issues that were dividing
them.

Our next step was to help them develop an agreement they could both
live with. With our assistance, Mindy and Stefan came up with an
agreement that they signed and dated. Here is what they wrote:

AGREEMENT

We agree to try one more IVF attempt. We are hopeful that it will succeed and that a resulting pregnancy will go to term. However, should we fail to get pregnant, or get pregnant and have a miscarriage, we agree that we will end our efforts to have our own biological child. Instead, we will begin to explore adoption as a way to expand our family.

_____   _____
Mindy Mateja (wife)   Stefan Mateja (husband)

_____   _____
Helane S. Rosenberg (witness)   Yakov M. Epstein (witness)

_____
Date

Like Mindy and Stefan, you may resolve your pregnancy quest with a decision to adopt if your next attempt does not succeed. Most importantly, you must find a way to deal with your infertility as a strong, loving team.

GOODBYE

In Chapter One, we noted that by the time you reach the end of this book you would have two books: the one you bought and the one you created as you photocopied pages and made your own personal notebook. This is the end of our book. But it may not yet be the end of yours. Perhaps you will need to add more pages as you keep using our activities in your quest to have a baby. But we sincerely hope that you will reserve, and someday be able to fill in, one final page in your book—the page with the picture of the baby you will cradle in your arms after getting pregnant when you thought you couldn't.

AFTERWORD:

BEYOND MEDICAL TREATMENT

NOTE FROM THE AUTHORS: No one but you can know when it is time to abandon infertility treatment and either begin the adoption process or decide to forgo having children altogether. Factors that come into play may include your age, financial situation, views on parenthood and childbirth, and your ability and willingness to find satisfaction in pursuits other than raising children. These are highly emotional, deeply personal issues. But we believe that most people instinctively begin to transform their mind-set during the treatment period and eventually make peace with one of the alternatives.

After reading this book, we hope you have learned how to make the best use of optimism, relaxation, medical partnerships, and persever-ance. Many people who want to stop treatment ask us how these newly acquired skills can be channeled into dealing with such choices as adoption or child-free living. Since we counsel couples to keep trying as long as possible (we finally conceived a baby with the help of a donor egg and a GIFT procedure), we were hard-pressed to help you should you choose a different path. So we turned to Charlotte Rosin, a friend and former president of our own Central New Jersey RESOLVE chapter. Here is her story:

For years I tried to become pregnant. To my profound regret, medical science was unable to help me conceive, even though we tried so hard. Finally, after many heartbreaking years, I closed the door on that chapter of my life.

When I finally did, I felt glad to give up the promise of pregnancy, the hope for a baby engineered somehow in the factory of my body, because that hope was just the flip side of disappointment. Medical science had given shape to my hope; it had also enclosed me in its space. I had not been seriously moving toward resolution because I had been stuck in the repetition of hope/loss.

Now without the support of reproductive technology, I felt unexpectedly light-headed with the prospect of free time, with the limitless present, with the open-ended choice of the future. I was relieved to escape the cyclical ups and downs of mind and body. At the same time, however, giving up my single-minded pursuit had cast me adrift, without a clue about what would give my life meaning. I had begun the process of resolution.

No one can know the moment when another should move on to considering adoption, or finding satisfaction in pursuits other than raising children—but I think that most people have a sense for themselves when they've arrived at this stage. Whether that moment comes now or later seems to matter little in the grand scheme of things.

Adoption is no longer limited to the young; child-free living can be enjoyed at any age. Some take the view that they will budget their limited resources (their money, their energy for dealing with children, their emotional well-being, and so on) by choosing adoptive parenthood now and working on giving birth again sometime in the future, if they still have the motivation. Others take a break from or stop medical treatment to renew their marriages and/or careers, which have been sorely stressed by infertility. Still others carry on resolutely, becoming experts in all aspects of reproductive endocrinology.

The overwhelming majority of infertile couples who desire children will conceive and give birth eventually. The treatments do work, albeit selectively; and of course nature's roulette wheel is still spinning for some, as we occasionally see couples who have tried for years to bear a child become pregnant when they least expect it.

But survival is possible, even when it appears that pregnancy and childbirth are not. I do not say this lightly, because I experienced the slow death of my dream.

When the death is intangible, it is difficult to put boundaries on the loss. Where is the grave for a child who never lived or died, a pregnancy that never was, an event that hasn't happened? My heart burst with the love I had to give to the child my husband and I did not conceive.

And when did I acknowledge the end of possibility? My sadness was overwhelming. I couldn't move on until I could focus my grief and accept the death of my dream.

When that time came, I found that I could survive and heal. Not that I have forgotten, nor that I don't have a memory of feeling cheated in life's game, but it no longer gives me pain in the present.

My husband and I created our destiny, as much as anybody can, when we decided to adopt a child. Today, I feel free and strong. My resolution is a success.

Charlotte Rosin,
past president of
RESOLVE of Central New Jersey

WE'D LIKE TO HEAR FROM YOU

As we were writing this book, we felt as if we were really talking to you, our reader. Now that you have actually read our book, we'd like to learn more about you and about the details of your experience with infertility. And we'd like to learn whether you used the activities in *Getting Pregnant* and whether they helped you. Your feedback and comments will be invaluable as we revise activities to use with our clients and share with our readers in any revised editions of this book. Please feel free to write to us at the following address:

Helane Rosenberg and Yakov Epstein
IVF New Jersey
1527 Highway 27
Suite 2100
Somerset, NJ 08873

And if you succeed in having a baby, we'd be delighted to receive a picture of her, him, or them. Or hear your story. We look forward to your response.

RESOURCES

Support groups for parents who have experienced a pregnancy loss:

Reach Out to Parents of an Unknown Child
c/o Health House
One High Street
Port Jefferson, NY 11777
516-474-5300

Compassionate Friends Inc.
PO Box 3696
Oak Brook, IL 60522
708-990-0010

Personal Care
c/o Sister Mary Alice
Mercy Hospital
North Village Avenue
Rockville Centre, NY 11570
516-255-2241

National Infertility advocacy and education organization:

RESOLVE Inc.
1310 Broadway
Somerville, MA 02174
617-623-0744 (for counseling)
617-623-1156 (business office)

Tapes of talks and workshops at New York City RESOLVE symposia can be ordered from:

RESOLVE NYC
PO Box 185, Gracie Station
New York, NY 10028
212-971-8538

Support organization for DES offspring:

DES Action
1615 Broadway
Oakland, CA 94612
510-465-4011

Medical society for fertility professionals:

(Publisher of the journal *Fertility and Sterility*)
American Fertility Society
2140 11th Avenue South, Suite 200
Birmingham, AL 35205
205-933-8494

Medical society for obstetricians and gynecologists:

American College of Obstetricians and Gynecologists (ACOG)
409 12th Street SW
Washington, DC 20024
202-638-5577

Medical societies for specialists in male infertility:

American Society of Andrology
309 West Clark Street
Champaign, IL 61820
217-356-3182

American Urological Association Inc.
1120 North Charles Street
Baltimore, MD 21201
301-727-1100

Source of pamphlets about various aspects of infertility as well as information about insurance coverage:

SERONO Symposia, U.S.A.
100 Longwater Circle
Norwell, MA 02061
617-982-9000

Surrogate parenting information is available from these organizations:

ICNY
14 East 60th Street, Suite 1204
New York, NY 10022
212-371-0811

Center for Surrogate Parenting
8383 Wilshire Boulevard, Suite 750
Beverly Hills, CA 90211
213-655-1974

The Surrogate Parent Program
11110 Ohio Avenue, Suite 202
Los Angeles, CA 90025
310-473-8961

The Surrogate Mother Program Inc.
c/o Dr. Betsy P. Aigen
220 West 93rd Street
New York, NY 10025
212-496-1070

Adoption information is available from the following sources:

Adoptive Families of America
3333 Highway 100 North
Minneapolis, MN 55422
612-535-4829

(NOTE: This group publishes *OURS*, a magazine for adoptive families. They maintain a listing of adoption support groups in states throughout the United States. They also publish a list of adoption agencies.)

Child Welfare League of America
440 First Avenue NW
Washington, DC 20001
202-638-2952

National Adoption Exchange
1218 Chestnut Street, Suite 404
Philadelphia, PA 19107
215-925-0200

National Adoption Information
  Clearinghouse
11426 Rockville Pike, Suite 410
Rockville, MD 20852
301-231-6512

Support organizations for persons with endometriosis:

Endometriosis Association
8585 North 76th Place
Milwaukee, WI 53223
414-355-2200
800-992-ENDO

The Endometriosis Alliance of Greater
  New York Inc.
PO Box 634, Old Chelsea Station
New York, NY 10113-0634
212-533-ENDO

Advice about infertility caused by an IUD (intrauterine device):

IUD Litigation Information Service
National Women's Health Network
1325 G Street NW
Washington, DC 20005
202-347-1140

Periodicals and newsletters about infertility:

Fertility and Sterility
Contact the American Fertility Society
for information about obtaining copies.

Infertility: Medical and Social Choices
Document No. OTA-BA-358, May
  1988
Obtained from:
Superintendent of Documents
U.S. Government Office of
  Technology Assessment
Dept. 36-AW
Washington, DC 20402-9325

Loving Arms
Pregnancy and Infant Loss Center of
  Minnesota
1415 East Wayzata Boulevard,
  Suite 22
Wayzata, MN 55391

Stepping Stones
PO Box 11141
Wichita, KS 67211
(This is a free bimonthly newsletter
for Christian infertile couples.)

The following is a list of clinics performing assisted reproductive procedures. The list is taken from clinics that completed a 1989 survey conducted by the Society for Assisted Reproductive Technology (SART). SART publishes similar surveys each year. The survey lists the number of IVF and GIFT procedures each clinic performed and their success rates. A copy of the survey report can be purchased from the American Fertility Society. Call them at 205-933-8494 for details about acquiring a copy. The listing we provide is organized on a state-by-state basis.

ALABAMA

ART Program
(Dr. Kathryn Honea, Director)
2006 Brookwood Medical Center Drive
Birmingham, AL 35209
205-870-9784

University of Alabama at Birmingham
(Dr. Michael P. Steinkampf, Director)
Dept. of Obstetrics and Gynecology
Birmingham, AL 35294
205-934-3394

University of South Alabama
(Dr. Sezer Aksel, Director)
Dept. of Obstetrics and Gynecology
Division of Reproductive Endocrinology
CCCB, Room 324
Mobile, AL 36688
205-460-7173

ARIZONA

Arizona Fertility Institute
(Dr. Robert H. Tamis, Director)
2850 North 24th Street, Suite 500-A
Phoenix, AZ 85008
602-468-3840

Southwest Fertility Center
(Dr. Sujatha Gunnala, Director)
3125 North 32nd Street, Suite 200
Phoenix, AZ 85018
602-956-7481

Arizona Center for Fertility Studies
(Dr. Jay S. Nemiro, Director)
8997 East Desert Cove Avenue,
  2nd Floor
Scottsdale, AZ 85260
602-860-4792

CALIFORNIA

Alta Bates In Vitro Fertilization Program
(Dr. Ryszard J. Chetkowski, Director)
Alta Bates-Herrick Hospital
3001 Colby Street
Berkeley, CA 94705
510-204-1416

East Bay Fertility
(Dr. F. J. Beernink, Director)
OB-GYN Medical Group
2999 Regent Street
Berkeley, CA 94705
510-841-5510

Encino and Beverly Hills Fertility
  Institutes
(Dr. Jeffrey Steinberg, Director)
16500 Ventura Boulevard, Suite 220
Encino, CA 91436
818-501-6674

Central California IVF Program
(Dr. Carlos E. Sueldo, Director)
6215 North Fresno, Suite 106
Fresno, CA 93710
209-439-1913

Scripps Clinic Fertility Center
(Dr. Jeffrey S. Rakoff, Director)
10666 North Torrey Pines Road
La Jolla, CA 92037
619-455-9100

Loma Linda Fertility Center
(Dr. Donald R. Treadway, Director)
11370 Anderson Street, Suite 3950
Loma Linda, CA 92357
714-796-4806

Long Beach Memorial
(Dr. Bill Yee, Director)
2880 Atlantic Avenue, Suite 220
Long Beach, CA 90806
310-595-2000

Cedars Sinai Medical Center
(Dr. John F. Kerin, Director)
444 South San Vicente Boulevard,
Suite 1101
Los Angeles, CA 90048
310-855-5000

Century City Hospital
(Dr. David L. Hill, Director)
2070 Century Park East
Los Angeles, CA 90067
310-553-6211

Institute for Reproductive Research
(Dr. Richard P. Marrs, Director)
1245 Wilshire Boulevard, Suite 905
Los Angeles, CA 90017
213-482-4552

Southern California Fertility Institute
(Dr. William G. Karow, Director)
12301 Wilshire Boulevard, Suite 415
Los Angeles, CA 90025
310-820-3723

Tyler Medical Clinic
(Dr. Jaroslav Marik, Director)
921 Westwood Boulevard
Los Angeles, CA 90014
310-208-6765

UCLA Fertility Center
(Dr. Joseph Gambone, Director)
10833 Le Comte Avenue
Los Angeles, CA 90024-1740
310-825-7955

USC-CAL Reproductive Health Institute
(Dr. Richard J. Paulson, Director)
1138 South Hope Street
Los Angeles, CA 90015
213-342-2000

Hoag Memorial Hospital
(Dr. L. B. Werlin, Director)
356 Hospital Road, Suite 316
Newport Beach, CA 92663
714-760-2395

Northridge Hospital Medical Center
(Dr. David Richards, Director)
18300 Roscoe Boulevard
Northridge, CA 91328
818-885-8500

Huntington Reproductive Center
(Dr. Paulo Serafini, Director)
39 Congress Street, Suite 202
Pasadena, CA 91105
818-440-9161

South Bay Hospital IVF
(Dr. David R. Meldrum, Director)
514 North Prospect Avenue
Redondo Beach, CA 90277
310-376-9474

IGO Medical Group of San Diego
(Dr. Joseph F. Kennedy, Director)
9339 Genesee Avenue, Suite 220
San Diego, CA 92121
619-455-7520

Pacific Fertility Center
(Dr. Geoffrey Sher, Director)
2100 Webster Street, Suite 506
San Francisco, CA 94115
415-923-3344

University of California, San Francisco
(Dr. Mary C. Martin, Director)
Dept. of Ob/Gyn, Room 1489
San Francisco, CA 94143-0132
415-476-2564

Fertility and Reproductive Health
  Institute
(Dr. G. D. Adamson, Director)
2516 Samaritan Drive, Suite A
San Jose, CA 95125
408-358-2500

Forest Fertility Center
(Dr. Vincent F. Nola, Director)
2110 Forest Avenue
San Jose, CA 95128
408-288-9933

Nova Fertility Center
(Dr. Francis F. Polansky, Director)
101 South San Mateo Drive
San Mateo, CA 94401
415-340-0500

Stanford University Medical Center
(Dr. Emmet J. Lamb, Director)
Room S-253
Stanford, CA 94305
415-723-4000

John Muir Medical Center
(Dr. Bernard Larner, Director)
1601 Ygnacio Valley Road
Walnut Creek, CA 94598
510-939-3000

COLORADO

Conceptions Reproductive Technology
  Consultants
(Dr. Bruce Albrecht, Director)
455 South Hudson Street
Denver, CO 80022
303-333-3378

Reproductive Genetics, In Vitro
(Dr. George P. Henry, Director)
455 South Hudson Street, Level 3
Denver, CO 80022
303-399-5393

Swedish Medical Center
(Dr. William Schoolcraft, Director)
701 East Hampden Avenue, Suite 310B
Englewood, CO 80110
303-788-5000

CONNECTICUT

University of Connecticut Health Center
(Dr. Anthony Luciano, Director)
263 Farmington Avenue
Farmington, CT 06030
203-679-1000

Hartford Hospital
(Dr. Augusto P. Chong, Director)
100 Retreat Avenue, Suite 900
Hartford, CT 06106
203-524-3011

Yale University School of Medicine
(Dr. Alan H. DeCherney, Director)
Dept. of Ob/Gyn
333 Cedar Street
New Haven, CT 06510-8063
203-432-0222

DISTRICT OF COLUMBIA

Columbia Hospital for Women
(Dr. Maurice J. Butler, Director)
IVF Program
2440 M Street NW, Suite 401
Washington, DC 20037
202-293-6500

George Washington University
  Medical Center
(Dr. Paul R. Gindoff, Director)
Dept. of Ob/Gyn
2150 Pennsylvania Avenue NW
Washington, DC 20037
202-994-4357

DELAWARE

Medical Center of Delaware
(Dr. Jeffrey B. Russell, Director)
Reproductive Endocrinology and
  Fertility Center
4755 Ogletown-Stanton Road
Newark, DE 19713
302-738-4600

FLORIDA

Fertility Institute of Boca Raton
(Dr. Moshe R. Peress, Director)
875 Meadows Road
Boca Raton, FL 33428
407-368-5500

Florida Institute of Fertility
(Dr. Eliezer J. Livnat, Director)
5000 West Oakland Park Boulevard
Fort Lauderdale, FL 33313
305-739-6222

University of Florida Shands Hospital
  Park Avenue Center
(Dr. Gregory T. Fossum, Director)
817 Northwest 56th Terrace, Suite C
Gainesville, FL 32605
904-392-6200

Fertility Institute of Northwest Florida
(Dr. R. C. Pyle, Director)
1110 Gulf Breeze Parkway
Gulf Breeze, FL 32561
904-934-3900

Memorial Medical Center of
  Jacksonville
(Dr. Marwan Shaykh, Director)
3625 University Boulevard South
Jacksonville, FL 32216
904-399-6996

IVF Florida
(Dr. Wayne S. Maxson, Director)
5800 Colonial Drive, Suite 200
Margate, FL 33063
305-975-4775

University of Miami Medical School
(Dr. Terry T. Hung, Director)
Dept. of Ob/Gyn (D-5)
P.O. Box 016960
Miami, FL 33101
305-547-5818

Mount Sinai Medical Center of Miami
(Dr. Bernard Cantor, Director)
4300 Alton Road
Miami Beach, FL 33140
305-674-2121

Sand Lake Hospital of Orlando
   IVF Program
(Dr. Frank C. Riggall, Director)
9430 Turkey Lake Road, Suite 204
Orlando, FL 32819
407-351-8504

Humana Women's Hospital
(Dr. George Maroulis, Director)
3030 West Martin Luther King
   Boulevard
Tampa, FL 33607
813-879-4730

Center for Infertility and
   Reproductive Medicine
(Dr. Gary W. DeVane, Director)
1936 Lee Road, Suite 100
Winter Park, FL 32789
407-740-0909

GEORGIA

Reproductive Biology Associates
(Dr. H. I. Kort, Director)
5505 Peachtree Dunwoody Road,
   Suite 400
Atlanta, GA 30342
404-843-3064

Augusta Reproductive Biology
   Associates
(Dr. Edouard J. Servy, Director)
812 Chafee Avenue
Augusta, GA 30904
706-724-0228

Medical College of Georgia
(Dr. Gail F. Whitman, Director)
Dept. of Ob/Gyn
Reproductive Endocrinology, CK-159
Augusta, GA 30912-3360
706-721-3434

HAWAII

Pacific IVF Institute
(Dr. Philip I. McNamee, Director)
1319 Punahou Street, Suite 525
Honolulu, HI 96826
808-946-2226

ILLINOIS

IVF Illinois
(Dr. A. Lifchez, Director)
836 West Wellington
Chicago, IL 60657
312-296-7221

Michael Reese Fertility Center
(Dr. Edward L. Marut, Director)
60 East Delaware, Suite 1400
Chicago, IL 60611
312-440-5100

Mount Sinai of Chicago Center for
   Human Reproduction
(Dr. Norbert Gleicher, Director)
750 North Orleans Street
Chicago, IL 60610
312-649-9686

Northwestern University Center for
Assisted Reproduction
(Dr. Anne Colston Wentz, Director)
680 North Lake Shore Drive
Chicago, IL 60611
312-908-7269

Rush Presbyterian Saint Luke's
Medical Center
(Dr. Zvi Binor, Director)
Dept. of Ob/Gyn
1653 West Congress Parkway
Chicago, IL 60612
312-942-3026

Glenbrook Hospital IVF
(Dr. John S. Rinehart, Director)
2050 Pfingsten Road, Suite 350
Glenview, IL 60025
708-657-5700

Center for Advanced Reproduction
(Dr. Charles E. Miller, Director)
1875 Dempster Street, Suite 180
Park Ridge, IL 60068
708-696-8217

INDIANA

Indiana University Coleman Clinic
(Dr. Marguerite K. Shepard,
Director)
Dept. of Ob/Gyn
University Hospital, N 250
Indianapolis, IN 46202
317-274-8231

Methodist Center for Reproduction
(Dr. Carolyn B. Coulam, Director)
1633 North Capitol Avenue,
Suite 488
Indianapolis, IN 46202
317-929-8893

Pregnancy Initiation Center
(Dr. John C. Jarrett, Director)
8091 Township Line Road
Indianapolis, IN 46260
317-875-5978

IOWA

McFarland Clinic
(Dr. Alan Munson, Director)
1215 Duff Avenue
Ames, IA 50010
515-239-4400

University of Iowa Hospital and Clinic
(Dr. Craig H. Syrop, Director)
Dept. of Ob/Gyn
Center for Advanced Reproductive Care
Iowa City, IA 52242
319-356-1767

KANSAS

Reproductive Resource Center
(Dr. Rodney Lyles, Director)
10600 Quivira Road, Suite 110
Overland Park, KS 66215
913-894-2323

Center for Reproductive Medicine
(Dr. B. W. Webster, Director)
2903 East Central
Wichita, KS 67214
316-687-2112

KENTUCKY

University of Kentucky Center for
Women's Health
(Dr. Robert J. Homm, Director)
800 Rose Street, Room C-312
Lexington, KY 40536
606-275-6970

University of Louisville Fertility
Program
(Dr. Christine L. Cook, Director)
Norton Hospital Women's Pavilion, 3S
200 East Chestnut Street
Louisville, KY 40202
502-629-8000

LOUISIANA

Fertility Center of Louisiana
(Dr. Heber Dunaway, Director)
4720 I-10 Service Road, Suite 100
Metairie, LA 70001
504-454-2165

Fertility Institute of New Orleans
(Dr. Richard P. Dickey, Director)
6020 Bullard Avenue
New Orleans, LA 70128
504-246-8971

MARYLAND

Johns Hopkins IVF Program
(Dr. Marian D. Damewood, Director)
The Johns Hopkins Hospital
600 North Wolfe Street, Houck 249
Baltimore, MD 21205
410-955-5000

University of Maryland
(Dr. Eugene Katz, Director)
405 West Redwood Street, 3rd Floor
Baltimore, MD 21201
410-328-6640

Women's Hospital Fertility Center
(Dr. Jairo E. Garcia, Director)
Greater Baltimore Medical Center
6565 North Charles Street, Suite 207
Baltimore, MD 21204
410-828-2597

Montgomery Infertility Institute
(Dr. Jay M. Grodin, Director)
10215 Fernwood Road, Suite 303-305
Bethesda, MD 20817
301-897-8850

MASSACHUSETTS

Brigham and Women's Hospital
IVF Program
(Dr. Andrew J. Friedman, Director)
75 Francis Street
Boston, MA 02115
617-732-4239

New England Medical Center/Tufts
(Dr. Steven Bayer, Director)
750 Washington Street, Box 36
Boston, MA 02111
617-956-5000

Boston IVF
(Dr. Selwyn Oskowitz, Director)
One Brookline Place
Brookline, MA 02146
617-735-9000

Fertility Institute of Western
Massachusetts
(Dr. Ronald K. Burke, Director)
130 Maple Street, Suite 246
Springfield, MA 01130
413-781-8220

New England Memorial Fertility Center
(Dr. Vito R. S. Cardone, Director)
Medical Office Building
Three Woodland Road, Suite 321
Stoneham, MA 02180
617-979-0122

IVF Australia Boston at
  Waltham-Weston Hospital
(Dr. Patricia M. McShane, Director)
Hope Avenue
Waltham, MA 02254
617-647-6000

MICHIGAN

University of Michigan
(Dr. William W. Hurd)
Dept. of Ob/Gyn, Division of
  Reproductive Endocrinology
1500 East Medical Center Drive
Ann Arbor, MI 48109-0718
313-936-4000

Oakwood Hospital Center for
  Reproductive Medicine
(Dr. David Magyar, Director)
Medical Office Building, Suite 100G
18181 Oakwood Boulevard
Dearborn, MI 48124
313-593-5880

Hutzel Hospital/Wayne State University
(Dr. Charla M. Blacker, Director)
4707 St. Antoine
Detroit, MI 48201
313-745-7555

Blodgett Memorial Medical Center
(Dr. Robert D. Visscher, Director)
1900 Wealthy SE
Grand Rapids, MI 49506
616-774-7444

Beaumont Fertility Center
(Dr. William R. Keye, Jr., Director)
3535 West Thirteen Mile Road,
  Suite 344
Royal Oak, MI 48072
313-551-5000

Saginaw Cooperative Hospitals
(Dr. M. Hasan Fakih, Director)
1000 Houghton Avenue
Saginaw, MI 48602
517-771-6742

IVF Ann Arbor
(Dr. Jonathan Ayers, Director)
4990 Clark Road, Suite 100
Ypsilanti, MI 48197
313-434-4766

MINNESOTA

University of Minnesota Hospital
(Dr. George E. Tagatz, Director)
Dept. of Ob/Gyn
Box 395 UMHC
Minneapolis, MN 55455
612-626-3232

Mayo Clinic
(Dr. Randle S. Corfman, Director)
100 First Street SW
Rochester, MN 55905
507-284-2511

MISSISSIPPI

University of Mississippi Medical
  Center
(Dr. Bryan D. Cowan, Director)
Dept. of Ob/Gyn
2500 North State Street
Jackson, MS 39216
601-984-1000

MISSOURI

International Center for Reproductive
   Research
(Dr. Nezaam Zamah, Director)
3101 Broadway, Suite 650B
Kansas City, MO 64111
816-931-2733

Jewish Hospital of St. Louis
(Dr. Ronald C. Strickler, Director)
216 South Kings Highway Boulevard
St. Louis, MO 63110
314-454-7000

Saint Luke's of St. Louis
(Dr. Sherman J. Silber, Director)
224 South Woods Mill Road,
   Suite 730
St. Louis, MO 63017
314-576-1400

NEBRASKA

Nebraska Methodist Hospital
(Dr. Marvin Dietrich, Director)
8303 Dodge
Omaha, NE 68104
402-390-4000

NEVADA

Northern Nevada Fertility Center
(Dr. Victor Knutzen, Director)
350 West 6th Street, Suite A-3
Reno, NV 89503
702-688-5600

NEW HAMPSHIRE

Dartmouth Hitchcock Medical Center
(Dr. Paul Manganiello, Director)
Clinic 500
2 Maynard Street
Hanover, NH 03756
603-650-8161

NEW JERSEY

IVF New Jersey
(Dr. Michael C. Darder, Director)
1527 Highway 27, Suite 2100
Somerset, NJ 08873
908-220-9060

UMDNJ Newark Center For Fertility
(Dr. Cecilia L. Schmidt, Director)
Medical Sciences Building, Room E506
185 South Orange Avenue
Newark, NJ 07103-2757
201-456-4300

UMDNJ Robert Wood Johnson
   Medical School IVF Program
(Dr. E. Kemmann, Director)
Dept. of Ob/Gyn
CN 19
New Brunswick, NJ 08903
908-937-7627

NEW MEXICO

Presbyterian Hospital
(Dr. Jim Thompson, Director)
1100 Central Southeast
Albuquerque, NM 87102
505-841-1234

NEW YORK

Albany Medical College IVF
(Dr. Peter M. Horvath, Director)
New Scotland Avenue
Albany, NY 12208
518-445-3125

Children's Hospital—Buffalo
(Dr. Kent Crickard, Director)
Dept. of Ob/Gyn
140 Hodge Avenue
Buffalo, NY 14222
716-878-7000

Montefiore Medical Center—Albert
  Einstein College of Medicine
(Dr. David Barad, Director)
20 Beacon Hill Road
Dobbs Ferry, NY 10522
212-430-2000

North Shore University Hospital
(Dr. Frances Taney, Director)
300 Community Drive
Manhasset, NY 11030
516-562-0100

Columbia Presbyterian Medical Center
(Dr. Christina R. Veit, Director)
622 West 168th Street
New York, NY 10032
212-305-2500

Cornell Medical Center
(Dr. Zev Rosenwaks, Director)
505 East 70th Street, HT 300
New York, NY 10021
212-746-5454

Mount Sinai Medical Center
  IVF Program
(Dr. Daniel Navot, Director)
1212 Fifth Avenue
New York, NY 10029
212-241-5927

New York Medical Services
(Dr. Niels H. Lauersen, Director)
784 Park Avenue
New York, NY 10021
212-744-4222

Saint Luke's Roosevelt Hospital
  IVF Program
(Dr. Dov S. Goldstein, Director)
1111 Amsterdam Avenue
New York, NY 10024
212-523-4000

IVF Australia at United Hospital
(Dr. John J. Stangel, Director)
406 Boston Post Road
Port Chester, NY 10573
914-939-5600

IVF Long Island Hospital
(Dr. David Kreiner, Director)
60 North Country Road
Port Jefferson, NY 11777
516-473-1320

Institute for Reproductive Health and
  Infertility
(Dr. Ko-En Huang, Director)
1561 Long Pond Road, Suite 410
Rochester, NY 14626
716-723-7470

University of Rochester
(Dr. John H. Mattox, Director)
601 Elmwood Avenue, Box 668
Rochester, NY 14642
716-275-2871

NORTH CAROLINA

Chapel Hill Fertility Center
(Dr. Gary S. Berger, Director)
109 Conner Drive, Suite 2104
Chapel Hill, NC 27514
919-968-4656

University of North Carolina
(Dr. Luther M. Talbert, Director)
Dept. of Ob/Gyn
CB #7570, Old Clinic Building
Chapel Hill, NC 27599-7570
919-962-2211

Duke University Medical Center
(Dr. William C. Dodson, Director)
Box 3143
Durham, NC 27710
919-684-8111

Bowman Gray Medical School
(Dr. Jeffrey L. Deaton, Director)
300 South Hawthorne Road
Winston-Salem, NC 27103
919-748-2011

NORTH DAKOTA

Centennial Medical Center
(Dr. David L. MacDonald, Director)
1500 24th Avenue SW
Minot, ND 68702-0040
701-852-0777

OHIO

Akron City Hospital IVF
(Dr. Nicholas J. Spirtos, Director)
525 East Market Street
Akron, OH 44309
216-375-3000

Bethesda City Hospital Fertility Center
(Dr. NeeOo W. Chin, Director)
619 Oak Street
Cincinnati, OH 45206-1690
513-569-6161

University Hospital of Cleveland
(Dr. James Goldfarb, Director)
2072 Abington Road
Cleveland, OH 44106
216-844-3896

Grant Reproductive Center
(Dr. Nichols Vorys, Director)
340 East Town Street, 8-400
Columbus, OH 43215
614-253-8383

Riverside Reproductive Services
(Dr. Grant Schmidt, Director)
3726 K Olentangy River Road
Columbus, OH 43214
614-566-5100

Miami Valley Fertility Center
(Dr. P. Daneshjoo, Director)
One Wyoming Street
Dayton, OH 43409
513-435-1445

OKLAHOMA

Bennett Fertility Center
(Dr. David A. Kallenberger, Director)
3300 Northwest Expressway
Oklahoma City, OK 73112
405-949-6060

Hillcrest Fertility Center
(Dr. Stanley G. Prough, Director)
1145 South Utica, Suite 1209
Tulsa, OK 74104
918-584-2870

OREGON

Northwest Fertility Center
(Dr. Eugene M. Stoelk, Director)
River Place Office Building, Suite 200
1750 Southwest Harbor Way
Portland, OR 97201
503-227-7799

Oregon Reproductive Research and
   Fertility Program
(Dr. Phillip E. Patton, Director)
3181 Southwest Sam Jackson Park Road
Portland, OR 97201
503-494-6307

PENNSYLVANIA

Abington Memorial Hospital
(Dr. G.W. Campbell, Director)
1200 Old York Road
Abington, PA 19001
215-576-2349

Christian Fertility Institute
(Dr. William I. Cooper, Director)
241 North 13th Street
Easton, PA 18042
215-250-9700

Endrocrine Histology Associates
(Dr. Jerome H. Check, Director)
7447 Old York Road
Melrose Park, PA 19126
215-635-4930

Albert Einstein Medical Center IVF-ET
(Dr. Martin Freedman, Director)
Klein Building, Suite 400
York and Tabor Roads
Philadelphia, PA 19141
215-456-9870

Pennsylvania Reproductive Associates
(Dr. Stephen L. Corson, Director)
Pennsylvania Hospital
Spruce Building, Room 786
800 Spruce Street
Philadelphia, PA 19107
215-829-3000

University of Pennsylvania Hospital
(Dr. Richard W. Tureck, Director)
#1 Dulles Building
3400 Spruce Street
Philadelphia, PA 19104
215-662-4000

Magee Women's Hospital
(Dr. Carolyn J. Kubik, Director)
Forbes Avenue and Halket Street
Pittsburgh, PA 15213
412-647-1000

Shadyside Hospital IVF
(Dr. Amir A. Ansari, Director)
5230 Centre Avenue
Pittsburgh, PA 15232
412-623-2121

Fertility Medical Labs
(Dr. Vincent Pellegrini, Director)
301 South Seventh Avenue
West Reading, PA 19611
215-374-2214

PUERTO RICO

Hospital San Pablo
(Dr. Pedro J. Beauchamp, Director)
Santa Cruz Medical Building No. 73,
   Suite 213
Bayamóu, PR 00619
809-740-4747

RHODE ISLAND

Women and Infants Hospital
(Dr. Ray V. Maning, Director)
Dept. of Reproductive Endocrinology
101 Dudley Street
Providence, RI 02905
401-274-1100

SOUTH CAROLINA

Southeastern Fertility Center
(Dr. Gary L. Moltz, Director)
900 Bowman Road, Suite 108
Mount Pleasant, SC 29464
803-881-3900

TENNESSEE

Humana East—Ridge Hospital Infertility
  Center
(Dr. John A. Lucas, Director)
941 Spring Creek Road
Chattanooga, TN 37412
615-894-7870

East Tennessee State University
(Dr. Samuel S. Thatcher, Director)
Dept. of Ob/Gyn
Box 19, 570A, James M. Quillen
  College of Medicine
Johnson City, TN 37614
615-929-6335

University of Tennessee Medical Center
(Dr. Michael C. Doody, Director)
1924 Alcoa Highway
Knoxville, TN 37920
615-544-9306

University of Tennessee Medical Group
  Pair
(Dr. Sandra A. Carson, Director)
66 North Pauline Street, Suite 424
Memphis, TN 38105
901-528-6610

Vanderbilt University Medical Center
(Dr. Jamie M. Vasquez, Director)
Center for Fertility and Reproductive
  Research
C-1100 Medical Center North
Nashville, TN 37232
615-322-5000

TEXAS

Saint David's Hospital IVF Program
(Dr. Thomas Vaughn, Director)
P.O. Box 4039
Austin, TX 78765
512-476-7111

Trinity IVF-ET Program
(Dr. W. F. Howard, Director)
4333 North Josey Lane, Suite 200
Carrollton, TX 75010
214-394-8483

Baylor Center for Reproductive Health
(Dr. J. Michael Putman, Director)
3707 Gaston Avenue, Suite 310
Dallas, TX 75246
214-821-2274

Presbyterian Hospital of Dallas
(Dr. James D. Madden, Director)
8160 Walnut Hill Lane, Box 17
Dallas, TX 75231
214-345-6789

University of Texas Dallas
Southwestern Medical Center IVF
(Dr. Karen Bradshaw, Director)
5323 Harry Hines Boulevard
Dallas, TX 75235
214-688-2022

Harris Methodist Fort Worth Infertility
Center
(Dr. Kevin J. Doody, Director)
1325 Pennsylvania Avenue, Suite 440
Fort Worth, TX 76104
817-878-5360

Baylor IVF Program
(Dr. James N. Wheeler, Director)
One Baylor Plaza
Houston, TX 77030
713-798-4951

Houston Reproductive Center
(Dr. Irvin Reiner, Director)
1615 Hillendahl
Houston, TX 77055
713-932-5679

OB/GYN Associates
(Dr. George M. Grunert, Director)
Laboratory for Assisted Reproduction
7550 Fannin Street
Houston, TX 77054
713-797-9163

Southwest Fertility Center
(Dr. Joseph McWherter, Director)
1717 Precinct Line Road
Hurst, TX
817-498-1123

Texas Tech University IVF Program
(Dr. Janelle Dorsett, Director)
Dept. of Ob/Gyn
Lubbock, TX 79430
806-743-2335

Methodist Hospital Fertility Program
(Dr. Thomas B. Pool, Director)
4499 Medical Drive, Suite 160
San Antonio, TX 78229
512-692-4000

University of Texas Health Science
Center
(Dr. Robert S. Schenken, Director)
7703 Floyd Curl Drive
San Antonio, TX 78284-7836
512-567-7000

UTAH

University of Utah Fertility Center
(Dr. Kirtly Parker Jones, Director)
50 North Medical Drive
Salt Lake City, UT 84132
801-581-2121

VERMONT

University of Vermont IVF Program
(Dr. Mark Gibson, Director)
Dept. of Ob/Gyn
One South Prospect Street
Burlington, VT 05401
802-656-2272

VIRGINIA

Institute for Reproductive Medicine
(Dr. John D. Paulson, Director)
4324-C Evergreen Lane
Annandale, VA 22003
703-658-9300

Dominion Fertility and Endocrinology
   Institute
(Dr. Michael DiMattina, Director)
46 South Glebe Road, Suite 301
Arlington, VA 22204
703-920-3890

Genetics and IVF Institute
(Dr. Joseph D. Schulman, Director)
3020 Javier Road
Fairfax, VA 22031
703-698-7355

Jones Institute for Reproductive
   Medicine
(Dr. Suheil J. Muasher, Director)
825 Fairfax Avenue, 6th Floor
Norfolk, VA 23507
703-446-8948

Henrico Doctors Hospital IVF Program
(Dr. Sanford M. Rosenberg, Director)
7603 Forest Avenue, Suite 301
Richmond, VA 23229
804-289-4500

Medical College of Virginia
(Dr. Kenneth A. Steingold, Director)
Box 34, MCV Station
Richmond, VA 23298
804-786-9000

WASHINGTON

Reproductive Genetics Laboratory
(Dr. Laurence E. Karp, Director)
Swedish Hospital
747 Summit
Seattle, WA 98104
206-386-2101

University of Washington Fertility
   Center
(Dr. Paul W. Zarutskie, Director)
4225 Roosevelt Way NE, Suite 101
Seattle, WA 98105
206-548-4225

WISCONSIN

Appleton Medical Center
(Dr. John S. Harris, Director)
Family Fertility Clinic
1818 North Meade Street
Appleton, WI 54911
414-731-4101

University of Wisconsin Medical
   Clinics IVF Program
(Dr. Sander S. Shapiro, Director)
Room H4/635
Madison, WI 53792
608-263-6400

Medical College of Wisconsin
(Dr. E. James Alman, Director)
8700 West Wisconsin Avenue
Milwaukee, WI 53226
414-257-8296

Waukesha Memorial Hospital
(Dr. K. Paul Katayama, Director)
725 American Avenue
Waukesha, WI 53188
414-544-2011

The following is a list of sperm banks that are associated with the American Association of Tissue Banks (AATB). All of the banks are directed by individuals who, as AATB members, practice AATB standards and participate in AATB questionnaires on clinical applications and results with cryobanked semen. However, only the banks listed in Group I are AATB accredited facilities.

GROUP I

Biogenetics Corporation
(Albert Anouna, Director)
P.O. Box 1290
1330 Route 22 West
Mountainside, NJ 07092
800-942-4646

California Cryobank
(Charles Simms, Director)
1019 Gayley Avenue
Los Angeles, CA 90024
800-231-3373

Cryogenic Laboratories Inc.
(Dr. John H. Olson, Director)
2233 Hamline Avenue North
Roseville, MN 55113
612-636-3792

Genetic Semen Bank
(Warren Sanger, Director)
University of Nebraska Medical Center
82nd Street and Dewey Avenue
Omaha, NE 68105
402-559-5070

Reproductive Associates
(Brenda Bordson, Director)
4740 I-10 Service Road, Suite 340
Metairie, LA 70001
800-227-4561

University of Texas
(William Byrd, Director)
Southwestern Medical Center
  Andrology and Reproductive
  Andrology Center
Dallas, TX 75235
214-588-2376

GROUP II

Arbor Park Reproductive Lab
(Dr. E. P. Peterson, Director)
4990 Clark Road, Suite 100
Ypsilanti, MI 48197
313-434-4766

Arizona Institute for Reproductive
  Medicine
(Robert Tamis, Director)
4602 North 16th Street, No. 201
Phoenix, AZ 85106
602-251-7440

Baylor Sperm Banking Program
(Dr. Larry Lipschultz, Director)
Scott Dept. of Urology
6560 Fannin, No. 1002
Houston, TX 77030
713-798-4001

Center for Reproduction and
  Transplantation Immunology
(John M. Critser, Director)
Methodist Hospital of Indiana
1701 North Sanata Boulevard
Indianapolis, IN 46202
317-929-6158

Cryobiology
(William Baird, Director)
4830-D Knightsbridge Boulevard
Columbus, OH 43214
614-451-4375

Cryo Laboratory Facility
(Alfred Morris, Director)
100 East Ohio, Suite 268
Chicago, IL 60601
312-751-2632

Desert Cryobank
(Dr. Sujatha Ounnala, Director)
3125 North 32nd Street, Suite 310
Phoenix, AZ 85108
602-956-7481

Division of Reproductive Technology
(Mary Forster, Director)
Swedish Hospital
747 Summit Avenue
Seattle, WA 98104
206-386-2483

Evanston/Glenbrook Hospital
    IVF Program
(Marybeth Gerrity, Director)
2050 Pfingsten Road, Suite 350
Glenview, IL 60025
708-657-5700

Fairfax Cryobank
(Edward Fugger, Director)
3015 Williams Drive, Suite 110
Fairfax, VA 22031
703-698-3976

Fertility Institute of New Orleans
(Terry Olar, Director)
6020 Bullard Avenue
New Orleans, LA 70128
504-246-8871

Fertility Institute of Southern California
(Jean-Philipe F. Bailly, Director)
1125 East 17th Street
Santa Ana, CA 92701
714-953-5683

Grant Hospital of Chicago—
    Chicago IVF and Fertility Institute
(Dr. W. Paul Dmowski, Director)
550 Webster Avenue
Chicago, IL 60614
312-883-3866

Idant Laboratory
(Dr. Joseph Feldschuh, Director)
645 Madison Avenue
New York, NY 10022
212-935-1430

International Cryogenics Inc.
(Mary Ann Brown, Director)
189 Townsend, Suite 203
Birmingham, MI 48009
313-641-5822

Jefferson Sperm Bank
(Dr. Irvin Hirsch, Director)
Thomas Jefferson University Hospital
111 South 11th Street
Philadelphia, PA 19107
215-955-6961

Midwest Fertility Foundation and
    Laboratory
(Dr. Elwyn Grimms, Director)
3101 Broadway, Suite 650-A
Kansas City, MO 64111
816-756-0040

Midwest IVF/Andrology Laboratory
(Susan Sachdeva, Director)
4333 Main Street
Downers Grove, IL 60515
708-810-0212

National Health Guard, Inc.
(Robert E. Moon, Director)
6355 Northwest Ninth Avenue,
  Suite 107
Fort Lauderdale, FL 33309
305-772-2081

New England Andrology
(Dr. Robert A. Newton, Director)
Pratt Building
2014 Washington Street
Newton, MA 02162
617-332-1224

Northern California Cryobank
(Dr. Marvin Kamras, Director)
5821 Jameson Court
Carmichael, CA 95608
916-486-0451

Paces Cryobank and Infertility Services
(Vicki Ofma, Director)
124 Hammond Drive NE
Atlanta, GA 30328
404-252-7049

The Repository for Germinal Choice
(Robert Graham, Director)
PO Box 2876
Escondido, CA 92025
619-643-0772

Reproductive Lab
(Phillipe Bailly, Director)
336 East 30th Street
New York, NY 10016
212-779-3988

ReproMed Ltd.
(Dr. A. P. DeValle, Director)
2333 Dundas Street West, Suite 209
Toronto, Ontario
Canada M6R 3A6
416-537-6895

Rochester Regional Cryobank
(Grace Cantola, Director)
University of Rochester
  Department of Ob/Gyn
601 Elmwood Avenue
Rochester, NY 14642
716-275-1084

Rocky Mountain Cryobank
(William Racow, Director)
PO Box 3033
Jackson, WY 83001
307-733-9170

Drs. Sparr, Stephens, and Associates
(Dr. Stacy Stephens, Director)
8160 Walnut Hill Lane, Suite 384
Dallas, TX 75231
214-691-0924

The Sperm Bank of California
(Barbara Raboy, Director)
3007 Telegraph Avenue, Suite 2
Oakland, CA 94609
510-444-2014

University of Arkansas for Medical
  Sciences Semen Cryobank
(J. N. Sherman, Director)
4301 West Markham Street
Little Rock, AR 72205
501-686-8450

University McDonald Women's
  Hospital
(Leon Sheean, Director)
Andrology Laboratory
2074 Abington Road
Cleveland, OH 44106
216-844-1317

University of Missouri—Columbia
  Medical School
(Jawad Ali, Director)
Dept. of Urology
Health Sciences Center, N510
One Hospital Drive
Columbia, MO 65212
314-882-7176

University of Southern California
  Medical School
(Mark Siegel, Director)
Dept. of Ob/Gyn Andrology Lab
1321 North Mission Road
Los Angeles, CA 90033
213-343-9967

University of Wisconsin Clinical
  Sciences Center
(Dr. Sander Shapiro, Director)
Dept. of Ob/Gyn
600 Highland Avenue
Madison, WI 53705
608-263-1217

Washington Fertility Study Center
(Sal Leto, Director)
2600 Virginia Avenue NW, Suite 500
Washington, DC 20037
202-333-3100

Western Cryobank
(Charles Johnson, Director)
2010 East Bijou
Colorado Springs, CO 80909
719-578-9014

Xytex Corporation
(Armand Karow, Director)
1100 Emmett Street
Augusta, GA 30904
800-277-3210

Zygen Laboratory
(Dr. Cyrus Milani, Director)
16742 Stagg Street, Unit 105
Van Nuys, CA 91406
810-988-2500

The following is a pharmacy that can provide a complete inventory of supplies and medications for infertility. This establishment has laboratory facilities to produce certain medications that cannot be supplied by pharmacies without specialized facilities. They can ship medications to any area of the United States.

Boghen Pharmacy
1080 Park Avenue
New York, NY 10128
212-289-5866

GLOSSARY

abortion: The loss of a pregnancy before a fetus can survive on its own.

acrosin: An enzyme in the head of a sperm that dissolves the coating around the egg in order to allow the sperm to penetrate the egg.

acrosome reaction: The chemical changes that enable the sperm to penetrate the egg.

adhesions: Bands of scar tissue attached to the surface of organs such as the ovary, the bowels, or the fallopian tubes.

adrenaline: A hormone secreted by the adrenal medulla during strong emotion. This hormone causes bodily changes such as increased blood pressure.

agglutination of sperm: Sperm cells that clump or stick together.

AIH (Artificial Insemination by Husband): A procedure in which a wife is inseminated with her husband's sperm, in contrast to being inseminated by the sperm of a donor.

amenorrhea: Absence of menstrual cycles.

The American Fertility Society (AFS): An organization of more than 10,000 health care specialists interested in reproductive medicine.

ampulla: The outer end of the fallopian tube that is the widest part of the tube.

andrologist: A doctor specializing in male reproductive problems.

anesthesia (general): An agent that produces unconsciousness and complete loss of sensation throughout the body.

anesthesia (local): The use of medication to induce a loss of sensation in a specific part of the body without loss of consciousness.

anovulatory: A term describing a woman who rarely or never ovulates.

anticardiolipin antibodies: Proteins produced by the mother's body which are directed against the fat cells of the fetus. These antibodies are associated with repeated miscarriages.

antisperm antibodies: Protective agents produced by the body's immune system that attach to the sperm and prevent them from moving and fertilizing the egg.

ART: *See* Assisted reproductive technologies (ZIFT)

artificial insemination: The introduction of sperm into a woman's vagina or cervix using a special instrument rather than their introduction through intercourse.

artificial insemination by husband: A procedure in which a wife is inseminated with her husband's sperm, in contrast to being inseminated by the sperm of a donor.

Asherman's syndrome: A condition in which adhesions form inside the cavity of the uterus.

aspiration: The application of light suction to the ovarian follicle to remove the eggs.

assertiveness training: A behavior therapy technique for helping individuals become more self-assertive in their interpersonal relationships.

assisted reproductive technologies (ART): ART encompasses various techniques to stimulate the production of multiple eggs and enhance their likelihood of being fertilized. The list of techniques includes IVF, GIFT, ZIFT, TET, FET, and PROST.

automatic thoughts: Thoughts that occur in your stream of consciousness that are rarely questioned. They include "shoulds" and "musts" and are difficult to tune out.

azoospermia: The absence of sperm in the ejaculate.

bacteria: Microscopic single-celled organisms that can cause infections.

basal body temperature (BBT): The body temperature at rest. Some female infertility patients are asked to complete a BBT chart showing their temperature, taken orally, on consecutive days for one or more months.

behavior modification: Techniques to change specific behaviors.

behavioral medicine: An interdisciplinary field concerned with the relation between physical health and psychological aspects of individuals who have, or are at risk for, physical disease.

beta hCG: A pregnancy test that determines the presence of hCG in the woman's bloodstream.

bicornuate uterus: A congenital malformation of the uterus in which there are two small horn-shaped bodies each having one fallopian tube.

biochemical pregnancy: When a patient's pregnancy test is positive but no pregnancy is visible on ultrasound.

biofeedback: Treatment technique in which data regarding an individual's biological activity are collected, processed, and conveyed back so that one can modify that activity.

blastocyst: The stage of development in which the embryo consists of many cells packed inside a tough outer membrane.

bromocriptine (Parlodel): A drug used to suppress the production of prolactin.

catheter: A flexible tube used for aspirating or injecting fluids.

capacitation: The alteration of sperm during their passage through the female reproductive tract that gives them the capacity to penetrate and fertilize the egg.

cervical mucus: A secretion produced by the lining of the cervical canal.

cervicitis: An inflammation of the cervix.

cervix: The lower section of the uterus that protrudes into the vagina and dilates during labor to allow the passage of the infant.

chlamydia: A type of bacteria that is transmitted often between sexual partners.

chromosome: Strands of DNA in a cell's nucleus that transmit hereditary information.

cilia: Microscopic hairlike projections from the surface of a cell capable of beating in a coordinated fashion.

cleavage: The division of a fertilized egg. The egg size remains unchanged; the cleavage cells become smaller with each division.

clinical pregnancy: A pregnancy confirmed by an increasing level of hCG and the presence of a gestational sac detected by ultrasound.

clinical psychology: A field of psychology concerned with understanding, assessing, treating, and preventing maladaptive behavior.

Clomid: A brand name for clomiphene citrate.

Clomiphene citrate: An antiestrogen drug used to induce ovulation.

cognitive activation: Setting into motion mental processes including perception, memory, and reasoning by which a person acquires knowledge, solves problems, and makes plans.

cognitive psychotherapy: Treatment approach to psychological problems in which a patient identifies his "warped thinking" and learns more realistic ways to formulate his experiences.

conception: The fertilization of a woman's egg by a man's sperm resulting in a new life.

corpus luteum: The "yellow body" formed in the ovary following ovulation that produces the supply of progesterone needed to sustain a pregnancy.

CPT codes: Medical codes used to refer to a standard list of medical procedures. Insurance companies refer to these codes to determine the reasonable cost for a medical procedure.

creative visualization: *See* Guided Fantasy.

cryopreservation: Freezing at a very low temperature, such as in liquid nitrogen (-196°C), to keep embryos or sperm viable.

cycle synchronization: A procedure for ensuring that an egg donor and an egg recipient reach the middle of their menstrual cycle at the same time.

danzol: A drug used to treat endometriosis.

Danoccine: The trade name for danazol.

Day 3 FSH: A woman's FSH level taken on Day 3 of her cycle. This reading is an indication of the woman's ovarian reserve. A level greater than 20 indicates a possible fertility problem.

DES (diethylstilbestrol): A synthetic form of estrogen that was prescribed to prevent miscarriage. Tragically, this drug caused malformations of the reproductive system of women born to mothers who took this drug.

dilation and curettage (D&C): A procedure performed after a miscarriage. It involves opening the cervix, stretching (or dilating) it, and scraping (curetting) the lining of the uterus.

dominant follicle: The largest follicle among developing follicles in the ovary.

downregulation: The use of the drug Lupron to inhibit the woman's body from producing its own FSH and LH. Downregulation enables the doctor to have complete control over the woman's menstrual cycle.

doxycycline: An antibiotic used to prevent infection during an ART procedure.

ectopic pregnancy: A pregnancy in the fallopian tube or elsewhere outside the lining of the uterus. Also called a tubal pregnancy.

egg donation: Surgical removal of an egg from one woman for transfer into the fallopian tube or uterus of another woman.

egg harvest: The procedure by which eggs are obtained by inserting a needle into the ovarian follicle and removing the fluid and the egg by suction. Also called ova aspiration.

egg retrieval: The procedure for obtaining eggs by using a needle to puncture each ovarian follicle and suck out the fluid containing the egg.

ejaculate: The seminal fluid and sperm released from the penis during orgasm.

embryo: The early stages of fetal growth, from conception to the eighth week of pregnancy.

embryo transfer: Placement of the pre-embryos into the uterus or, in the case of ZIFT and TET, into the fallopian tube.

endocrine system: System of glands including the thymus, pituitary, thyroid, adrenals, testicles, or ovaries.

endometrial biopsy: Removal of a portion of the uterine lining in order to study the tissue under a microscope.

endometriosis: A disease in which normal endometrial tissue (the lining of the uterus) grows outside the uterus. It may be associated with infertility.

endometrium: The mucus membrane lining the uterus.

epididymis: An elongated organ in the male lying above and behind the testicles. It contains a highly convoluted canal, four to six meters in length, where, after production, sperm are stored, nourished, and ripened for a period of several months.

estradiol: A hormone released by follicles in the ovary. Plasma estradiol levels are used to help determine progressive growth of the follicle during ovulation induction.

estrogen: The female hormone largely responsible for thickening the uterine lining during the first half of the menstrual cycle.

fallopian tubes: A pair of tubes attached to the uterus, one on each side, where sperm and egg meet in normal conception.

fertilization: The penetration of the egg by the sperm and fusion of genetic materials to result in the development of an embryo.

FET (Frozen Embryo Transfer): Embryos not transferred during an IVF procedure can be frozen. During a subsequent cycle these frozen embryos are thawed and are replaced in the uterus in a procedure called FET (frozen embryo transfer).

fetus: The stage of development of a pregnancy from the third month until delivery.

fibroid: A benign (noncancerous) tumor found in the wall of the uterus.

fimbria: The fringed and fingerlike outer ends of the fallopian tubes.

follicle: A fluid-filled, cystlike structure or sac just beneath the ovary's surface in which the egg grows to maturity.

follicle stimulating hormone (FSH): The pituitary hormone responsible for the stimulation of the follicle cells around the egg.

follicular phase: The first portion of the menstrual cycle occurring from the time of menstruation to just prior to ovulation.

frozen embryo transfer (FET): The transfer to the uterus of an embryo that has been frozen (cryopreserved) and then thawed out.

fructose test: A test to determine whether fructose sugar is present in the semen. The test helps to determine whether an obstruction is preventing sperm from getting into the ejaculate.

gamete: The male or female reproductive cells—the sperm or the ovum (egg).

gamete intrafallopian transfer (GIFT): A method of assisted reproduction that involves surgically removing an egg from the woman's ovary; combining it with sperm; and immediately placing the egg and sperm into the fallopian tube. Fertilization takes place inside the tube.

gene: A structure within the nucleus of a cell that contains hereditary characteristics. Genes consist of DNA and are found at specific locations on chromosomes.

genetic abnormality: A disorder resulting from a chromosomal error or a mistake in the structure of a gene.

Gestalt psychotherapy: A type of psychotherapy that emphasizes the wholeness of the person and the integration of thought, feeling, and action.

gestational sac: A fluid-filled structure that develops within the uterine cavity early in pregnancy.

GIFT: *See* Gamete Intrafallopian Transfer.

gland: An organ that produces a hormone.

GnRH analogues: Synthetic hormones similar to the naturally occurring gonadotropin-releasing hormone (GnRH). Examples are Lupron and Synarel.

gonadotropin: A hormone capable of stimulating the testicles or the ovaries to produce sperm or an egg, respectively.

gonadotropin releasing hormone (GnRH): Hormone secreted by the hypothalamus, a control center in the brain, that prompts the pituitary gland to release follicle stimulating hormone (FSH) and luteinizing hormone (LH) into the bloodstream.

gonorrhea: A venereal disease characterized by inflammation of the mucus membrane of the genitourinary tract.

GPST (Getting Pregnant Self-Talk): Words a person says to him- or herself in the mind's ear to motivate the person to act. These self-statements combat the negative automatic thoughts that prevent the person from taking necessary actions.

guided fantasy: Mental images that help you relax, get motivated, and develop a positive, optimistic attitude.

gynecologist: A physician who specializes in treating female disorders.

hamster penetration test: A test to determine the penetrating ability of a man's sperm. The test uses a hamster egg rather than a human egg to assess the sperm's penetrating ability.

herpes: A sexually transmitted virus infection.

HSG: *See* Hysterosalpingogram.

Huhner test: A post-coital test (PCT) to determine whether sperm are surviving in the cervical mucus after intercourse.

human chorionic gonadotropin (hCG): A hormone produced by the placenta during pregnancy; its detection is the basis for most pregnancy tests. HCG is often used with clomiphene or hMG for the treatment of ovulation problems. HCG is also used during ovulation induction to trigger ovulation.

human menopausal gonadotropin (hMG): An ovulation drug, containing follicle stimulating hormone (FSH) and luteinizing hormone (LH), derived from the urine of post-menopausal women. Pergonal is a brand name.

hydrosalpinx: A fluid-filled, club-shaped fallopian tube that is closed at its end near the ovary. This condition is a contributor to infertility.

hyperstimulation syndrome: A possible side effect of treatment with human menopausal gonadotropin in which the ovaries become painful and swollen and fluid may accumulate in the abdomen and chest.

hypothalamus: A thumb-sized area in the base of the brain that controls many body functions and regulates the pituitary gland.

hysterosalpingogram (HSG): A test to determine whether the fallopian tubes are open (patent). The test involves injecting dye and taking an X ray of the tubes and the uterus.

hysteroscopy: Examination of the inner part of the uterus by means of a telescopic instrument inserted through the vagina and the cervical canal.

immune system: The body's means of defending itself against injury or invasion by foreign substances.

immunobead test: A test to check for the presence of antibodies on the sperm.

immunologist: One who studies the functioning of the immune system.

implantation: The embedding of the fertilized egg in the endometrium of the uterus.

infertility: The inability of a couple to achieve a pregnancy after one year of regular unprotected sexual relations, or the inability of the woman to carry a pregnancy to live birth.

insemination: The introduction of semen into a woman's vagina for the purpose of conception.

intracervical insemination: Artificial insemination of sperm into the cervical canal.

intrauterine insemination (IUI): Artificial insemination of sperm into the uterine cavity, bypassing the cervix.

insomnia: The inability to sleep.

in vitro fertilization (IVF): A method of assisted reproduction that involves surgically removing an egg from the woman's ovary and combining it with sperm in a laboratory dish. If the egg is fertilized, resulting in a pre-embryo, the pre-embryo is transferred to the woman's uterus.

isthmus: The narrow portion of the fallopian tube that is attached to the uterus.

IUI: *See* Intrauterine Insemination.

Laparoscope: A small telescopic instrument used to perform a laparoscopy.

laparoscopy: The direct visualization of the ovaries and the exterior of the fallopian tubes and uterus by means of inserting a surgical instrument through a small incision below the navel.

legitimation: The feeling that your partner (or anyone) considers your concerns to be legitimate and valid.

leveling: Sharing one's inner world with one's partner during communication.

LH: *See* Luteinizing Hormone.

listening: Actively trying to understand one's partner's inner world of experience.

Lisuride: a drug having properties similar to those of Parlodel.

Lupron: The trade name for leuprolide acetate, a GnRH analog. This medicine is injected daily during superovulation to prevent premature ovulation and to allow the doctors to control the follicular phase of the menstrual cycle.

luteal phase: The phase of the menstrual cycle occurring after ovulation.

luteal phase defect (LPD): Inadequate functioning of the corpus luteum that can hamper the fertilized egg's ability to implant in the endometrium.

luteinizing hormone (LH): A hormone secreted by the anterior lobe of the pituitary throughout the menstrual cycle. Secretion of LH increases in the middle of the cycle to induce release of the egg.

meditation: A practice of uncritically attempting to focus attention on one thing at a time. The technique is used to reduce stress.

meiosis: When gametes lose half their chromosomes before fertilization.

menses: A woman's menstrual flow or period.

menstrual cycle: A cycle involving the development of an egg, its ovulation, and terminating in the shedding of the lining of the uterus.

menstruation: The regular shedding of the lining of the uterus, usually occurring each month.

mental imaging: The ability to reproduce internally a variety of sensations when the object that stimulated them is no longer physically present.

mental rehearsal: Constructing a "movie in your mind" of a future event and rehearsing your behavior in that situation.

Metrodin: A fertility drug consisting of pure follicle stimulating hormone (FSH).

miscarriage: A spontaneous abortion.

mitosis: When cells divide in half as the embryo grows.

motility of sperm: The ability of the sperm to move about.

mycoplasma: An agent causing a sexually transmitted infection.

Neuromuscular relaxation: A process by which an individual can perform a series of exercises to reduce neural activity and contractile tension in skeletal muscles.

neuropeptides: Peptide hormones produced by the immune system that influence immune activity.

olfactory: Involving the sense of smell.

oligospermia: An abnormally low number of sperm in the ejaculate of the male.

oocyte: The egg.

oocyte retrieval: A surgical procedure, usually under local anesthesia, to collect the eggs contained within the ovarian follicles. A needle is inserted into the follicle, the fluid and egg are aspirated into the needle, and then placed into a culture-medium-filled dish.

orgasm: The sexual climax involving male ejaculation and female experience of intense sexual pleasure and excitement.

ovary: The sexual gland of the female that produces the hormones estrogen and progesterone, and in which the ova are developed. There are two ovaries, one on each side of the pelvis, and they are connected to the uterus by the fallopian tubes.

ovulation: The release of a mature egg from the surface of the ovary.

ovum donation: A procedure in which eggs are retrieved from a fertile donor, fertilized in a laboratory dish by a husband's sperm, and the resulting embryo is replaced in the recipient woman's uterus.

panic attacks: A situation in which a person experiences intense anxiety and feels immobilized.

Pap smear: a procedure by which cells are removed from the surface of the cervix and studied under a microscope.

PCT: *See* Post-Coital Test.

Parlodel: a drug (also known as Bromocriptine) used to suppress prolactin secretion.

Pelvic Inflammatory Disease (PID): a condition in which a female pelvic organ becomes inflamed, usually as a result of a sexually transmitted disease.

Pergolide: A drug, similar to Parlodel, used to suppress prolactin secretion.

Pergonal: A fertility drug consisting of a combination of FSH and LH.

PID: *See* Pelvic Inflammatory Disease.

pituitary gland: An organ lying at the base of the brain that secretes hormones. This particular gland is known as the master gland. The pituitary gland controls most of the other endocrine glands in the body.

placenta: A spongy organ attached to the wall of the uterus.

polycystic ovarian syndrome (PCO): Development of multiple cysts in the ovaries due to arrested follicular growth. There is an imbalance in the amount of LH and FSH released during the ovulatory cycle.

polyp: A small growth in the uterus or cervix.

polyspermia: Fertilization of the egg by more than one sperm.

Post-coital test (PCT): An examination under the microscope of cervical mucus during the time of maximum fertility to determine the number of sperm surviving in the mucus following intercourse.

primary infertility: The inability of a couple to achieve a pregnancy after one year of unprotected sexual intercourse, or the inability of a woman to carry a pregnancy to live birth.

Profasi: The trade name for hCG (human chorionic gonadotropin).

Progesterone: A hormone secreted by the corpus luteum of the ovary after ovulation has occurred. Also produced by the placenta during pregnancy.

progestin: A synthetic substance that chemically resembles progesterone.

progressive relaxation: A deep muscle relaxation technique in which the individual identifies anxiety by noticing muscle tension and reduces anxiety by relaxing the tense muscles.

prolactin: The pituitary hormone that in large amount stimulates milk production.

PROST (pronuclear stage transfer): Embryos that are transferred at the pronuclear stage. Another name for a ZIFT procedure. See ZIFT.

prostaglandin: Hormonelike substances that can be responsible for cramping if they are not washed away from sperm samples used for intrauterine inseminations.

psychoneuroendocrinology: A branch of medicine based on the interaction of the brain, the endocrine system, and the immune system.

psychotherapy: Treatment of mental disorders by psychological methods.

radiologist: A physician who takes X rays and specializes in their interpretation.

RESOLVE Inc.: The national organization devoted to education and advocacy about infertility.

secondary infertility: The inability to conceive or carry a pregnancy after having successfully conceived and carried one or more pregnancies.

semen: The sperm and seminal secretions ejaculated during orgasm.

semen analysis: The study of fresh ejaculate under the microscope to count the number of million sperm per milliliter or cubic centimeter, to check the shape and size of the sperm, and to note their ability to move (motility).

semen density: How many sperm are present per milliliter of volume.

semen viscosity: How thick or watery the semen sample is.

semen volume: How much liquid is produced in the semen sample. Normal is 2 to 8 milliliters.

seminal vesicles: Two glands in the male that produce the secretion of a fluid containing fructose and store some sperm prior to ejaculation.

septum: A wall in the uterus that should not be there.

Serophene: A commercial name for the drug clomiphene citrate.

social support: The resources that are provided by other people to help an individual cope with a stressful situation. These resources can be informational (such as how to get insurance claims reimbursed), emotional (such as comforting a woman when her treatment did not succeed), or tangible (such as lending money to pay for a procedure that a couple could not otherwise afford).

sperm: A male reproductive cell.

sperm morphology: The shape of a sperm cell.

sperm precursors: Sperm that are not fully developed and still have twice the number of chromosomes (forty-six rather than twenty-three) that they should have when they attempt to fertilize an egg.

sperm washing: A technique that separates the sperm from the seminal fluid.

spontaneous abortion: A miscarriage.

stress: A dynamic relationship between a person and the environment in which the person judges that the demands of a situation exceed his or her resources for coping with the situation. Because the demands seem overwhelming, the person's sense of well-being feels endangered.

superovulation: Another name for controlled ovarian hyperstimulation, which is the method of using fertility drugs to stimulate the production of many egg cells.

surrogate gestational: Carrier woman who gestates an embryo that is not genetically related to her, and then turns over the child to its genetic parents.

swim up technique: A technique for extracting the best sperm from a sperm sample. After a sperm sample has been washed, a small amount of culture media is placed in a test tube, which is placed in an incubator. The most actively mobile sperm swim up from the bottom of the tube and the sluggish ones as well as any debris remain on the bottom.

Synarel: The commercial name for a GnRH analogue, similar to Lupron.

syphilis: A sexually transmitted disease that can lead to paralysis, insanity, and death.

TDI: *See* Therapeutic Donor Insemination.

testes: The male sexual glands of which there are two. Contained in the scrotum, they produce the male hormone testosterone and produce the male reproductive cells, the sperm.

testicular biopsy: The removal of a piece of testis by a surgical procedure in order to study it microscopically.

testosterone: The most potent male sex hormone, produced in the testicles. It stimulates the development of secondary sex characteristics such as beard growth during puberty.

TET (tubal embryo transfer): A procedure in which an early stage embryo is transferred to the fallopian tubes.

therapeutic donor insemination (TDI): Artificial insemination by donor.

tubal patency: Unobstructed fallopian tubes.

ultrasound: A technique for visualizing the follicles in the ovaries and the fetus in the uterus, allowing the estimation of size.

unexplained infertility: The diagnosis given to a couple who have had extensive diagnostic tests that fail to determine a cause for their infertility.

urologist: A physician who specializes in diseases of the urinary tract.

uterus: A hollow muscular structure that is part of the female reproductive tract. The major function of the uterus is to protect and nourish the developing fetus.

vagina: A tubular passageway in the female connecting the external sex organs with the cervix and uterus.

varicocele: A varicose vein in the testicles, sometimes a cause of male infertility.

varicocelectomy: A surgical procedure to correct a varicocele.

vas deferens: A pair of thick-walled tubes about forty-five centimeters long in the male that lead from the epididymis to the ejaculatory duct in the prostate. During ejaculation, the ducts make wavelike contractions to propel sperm forward.

ZIFT: *See* Zygote Intrafallopian Transfer.

zona pellucida: The outer covering of the ovum that the sperm must penetrate before fertilization can occur.

zygote: An embryo in early development state.

zygote intrafallopian transfer (ZIFT): The transfer of a fertilized egg in an early stage of development (called a zygote) into the fallopian tube so that it can migrate to the uterus and implant. ZIFT is also sometimes referred to as PROST.

NOTES

INTRODUCTION

1. Estimates of the number of infertile women in the United States vary. In a survey conducted by the United States Department of Public Health and Human Services (Mosher, W., and Pratt, W., "Fecundity and Infertility in the United States, 1965-88, *Vital and Health Statistics of the National Center for Health Statistics,* December 4, 1990, Number 192), the investigators concluded: "In 1988, about 4.9 million women 15-44 years of age had an impaired ability to have children. These women comprised 8.4 percent or about 1 in 12 of the 57.9 million women 15-44 years of age.... In some popular descriptions of infertility, it has been suggested that there are 9 or 10 million infertile couples, that 1 in 6 couples is infertile.... The findings of this report indicate that these perceptions are inaccurate" (p. 1). Despite the contentions in this report, there have been continued statements disputing the estimate of 1 in 12. For example, in a recent book (Greil, A. 1991. *Not Yet Pregnant.* New Brunswick, NJ: Rutgers University Press), researcher Arthur Greil comments: "Mosher's estimate of 2.4 million infertile couples is almost certainly too low because he does not account for the existence of hidden infertility; that is, some women, especially in lower age brackets, have never had intercourse unprotected by contraceptive devices and have therefore never tested their fertility" (p. 27). In light of this controversy, we will continue to use the 1 in 6 statistic that is most often mentioned in discussions of infertility.

2. You may notice that this book is addressed to women readers. We made this stylistic decision to create a book that is more readable. By talking to the woman we do not mean to imply that men are not interested in this material or that the burden of action should fall only on the woman's shoulders. Quite to the contrary, we advocate working as a team. In that vein, we hope that both members of the team will read this book.

CHAPTER 1

1. Scher, J., and Dix, C., 1990. *Preventing Miscarriage: The Good News*. New York: Harper Perennial.

2. Menning, B. *Infertility: A Guide for the Childless Couple*. 1988. 2nd ed. New York: Prentice Hall.

3. Liebmann-Smith, J. 1989. *In Pursuit of Pregnancy*. New York: Newmarket Press.

4. Sandelowski, M. "The Color Gray: Ambiguity and Infertility," 1987. *IMAGE: Journal of Nursing Scholarship*, 19, 2, 70-74.

5. Sandelowski, M. "Women's Experiences of Infertility," 1986. *IMAGE: Journal of Nursing Scholarship*, 19, 4, 140-44.

6. Ellis, A., and Harper, R. 1979. *A New Guide to Rational Living*. Englewood Cliffs, NJ: Prentice Hall.

7. Cohen, S., and Syme, S., eds. 1985. *Social Support and Health*. New York: Academic Press.

8. Jourard, S. 1964. *The Transparent Self*. Princeton, NJ: Van Nostrand Reinhold.

9. Our advice differs from the position taken by Anthony Reading who contends that "avoiding a baby shower may generalize to avoiding contact with friends who attend it and to places where children or pregnant women are likely to be seen. Such avoidant behaviors can limit sources of pleasure, distraction, and social support thereby increasing vulnerability to depression. Such a pattern needs to be recognized early and treated by graded exposure to distress provoking situations, combined with coping statements to overcome self-defeating thoughts about the situation." See Reading, A., Psychological Interventions and Infertility in A. Stanton and C. Dunkel-Schetter (eds.) 1991. *Infertility: Perspectives from Stress and Coping Research*. New York: Plenum Press, p. 191.

10. Greil, A. 1991. *Not Yet Pregnant*. New Brunswick, NJ: Rutgers University Press, p. 11.

11. Alberti, R., and Emmons, M. 1990. *Your Perfect Right: A Guide to Assertive Living*. San Luis Obispo, CA: Impact Books.

12. Suinn, R. 1983. "Imagery and Sports." In Sheikh, A., ed., *Imagery: Current Theory, Research, and Application*. New York: Wiley, pp. 507-34.

Chekhov, M. 1953. *To the Actor*. New York: Harper and Row.

Rosenberg, Helane S. "Visual Artists and Imagery," *Imagination, Cognition, and Personality*, 7(1), 1987-8, 77-93.

CHAPTER 2

1. Salzer, L. 1991. *Surviving Infertility*. New York: HarperCollins.

2. Lazarus, R. 1966. *Psychological Stress and the Coping Process*. New York: McGraw Hill.

3. Tunks, E., and Bellissimo, A. 1991. *Behavioral Medicine: Concepts and Procedures.* New York: Pergamon Press, p. 13.

4. Pert, C. 1990. "The Wisdom of the Receptors: Neuropeptides, the Emotions, and Body-Mind," in Ornstein, R., and Swencionis, C., eds., *The Healing Brain: A Scientific Reader.* New York: Guilford Press, pp. 147-58.

Siegel, B. 1986. *Love, Medicine & Miracles.* New York: Harper and Row.

Cousins, N. 1989. *Head First: The Biology of Hope and the Healing Power of the Human Spirit.* New York: Penguin Books.

5. Solomon, G. 1990. "Emotions, Stress, and Immunity," pp. 174-81.

6. D'Zurilla, T. 1986. *Problem-Solving Therapy.* New York: Springer.

7. Jacobson, E. 1938. *Progressive Relaxation.* Chicago: University of Chicago Press.

8. Woolfolk, R. and Richardson, F. 1978. *Stress, Sanity, and Survival.* New York: Monarch Books, p. 179.

9. Beck, A. 1976. *Cognitive Therapy and the Emotional Disorders.* New York: New American Library.

10. Meichenbaum, D. 1985. *Stress Inoculation Training.* New York: Pergamon Press.

11. Greil. 1991. *Not Yet Pregnant,* p. 63.

12. Ibid., p. 64.

13. Schwan, K. 1988. *The Infertility Maze: Finding Your Way to the Right Help and the Right Answers.* New York: Contemporary Books.

14. Edwards, W. 1961. "Behavioral Decision Theory." *Annual Review of Psychology, 12,* 473-98.

Tversky, A., and Kahneman, D. 1981. "The Framing of Decisions and the Psychology of Choice," *Science, 211,* 453-58.

15. Wilson-Barnett, J. 1990. "Diagnostic Procedures," in Johnson, M., and Wallace, L., eds., *Stress and Medical Procedures.* New York: Oxford University Press, p. 91.

16. Zoldbrod, A. 1990. *Getting Around the Boulder in the Road: Using Imagery to Cope with Fertility Problems.* Lexington, MA: Center for Reproductive Problems, p. 23.

CHAPTER 3

1. Speroff, L., Glass, R., and Kase, N. 1989. *Clinical Gynecologic Endocrinology and Infertility.* Baltimore: Williams and Wilkins, p. 124.

2. The interval between pulses actually varies considerably depending upon the phase of the menstrual cycle. For a discussion of this issue see ibid., p. 58.

3. *On average,* many women ovulate about half the time from the left ovary and half the time from the right ovary. Some women may alternate sides each month. Other women may have several consecutive ovulations from the right side followed by several consecutive months of ovulation from the left side.

4. Dr. Sherman Silber likens the sperm production process to an assembly line procedure. He states: "If one can imagine an automobile assembly line with a slow, steady, unstoppable movement from one stage to progressively more complex stages of production until the final car comes out for inspection, then one will have a pretty good understanding of how sperm are produced and indeed how sloppy the results can often

be. In fact, one might speculate that one reason for the extravagant number of sperm produced by the testicles is that only a small percentage will actually have all their nuts and bolts in the right place.'' See Silber, S. 1991. *How to Get Pregnant With the New Technology*. New York: Warner, p. 116.

5. According to Dr. Jonathan Scher, an expert on miscarriage, ''Because we know so little about miscarriage and the real number of occurrences, most people ask this question [(i.e., how often do miscarriages happen)]. The answer, unfortunately, is that no one knows for certain. Every scientific article that comes out, every magazine article, offers a different statistic. What we do know is that every day many more miscarriages happen than we record, because some may appear as just a heavy period.'' Scher and Dix. *Preventing Miscarriage*, p. 8.

6. Statistics about the proportion of the population who are unable to conceive because of various problems differ from one study to another. We base our figure on data provided by Mosher (1985), which used a sample size of 4,500,000 infertile couples in the United States.

CHAPTER 4

1. Drs. Speroff, Glass, and Kase believe ovulation occurs between 34 and 36 hours after LH surge. See Speroff, Glass, and Kase. *Clinical Gynecologic Endocrinology and Infertility*, p. 107.

2. According to Drs. Bill Yee and Gregory Rosen, it is important to identify the first day of the LH surge ''because LH can still be detected 24 hours after its onset.'' See Yee, B. and Rosen, G. 1990. ''Monitoring Stimulated Cycles'' in Yee, B. *Infertility and Reproductive Medicine: Clinics of North America*, 1, *1*, 15-36. Recall that ovulation will occur about thirty-six hours after the beginning of the surge. So if you perform the test just as the surge is beginning, ovulation will take place thirty-six hours later. But if you perform the test twelve hours after the surge began, then ovulation will take place about twenty-four hours later.

3. Research by Wilson-Barnett has shown that patients find diagnostic testing even more stressful than treatment itself. Surveys have found that the following information about testing can make them feel less anxious: the purpose of the test, what will happen, how long it will take, where it will be performed, who will do the test, what they will feel physically, and what they will feel emotionally. For a discussion of the stress of diagnostic testing see Wilson-Barnett, ''Diagnostic Procedures.''

4. The values for hormonal levels reported in this chapter are taken from Speroff, Glass, and Kase. *Clinical Gynecologic Endocrinology and Infertility*, pp. 628-29.

5. Progesterone and prolactin level values are taken from Berger, G., Goldstein, M., and Fuerst, M. 1989. *The Couple's Guide to Fertility*. New York: Doubleday, p. 117.

6. Values are taken from Speroff, Glass, and Kase. *Clinical Gynecologic Endocrinology and Infertility*, p. 568.

7. Drs. Speroff, Glass, and Kase discuss a controversy among physicians as to the best time to perform the PCT. On the one hand, testing after two hours may provide maximal information but it may also be deceptive because factors in the mucus that can immobilize sperm may not show up until sometime later. Therefore, other physicians recommend doing the test sixteen to twenty-four hours after intercourse. See Speroff, Glass, and Kase. *Clinical Gynecologic Endocrinology and Infertility,* p. 519.

8. For a discussion of the falloscopy procedure see Kerin, J., and Surrey, E. (1992). "Clinical Applications of the Falloscope," *Seminars in Reproductive Endocrinology (New Technologies in Reproductive Endocrinology),* 10, *1,* 51-57.

9. Scher and Dix. *Preventing Miscarriage.*

CHAPTER 5

1. For a complete description of the drugs of infertility, proper dosage, methods of administration, and side effects, see Rivlin, M. (1990). *Handbook of Drug Therapy in Reproductive Endocrinology and Infertility.* Boston: Little Brown.

2. Adashi, E. 1990. "Ovulation Initiation: Clomiphene Citrate," in Seibel, M. *Infertility: A Comprehensive Text.* Norwalk, CT: Appleton and Lange, p. 308.

3. Gysler, M. et al. 1982. "A Decade's Experience with an Individualized Clomiphene Treatment Regimen Including Its Effect on the Postcoital Test," *Fertility and Sterility,* 37, 161.

4. Taymor, M. 1990. "The Use and Misuse of Ovulation-Inducing Drugs." In Yee, B. *Infertility and Reproductive Medicine: Clinics of North America,* 1, *1,* 165-86.

5. Lunenfeld, B., and Lunenfeld, E. 1990. "Ovulation Induction: HMG," in Seibel. *Infertility,* p. 370.

6. Taymor, M. 1990. *Infertility: A Clinician's Guide to Diagnosis and Treatment.* New York: Plenum Medical Books, p. 194.

7. Allen, N., et al. 1985. "Intrauterine Insemination: A Critical Review," *Fertility and Sterility,* 44, *5,* 569-80.

8. Huszar, G., and DeCherney, A. 1987. "The Role of Intrauterine Insemination in the Treatment of Infertile Couples: The Yale Experience," in Quagliarello, J. *Seminars in Reproductive Endocrinology,* 5, *1,* 11-21.

9. This review consulted the following studies with the following results:

Irianni, F. et al. 1990. "Therapeutic Intrauterine Insemination (TII)—Controversial Treatment for Infertility," *Archives of Andrology,* 25, *2,* 147-67. Overall *per cycle:* 3 percent; unexplained infertility with stimulation: 8.3 percent *per cycle.*

Francavilla, F. et al. "Effect of Sperm Morphology and Motile Sperm Count on Outcome of Intrauterine Insemination in Oligozoospermia and/or Asthenozoospermia," *Fertility and Sterility,* 53, *5,* 892-97. Overall male factor: 22 percent; overall cervical factor: 38.9 percent.

Galle, P. et al. 1990. "Sperm Washing and Intrauterine Insemination for Cervical Factor, Oligospermia, Immunologic Infertility and Unexplained Infertility," *Journal of Reproductive Medicine,* 35, *2,* 116-22. Overall: 21.4 percent; cervical: 25 percent; women with antibodies: 60 percent; men with antibodies: 20 percent; male factor: 7 percent.

Horvatta, O. et al. 1990. "Direct Intraperitoneal or Intrauterine Insemination and Superovulation in Infertility Treatment: A Randomized Study," *Fertility and Sterility,* 54, *2,* 339-41. Overall: 31 percent.

Tucker, M. et al. 1990. "Intrauterine Insemination as Front-Line Treatment for Non-tubal Infertility," Asia-*Oceania Journal of Obstetrics and Gynaecology*, 16, *2*, 137-43. Overall: 33 percent; *per cycle*: 12 percent.

Valkenburg, M., Evers, J., and Dumoulin, J. 1990. "Pregnancies During and After Homologous Intrauterine Insemination Cycles," *Gynecological Obstetrics*, 29, *4*, 250-54. Overall: 23.1 percent.

Byrd, W. et al. 1990. "A Prospective Randomized Study of Pregnancy Rates Following Intrauterine and Intracervical Insemination Using Frozen Donor Sperm," *Fertility and Sterility*, 53, *3*, 521-27. Overall: 9.7 percent *per cycle* (with frozen donor sperm).

Treadway, D. et al. 1990. "Effectiveness of Stimulated Menstrual Cycles and Percoll Sperm Preparation in Intrauterine Insemination," *Journal of Reproductive Medicine*, 35, *2*, 103-108. Overall: 28 percent.

10. Wolmer, D., and Dodson, W. 1990. "Superovulation and Intrauterine Insemination," in Yee. *Infertility and Reproductive Medicine*. 135-44.

11. See Bayer, S., and Seibel, M. 1990. "Endometriosis: Pathophysiology and Treatment," in Seibel. *Infertility*, p. 124.

12. For a discussion of the importance of Day 3 FSH in predicting the success of infertility treatment see the following articles:

Toner, J. et al. 1991. "Basal Follicle-Stimulating Hormone Level is a Better Predictor of In Vitro Fertilization Performance than Age," *Fertility and Sterility*, 56, *4*, 784-91.

Rosenwaks, Z. 1991. "The Use of Gonadotropin and Estradiol Levels in Prediction of Stimulation Response and IVF Results," in American Fertility Society. *Course II: Assisted Reproductive Technologies—An Advanced Course*. Orlando, FL. October 19-20, 1991.

13. Diamond, M., Lavy, G., and DeCherney, A. 1990. "Diagnosis and Management of Ectopic Pregnancy," in Seibel. *Infertility*, p. 451.

14. McArdle, C. "Ultrasound in Infertility," in Seibel. 1990. *Infertility*, p. 274.

15. Wisot, A., and Meldrum, D. 1990. *New Options for Fertility*. New York: Pharos Books, p. 80.

16. Silber. *How to Get Pregnant with the New Technology*, p. 261.

17. Ibid., p. 51.

18. Franklin, R., and Brockman, D. 1990. *In Pursuit of Fertility*. New York: Henry Holt, p. 5.

19. Berger, Goldstein, and Fuerst. *The Couple's Guide to Fertility*, p. 5.

20. Corson, S. 1990. *Conquering Infertility*. New York: Prentice Hall, p. 41.

21. Silber. *How to Get Pregnant*, p. 52.

22. Diamond, E. 1991. "DI Achieves Extraordinary Breakthrough Combining Cervical Cap and Intrauterine Insemination," *Diamond Reports*, 1, *1*, 3.

We were unable to locate any research literature that corroborated Diamond's contention that the sperm can only survive for six hours. However, in a review of the literature on intrauterine insemination, Allen et al. claim that "timing [of IUI] may be especially important if most sperm are rapidly transported from the point of insemination to the peritoneal cavity." Allen et al. "Intrauterine Insemination," p. 573. Thus, whether sperm can live for only six hours may not be the critical matter; if they exit rapidly into the peritoneal cavity, they will no longer be available to fertilize the egg.

23. Kerin, J., and Quinn, P. 1987. "Washed Intrauterine Insemination in the Treatment of Oligospermic Infertility," in Quagliarello. *Seminars in Reproductive Endocrinology,* 23-33.

24. See Allen, N. et al. "Intrauterine Insemination, p. 570. Several other researchers also discuss this issue. Cruz, Kemmann, and their colleagues recommend that the insemination be done twenty-eight hours after hCG. See Cruz, R. et al. 1986. "A Prospective Study of Intrauterine Insemination of Processed Sperm from Men with Oligoasthenospermia in Superovulated Women," *Fertility and Sterility,* 46, *4,* p. 674. Taymor advises that insemination should be done thirty-two to thirty-five hours after hCG. See Taymor. *Infertility: A Clinician's Guide,* p. 198.

CHAPTER 6

1. For information about obtaining a copy of the *Membership Directory* of the American Fertility Society contact this organization at 2140 11th Avenue South, Suite 200, Birmingham, AL 35205-2800. Tel: 205-933-8494.

2. Speroff, Glass, and Kase. *Clinical Gynecologic Endocrinology and Infertility,* p. 517.

3. This activity is based upon an exercise described by Virginia Satir. See Satir, V. 1988. *The New Peoplemaking.* Mountain View, CA: Science and Behavior Books, pp. 71-72. It also draws upon ideas about productive dialogue and empathic communication discussed by Cohen and Epstein. See Cohen, B., and Epstein, Y. 1981. "Empathic Communication in Process Groups," *Psychotherapy: Theory, Research, and Practice,* 18, *4,* 493-500.

4. The presumption is made that Amanda and Al do *not* have a problem that would *never* allow them to get pregnant. The formula for computing their odds of getting pregnant after X attempts is:

$1-(1-y)^x$ where y = probability of success on any given month and ^{x} represents the number of attempts. In Amanda and Al's example, they were using the Duke University procedure that had a 14%/month success statistic for 6 months. Therefore, the odds for their success is $1-(1-.14)^6$, which equaled 1-(.404) = .595 or 60%.

5. For a discussion of Gestalt psychotherapy and the concept of human polarities see Polster, E., and Polster, M. 1973. *Gestalt Therapy Integrated: Contours of Theory and Practice.* New York: Brunner/Mazel, p. 62.

CHAPTER 7

1. The American Fertility Society publishes an annual report entitled *Annual Clinic Specific Report for the Year* _____. This report contains the names and addresses of each clinic on a state-by-state basis. For each clinic, it lists the number of IVF and GIFT procedures performed and the success statistics. For a copy of this report contact the

American Fertility Society, 2140 11th Avenue South, Suite 200, Birmingham, AL 35205-2800. Tel: 205-933-8494.

2. In addition to IVF, GIFT, and ZIFT, there are several other alphabet soup variations. These include TET (tubal embryo transfer), FET (frozen embryo transfer), and PROST (pronuclear stage transfer).

3. Medical Research International. 1992. The Society for Assisted Reproductive Technology, the American Fertility Society: In Vitro Fertilization and Embryo Transfer in the United States: 1990 Results from the IVF-ET Registry, *Fertility and Sterility,* 57, 15-24.

4. Waterstone, J., and Parsons, J. 1992. "A Prospective Study to Investigate the Value of Flushing Follicles During Transvaginal Ultrasound Directed Follicle Aspiration," *Fertility and Sterility,* 57, *1,* 221-23.

5. For a discussion of these techniques, see Schmidt, C. 1991. "Cycle of Replacement for Frozen Embryos: Natural or Artificial," in *In Vitro Fertilization and Embryo Transfer: A Comprehensive Update.* Santa Barbara, CA; UCLA School of Medicine, pp. 174-206.

6. Medical Research International. 1992. The Society for Assisted Reproductive Technology, the American Fertility Society: In Vitro Fertilization and Embryo Transfer in the United States: 1990 Results from the IVF-ET Registry, *Fertility and Sterility,* 57, 15-24.

7. Kovacs, G. et al. 1991. "Triplets or Sequential Siblings?: A Case Report of Three Children Born After One Episode of In Vitro Fertilization," *Fertility and Sterility,* 56, *5,* 987-88.

8. Doctors are currently experimenting with nonsurgical gamete transfer procedures.

9. Medical Research International. 1992. The Society for Assisted Reproductive Technology, the American Fertility Society: In Vitro Fertilization and Embryo Transfer in the United States: 1990 Results from the IVF-ET Registry, *Fertility and Sterility,* 57, 15-24.

10. These cost estimates are based on 1992 figures at one Northeastern clinic.

CHAPTER 8

1. Social psychologist Kurt Lewin pioneered the use of field theory to apply psychological concepts to the process of changing attitudes and behavior. Discussing Lewin's concepts, social psychologists Morton Deutsch and Robert Krauss note that "Lewin's analysis of the *status quo* as a quasi-stationary equilibrium . . . points out that change from the *status quo* can be produced either by adding forces in the desired direction or by diminishing opposing forces." Deutsch and Krauss point out that of the two approaches, removing impediments to change is the more desirable strategy. For a discussion of field theory and the way its concepts are applied to the process of change, see Deutsch, M., and Krauss, R. 1965. *Theories in Social Psychology.* New York: Basic Books, pp. 37-76.

2. Seligman writes about learned optimism as an antidote to learned helplessness. He discusses the health benefits that result from maintaining an optimistic attitude. Seligman indicates that social support and attempts to exert control over the difficult situation can promote an optimistic attitude. Our pointers are designed to increase the likelihood of getting support and of exerting control. For a discussion of Seligman's important ideas we urge you to read his book: *Learned Optimism: How to Change Your Mind and Your Life*. New York: Pocket Books, 1990.

3. Bonnicksen, A. 1989. *In Vitro Fertilization: Building Policy from Laboratories to Legislatures*. New York: Columbia University Press.

4. Godwin, R. 1992. "Advocacy Corner: Infertility Insurance Legislation," *RESOLVE of Central Jersey Newsletter,* January-February, p. 9.

5. Damewood, M. 1991. "In Vitro Fertilization: Insurance and Financial Considerations," *Assisted Reproduction Reviews*, 1, *1*, 38-49.

6. Johnson, J. "Insurance and the Cost of Infertility," *New York Times*, March 5, 1989.

7. Much of the material we have written about models of hope is based on the work of Israeli psychologist Shlomo Bresnitz. For a discussion of these ideas see Bresnitz, S. 1986, "The Effect of Hope on Coping with Stress," in Appley, M., and Trumbell, R., eds., *Dynamics of Stress: Physiological, Psychological, and Social Perspectives*. New York: Plenum Press, pp. 295-306. The concept of hope is also central to Seligman's ideas about learned optimism. For a discussion of the importance of hope in coping with stress see Seligman, *Learned Optimism*.

CHAPTER 9

1. Until recently, the procedure by which a woman is inseminated with sperm from a person not her husband was termed artificial insemination with donor sperm (AID) or donor insemination (DI), but both terms fell out of favor because each acronym caused confusion or fear. AID sounded too much like AIDS and DI was already the medical abbreviation for diabetes insipidus. To be most current, we encourage you to use the term TDI. Yet be aware that in earlier books, AID and DI often describe the same procedure.

2. In an article tracing the history of artificial insemination the authors relate, "In 1884, William Pancoast of Jefferson Medical College, Philadelphia, used AID (artificial insemination by donor) to treat a case of postgonococcal azoospermia. The insemination apparently came about as a result of jokes made by medical students, one of whom, the 'best looking member of the class,' was the semen donor. An intrauterine insemination was performed without the knowledge of the couple. When a pregnancy resulted, the husband was informed. Fortunately, he was pleased, although he asked that his wife not be told. The insemination was not reported until 25 years later by one of the medical students involved." See Arny, M., and Quagliarello, J. 1987. "History of Artificial Insemination: A Tribute to Sophia Kleegman, M.D." *Seminars in Reproductive Endocrinology,* 5, *1*, 1-3.

3. This figure is based on information discussed by Dr. Sherman Silber. See Silber. *How to Get Pregnant*, p. 216.

4. Batzer, F., and Corson, S. 1987. "Indications, Techniques, Success Rates, and Pregnancy Outcome: New Directions with Donor Insemination," *Seminars in Reproductive Endocrinology* 5, *1*, 45-57.

5. Several doctors discuss the medical and psychological pros and cons of mixing the donor's sperm with the husband's sperm. See Batzer and Corson. "Indications,

Techniques, Success Rates, and Pregnancy Outcome." Also see Taymor. *Infertility: A Clinician's Guide,* pp. 207-8.

6. American Fertility Society. 1990. "New Guidelines for the Use of Semen Donor Insemination: 1990," *Fertility and Sterility,* 53, *3,* Supplement 1.

7. Although the American Fertility Society suggests limiting pregnancies created by a single donor to ten, there is no enforcement of this suggestion. Perhaps this is because the doctor doesn't always report to the sperm bank whether a patient got pregnant using a given donor. Different banks vary in the upper limit of pregnancies they allow from each donor. Some banks limit donors to ten, whereas others permit twenty pregnancies.

8. A survey of donor insemination practices found that the majority of donors tend to be students in the health sciences who are usually unmarried, middle-class, and white, twenty to twenty-seven years of age, who have been examined by physicians and given an intelligence test. See Curie-Cohen, M., Luttrell, L., and Shapiro, S. 1979. "Current Practice of Artificial Insemination by Donor in the United States," *New England Journal of Medicine,* 300, 585.

9. One study examined the personality of seventy-five sperm donors using the Cattell 16 PF test. These donors were found to be intelligent, willing to take risks, and bold in contrast to similar men who were not sperm donors. These personality differences may reflect the donors' desire to perform a task that is important though unconventional. See Handelsman, D. et al. 1985. "Psychological and Attitudinal Profiles in Donors for Artificial Insemination," *Fertility and Sterility,* 43, 95.

10. Loy, R., and Seibel, M. 1990. "Therapeutic Insemination," in Seibel. *Infertility,* pp. 208-9.

11. It is difficult to give exact statistics for ovum donor success rates. We based our estimate on a compilation of statistics cited by various programs. For example, Dr. Mark Sauer of the USC program cites four studies involving 121 patients undergoing a total of 128 cycles. There were forty-two clinical pregnancies from these 128 cycles for an average success rate of 33 percent. The rates for each of the four studies were 37 percent, 75 percent, 15 percent, and 39 percent. See Sauer, M. 1991. "Oocyte Donation to Women of Advanced Reproductive Age," *Course II: Assisted Reproductive Technologies—An Advanced Course.* Orlando, FL: American Fertility Society Meetings.

Dr. Zev Rosenwaks of the Cornell IVF program reports statistics for his program. Twenty-three pregnancies resulted from eighty-nine transfers for a 26 percent success rate. However, Rosenwaks points out that the chance of success depends upon the timing of the transfer. See Rosenwaks, Z. 1991. "Present Status of Oocyte Donation," *Course II: Assisted Reproductive Technologies—An Advanced Course,* Orlando, FL: American Fertility Society Meetings.

12. Rosenwaks reports a window of opportunity for transfer of embryos. If the procedure is done outside this window of time, the success rate is zero. But when properly timed, success rate climbs to 35 percent. See Rosenwaks. "Present Status of Oocyte Donation."

13. Dr. Cecilia L. Schmidt, Director of Reproductive Endocrinology and Infertility at NYU Medical Center, discusses the pros and cons of oral micronized estradiol versus estradiol administered with transdermal patches. She conducted research that demonstrated that transdermal patches produced serum estradiol levels that were very similar to those seen in normal menstrual cycles. She therefore favors this mode of administration. See Schmidt, C. 1991. "Cycle of Replacement for Frozen Embryos."

14. See Sauer. "Oocyte Donation."

15. Although there have been very few reported serious complications arising from the stimulation protocol or the egg retrieval procedure, such complications are always a possibility. The recipient must be aware that should the donor suffer from a *serious* case of hyperstimulation, she will have to be hospitalized. The cost of such hospitalization could exceed $50,000 and would *not* be covered by the recipient's medical insurance. In that event, the recipient couple might have to cover these expenses out of their own pocket.

16. Ethics Committee of the American Fertility Society. 1990. "Surrogate Mothers," *Fertility and Sterility,* Supplement 2, 53, *6,* 68S.

17. Information taken from *Facts About Surrogate Parenting* provided by Dr. Betsy. P. Aigen, Director, *Surrogate Mother Program Inc.* Address: 220 West 93rd Street, New York, NY 10025.

18. For a discussion of legal decisions concerning surrogacy see Crockin, S. 1992. Legally Speaking, *Fertility News,* 26, 3, p. 6.

19. Cited in Ethics Committee of the American Fertility Society. "Surrogate Mothers," pp. 68S-69S.

20. Reported in a pamphlet entitled *Alternatives for Childless Couples* (1991) produced by the Infertility Center of New York (ICNY), 14 East 60th Street, Suite 1204, New York, NY 10022.

CHAPTER 10

1. Gold, M. 1988. *And Hannah Wept: Infertility, Adoption, and the Jewish Couple.* Philadelphia: Jewish Publication Society.

2. Vatican. 1987. *Congregation for the Doctrine of the Faith: Instruction on the Respect for Human Life in Its Origin and on the Dignity of Procreation.* Vatican City: Vatican Press.

3. See Ethics Committee of the American Fertility Society. 1990. "Ethical Considerations of the New Reproductive Technologies," *Fertility and Sterility, Supplement 2,* 53, *6.*

4. *Doornbos* v. *Doornbos,* 23 USLW 2303 (Sup. Ct. ILL 1954), appeal dismissed on procedural grounds, 12 ILL App. 2s 473, 139 NE 2d 844 (1956).

5. *Gursky* v. *Gursky,* 39 Misc 2d 1083, 242 NYS 2d 406 (Sup. Ct. 1963).

6. The states having these laws are Alaska, Arkansas, California, Colorado, Connecticut, Florida, Georgia, Idaho, Illinois, Kansas, Louisiana, Maryland, Michigan, Minnesota, Missouri, Montana, Nevada, New Jersey, New York, North Carolina, Ohio, Oklahoma, Oregon, Tennessee, Texas, Virginia, Washington, Wisconsin, and Wyoming.

7. *Baby M,* 109 NJ 306, 537 A.2d 1227 (1988).

8. *Doe* v. *Kelly,* 106 Mich App. 169, 307 NW 2d 438 (1981); cert denied 459 US 1183 (1983); In *re Baby M,* 109 NJ 306, 537 A.2d 1227 (1988).

9. *Surrogate Parenting Associates* v. *Kentucky,* SW 2d (Ky, Feb. 6, 1986).

10. A column highlighting recent court decisions affecting the new reproductive technologies, particularly surrogacy, and the families they created appeared in *Fertility News,* 1991, 25, *4* (December). The column was written by Susan L. Crockin, a Boston area attorney specializing in legal aspects of reproductive technology and adoption. Ms. Crockin is also a member of the National Board of RESOLVE.

11. The genetic determinants of outward physical appearance are exceedingly complex. The concern you have is whether your baby will have physical characteristics that provoke questions from observers. You want to avoid giving medical lectures about the reality of genetic possibilities.

CHAPTER 11

1. Our definition for secondary infertility is essentially the same as that of the World Health Organization's scientific group. They define secondary infertility as "Couple has previously conceived, but is subsequently unable to conceive despite cohabitation and exposure to pregnancy for a period of two years."

2. Mosher, W., and Pratt, W., 1990. "Fecundity and Infertility in the United States, 1965-88," *Advance Data from the Vital and Health Statistics of the National Center for Health Statistics,"* 192, December 4, 1990.

3. Krech, D., and Crutchfield, R. 1948. *Theory and Problems of Social Psychology.* New York: McGraw Hill, p. 488.

4. Mosher and Pratt. "Fecundity and Infertility."

5. For additional help in developing good negotiation skills, we suggest that you read Harvard Law School professor Roger Fisher's excellent book, which teaches these skills. See Fisher, R., and Ury, W. 1981. *Getting to Yes.* New York: Penguin.

CHAPTER 12

1. Statistics about this problem and a definition of it are provided in Wheeler, J. 1991. "Epidemiologic Aspects of Recurrent Pregnancy Loss," in Freedman, A., ed., *Infertility and Reproductive Medicine: Clinics of North America,* 2, *1,* 1-18.

2. Wheeler. "Epidemiologic Aspects of Recurrent Pregnancy Loss," p. 2.

3. Rein, M. 1991. "Luteal Phase Defect and Recurrent Pregnancy Loss," in Freedman A., ed., *Infertility and Reproductive Medicine: Clinics of North America, 2, 1,* 123.

4. Lauersen, N., and Bouchez, C. 1991. *Getting Pregnant: What You Need to Know Right Now To . . .* New York: Rawson Associates, p. 217.

5. Ibid., p. 218.

6. A critical review of the literature does not support the claims that infections cause miscarriage or that antibiotics can prevent miscarriage. After examining numerous studies on the contribution of mycoplasma to miscarriage, Drs. Laura E. Riley and Ruth Tuomala conclude that "the existing data do not substantiate that Mycoplasma colonization causes recurrent pregnancy loss, or that eradication of colonization improves outcome." See Riley, L., and Tuomala, R. 1991. "Infectious Diseases and Recurrent Pregnancy Loss," *Infertility and Reproductive Medicine: Clinics of North America,* 2, *1,* 168.

7. Herbst, A., Senekjian, E., and Frey, K. 1989. "Abortion and Pregnancy Loss Among Diethylstilbestrol-Exposed Women," *Seminars in Reproductive Endocrinology,* 7, 124.

8. Opponents of the approach dispute these contentions. They claim that the treatment is not needed since there is no evidence that such genetic similarity is problematical. In his review of the causes of recurrent pregnancy loss, Dr. Wheeler points out that "Human Leukocyte Antigen (HLA) overcompatibility was once thought to be an extremely attractive theory of recurrent pregnancy loss. Unfortunately, further research failed to demonstrate causation." Wheeler. "Epidemiologic Aspects of Recurrent Pregnancy Loss," p. 8.

9. From Warburton, D. et al. 1986. "Cytogenic Abnormalities in Spontaneous Abortions of Recognized Conceptions," in Porter, I. and Wiley, A., eds. *Perinatal Genetics: Diagnosis and Treatment*. New York: Academic Press, p. 36. (Reprinted with permission.)

10. Scher and Dix. *Preventing Miscarriage*, p. 11.

11. Schweibert, P., and Kirk, P. 1985. *When Hello Means Goodbye: A Guide for Parents Whose Child Dies Before Birth, at Birth, or Shortly After Birth*. Available from Perinatal Loss, 2116 NE 18th Avenue, Portland, OR 97212. Tel: 503-284-7426.

INDEX